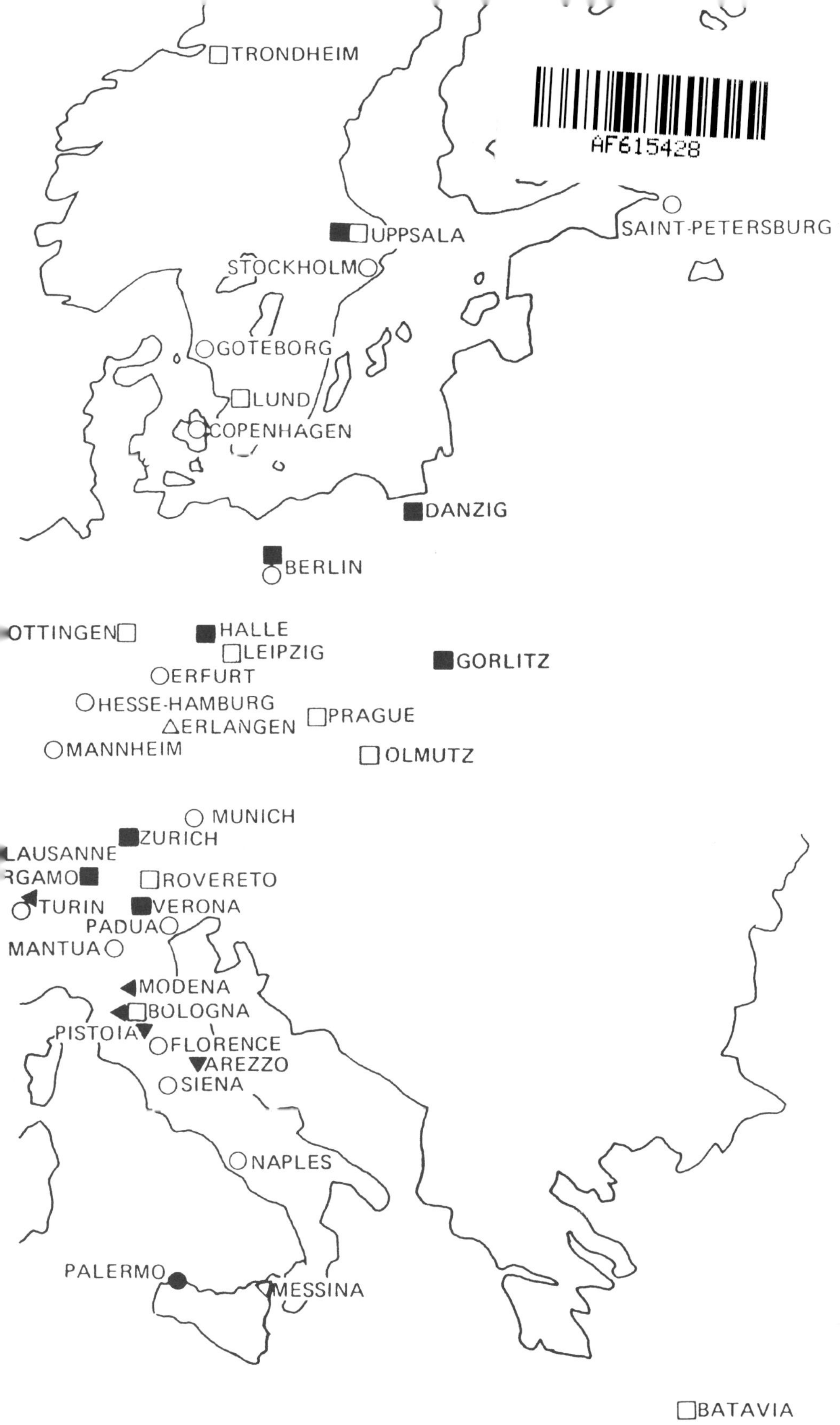
TRONDHEIM
UPPSALA
SAINT-PETERSBURG
STOCKHOLM
GOTEBORG
LUND
COPENHAGEN
DANZIG
BERLIN
OTTINGEN
HALLE
LEIPZIG
GORLITZ
ERFURT
HESSE-HAMBURG
ERLANGEN
PRAGUE
MANNHEIM
OLMUTZ
MUNICH
ZURICH
LAUSANNE
RGAMO
ROVERETO
TURIN
VERONA
PADUA
MANTUA
MODENA
BOLOGNA
PISTOIA
FLORENCE
AREZZO
SIENA
NAPLES
PALERMO
MESSINA
BATAVIA

MEDICINE IN THE ATHENS OF THE WEST 1799 - 1950

W. Porter Mayo, M.D., Ph.D.

MEDICINE IN THE ATHENS OF THE WEST 1799 - 1950

The History and Influence of the Lexington—Fayette County Medical Society

W. Porter Mayo, M.D., Ph.D.

Editor

Walker P. Mayo

Consultants

Camille Mayo Jernigan, Florence M. Witte and **Carolyn Kurz**

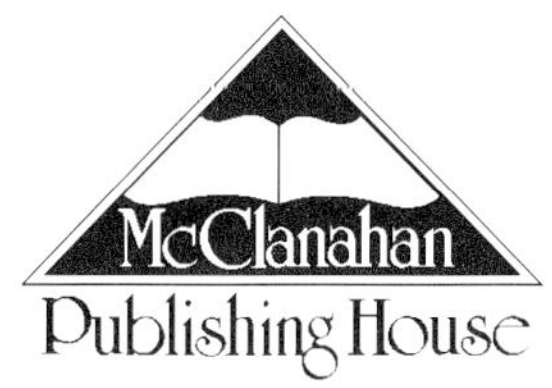

International Standard Book Number 0-913383-643
Library of Congress Catalog Card Number 9965231

Cover design and book layout by James Asher Graphics

Manufactured in the United States of America

All book order correspondence should be addressed to:

Fayette County Medical Society
2628 Wilhite Court, Ste. 201
Lexington, KY, 40503-3304
(606) 278-0569

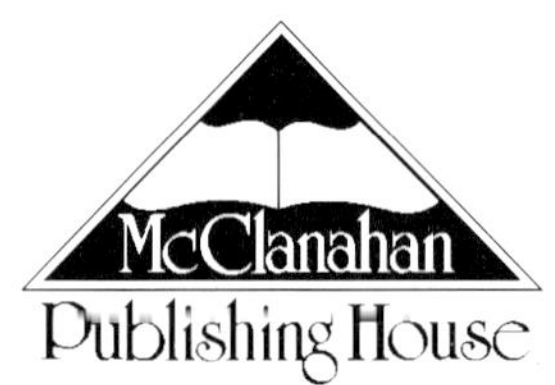

For
Helen (Pat) Prevost Mayo

Whatever may be the present status of Kentucky medicine-and I hold that it is high-the past at least is secure. When Kentucky was to a large extent a wilderness, and not yet wholly free from hostile incursions of the Indians, when the population was so sparse as scarcely to give encouragement to any educational enterprises except such as were necessary for the simplest branches of learning, the interests of medicine were not only not neglected but received conspicuous regard.

Lewis D. Rogers
Address of the President
Kentucky State Medical Society
1873

TABLE OF CONTENTS

Chapter I The Lexington Medical Society **21**

Chapter II Kappa Lambda Society **64**

Chapter III Disease and Therapy in Antebellum Lexington **90**

Chapter IV Medical Education in Antebellum Lexington **166**

Chapter V 1850 to 1900 ....**220**

Chapter VI The Twentieth Century 1901-1950 ....**262**

ILLUSTRATIONS

John Bradford 26
Samuel Brown, M.D....................29
Ridgely-Brown House....................33
Resolution of the Board of Trustees of Transylvania University
appointing Drs. Brown and Ridgely as professors of medicine 34,35,36
Representative pages of the
Lexington Medical Society Minutes (1803-1804)....................45
Ephraim McDowell, M.D. 47
The Transylvania Journal of Medicine and the Associate Sciences....................52
Samuel Brown, M.D....................67
Title page of the Constitution of the Kappa Lambda
Society of Hippocrates....................69
Transylvania University Thesis submitted by Henry Miller
for the degree of Doctor of Medicine....................81
Joseph Buchanan, M.D. 92
William "King" Solomon....................120
Lunsford P. Yandell, M.D. 129
Benjamin Winslow Dudley, M.D. 138
The Transylvania Journal of Medicine and the Associate Sciences....................140
Daniel Drake, M.D. 171
James Overton, M.D. 199
William Hall Richardson, M.D. 199
Horace Holley, A.M., A.A.S., President, Transylvania University....................200
Constantine S. Rafinesque....................201
Charles Caldwell, M.D. 202
Chart depicting the pupils and graduates of
Transylvania University Medical Department....................206
Robert Peter, M.D. 224
Frances Dallam Peter....................225
Ethelbert Dudley, M.D....................229
J. W. Pryor, M.D. 238
Waller O. Bullock, M.D. 238
Bush A. Hunter, M.D....................249
Samuel Gross, M.D. 251

The Training Nurses, The Good Samaritan Hospital, 1899 254
Archibald H. Barkley, M.D. 265
F. H. Clarke, M.D. 265
William B. McClure, M.D. 265
Benjamin F. Van Meter, M.D. 265
John W. Scott, M.D. 273
Nathaniel Lewis Bosworth, M.D. 275
Charles Crain Garr, M.D. 275
George P. Sprague, M.D. 276
Charles A. Vance, M.D. 276
"Button Up Coats and Cars" 281
Joseph A. Stucky, M.D. 303
Inauguration of the Fayette County Medical Society
Women's Auxiliary 1948 307
World War I Barrow Unit 309
David Barrow, M.D. 309
Fayette County physicians in service WW II 311
Matthew Cotton Darnell, M.D. 313
Fred Wharton Rankin, M.D. 315
Medical Staff St. Joseph Hospital, Lexington, Kentucky 316

PREFACE

The year 1999 marks the bicentennial year of the Lexington Medical Society and its successor, the Fayette County Medical Society. The formation of the Lexington Medical Society, its eminent early members and its close affiliation with the Transylvania Medical School culminated in the first and most influential center of medical practice and learning existing in America West of the Alleghenies during the first third of the nineteenth century. Two centuries ago, anyone who wished to practice medicine did so. There was no need for a degree or even a certificate. Even so, there were among the medical practitioners in Lexington during the 1790s qualified physicians with the desire to show to the public those traits and credentials that differentiated the regular physician (allopaths) from medical pretenders (irregulars). The regular physicians' need for respect and recognition led to the founding of a medical society with membership limited to those deemed qualified. Membership then was essentially a statement of the applicant's educational credentials. Education, not nobility nor place, set the society members apart from pretenders. So too, did the need for elevating medical education serve as one if not the primary stimulus in the formation of the American Medical Association a half century later (1846-47). The local and county medical societies are the indispensable elements of the more renowned American Medical Association, yet their history has not been as adequately told. That such societies were in existence in the American Colonies some one-hundred years before the founding of the American Medical Association demonstrates the need for further investigation and appreciation of their role and place in the birth of American Medicine.

Since this project began about six years ago, the scope of

the subject has grown far beyond the documentation of men and events of a local medical society, even one some two hundred years of age. Chapter One covers the founding of a medical society in the wilderness and how the social and economic conditions of Lexington played a significant role in erecting the first and foremost medical center West of the Alleghenies. The founding of the Lexington Medical Society in 1799 preceded the establishment of the Medical Department of Transylvania University, also in 1799. The two institutions grew side-by-side for almost thirty five years. The founder of the Lexington Medical Society, Dr. Samuel Brown (brother of John Brown, Kentucky's first United States Senator), was the first professor of medicine appointed by Transylvania University and a member of the American Philosophical Society. Dr. Brown made many scientific contributions. One of his major endeavors was the founding of the first national medical society in America, Kappa Lambda of Hippocrates, and an associated national medical journal *The North American Medical and Surgical Journal.* Chapter Two is devoted to the relationship between the Kappa Lambda Society and the subsequent founding of the American Medical Association. As expressed in the chapter, the American Medical Association is the flowering of Kappa Lambda.

The accomplishments of a later president of our society (1824), Dr. Daniel Drake, the foremost American medical educator of the nineteenth century, is likewise detailed in Chapters Three and Four, relating respectively to diseases of antebellum Lexington, essentially those of the Mississippi Valley, and to the theme of medical education in the West, initiated in Lexington but later transferred to Louisville and Cincinnati. Chapters Five and Six relate the re-emergence of the Lexington Medical Society in 1869 and 1882, following its earlier demise, a characteristic feature of early American medical societies.

Chapter Five also furnishes the reader with pictorial clips of medicine and other local affairs in Civil War Lexington as seen through the eyes of a young woman, Frances Dallam Peter, an avowed Yankee and daughter of the last dean of the Transylvania

University Medical School, Dr. Robert Peter. In addition, the struggle of women and African-Americans to join the ranks of practitioners and medical societies is documented. Chapter Six depicts the twentieth century shift of emphasis from that of the general practitioner to specialist, the influence of the car, telephone and modern hospital on medical delivery and cost. Records of the month-to-month deliberations of the Medical Society prove an invaluable witness to the province of medicine, both the good and the bad.

When the author began the collection of data to initiate a review of the Medical Society many questions came to mind. First, does a history of the Medical Society exist? Who founded the Society? When? Why? Do we know the names and the number of its members? Where and how often did the Society meet? How were the members selected? Did the Society have a Constitution? Minutes? What historical information exists in the archives of the Fayette County Medical Society? The State Medical Society? What other sources are available to the historian? The few records available in the archives of the Fayette County Medical Society reflect principally those of the twentieth century. Regrettably, documents were lost long ago, including notes concerning the Lexington College of Medicine and Surgery (1836), the entire minutes of the Society from 1882 until December 1903, and the minutes from 1913-16. How then in the absence of so many primary sources was one to write a history of the Society, especially of its founding and its role in the history of the nineteenth century?

The author has sought to use primary sources and to this end many documents and conclusions not previously published have been discovered and entered into the book:

1. The names of fifteen presidents of the Society, all of the nineteenth century and previously unknown.

2. The oldest and possibly the first Constitution (1821) of the Lexington Medical Society. (It is not known whether or not a Constitution was crafted in 1799. The 1803-04 minutes of the society suggest that the constitution and by-laws possibly were an ongoing affair and not fully documented until 1821 at which time the Society was incorporated).
3. The founder of the Lexington Medical Society: Dr. Samuel Brown.
4. The date when founded: 1799.
5. The identification of the Lexington Medical Society as the first student/physician medical society West of the Alleghenies and the second such society in the United States. It is the first student-physician medical society in the United States in which students were elected as officers of the Society.
6. The identification of three medical students (apprentices) as presidents of the Lexington Medical Society.
7. The first presidential address extant, given by Dr. Daniel Drake in December 1823.
8. The Constitution of the Lexington College of Physicians and Surgeons (1836).
9. The chronology of the offspring of the parent Lexington Medical Society, namely the Lexington College of Physicians and Surgeons (1836), the Lexington and Fayette County Medical Society (1869, 1882) and the Fayette County Medical Society (circa 1894-95).
10. The inclusion of the world renowned Dr. Ephraim McDowell, Father of Abdominal Surgery as a member of the Lexington Medical Society
11. A rendition of the achievements of Dr.

Samuel Brown, the Lexington Medical Society's founder, with documentation and interpretation of his role in establishing the first national medical society in America, Kappa Lambda of Hippocrates, and its influence in the structure of the American Medical Association.

12. Inclusion of selected and original dialogue from the minutes of the Fayette County Medical Society.

Of the many institutions visited in the preparation of this book, the Transylvania University Medical Archives proved to be invaluable. I am indebted to the able Special Collections Librarian and Transylvania University Archivist, B. J. Gooch. The Kentucky Room of the Lexington Downtown Library provided many sources, including the repertoire of newspapers referenced, namely the *Kentucky Gazette, Lexington Observer Reporter and Observer*, and *The Lexington Reporter* and the *Lexington Herald-Leader*, as well as city directories, telephone directories, and many books on Lexington's and Kentucky's history, including the *History of Kentucky* (two volumes) by Collins. The author also made use of the collections of the Special Collections of the University of Kentucky, the Filson Club, Louisville, the Kornhauser Library of the University of Louisville, the Kentucky Historical Society, Frankfort, and The Medical Archives of the University of Cincinnati, as well as correspondence with the College of Physicians, Philadelphia. The helpful hand of Billie Broaddus, Director of the Drake Collection, Cincinnati, deserves special recognition.

I would like to express my gratitude to a number of people who gave counsel and encouragement in the preparation of this book. In 1991 a special committee of the Fayette County Medical Society co-chaired by Dr. Thomson R. Bryant, Jr. and the author, Dr. Porter Mayo, was appointed to lay plans for a commemoration of the Society. At that time I was commissioned by the FCMS

Executive Committee to write a history of the Society. The author began the process of research in 1993 and writing of the text in 1996. Once the founding year of the Society (1799) was confirmed, the Society's Executive Committee prepared for the 200th anniversary for 1999.

To the editor, Walker Mayo, and the consultants, Camille Mayo Jernigan, Flo Witte and Carolyn Kurz, the author is indebted for their valuable suggestions and encouragement. Professors Lance Banning and Eric Christianson of the University of Kentucky each read a substantial part of the manuscript offering indispensable advice and criticism. I am particularly grateful to Drs. W. Lisle Dalton and John D. Stewart, II, past presidents, and to the current president of the Medical Society, Dr. J. Michael Moore, for their support in the preparation and publication of the book and the use of the Society's office, equipment and the many administrative courtesies by the staff. Others who gave specific aid or support included Drs. N. Lewis Bosworth, Ellsworth C. Seeley, and Walter L. Boswell; Claire R. McCann, Manuscript Librarian, Special Collections, University of Kentucky, and Jim Kurz. A special assistant, Shirley Boyd, gave vital support and long hours in the tedious and demanding editing of footnotes. Others, namely FCMS staff members Kathy Bethel, Cindy Madison and Sona Jewell, likewise aided the author in the daily essentials of typing and restoration of order in the references.

During the past twelve months the manuscript has been through seemingly endless revisions. In this final effort to ready the book for the publisher three people have been so vital, so committed to the project that a special recognition is in order. First, Vicki Hoven of the FCMS staff played a major role not only in the arduous task of proofreading but served admirably in the construction of figures, labels, and publication releases. Even more, she made numerous contacts by phone, fax and e-mail to the many librarians and publisher. Carolyn Kurz, Executive Vice President and Chief Executive Officer of the Society, played many roles in bringing the book to publication. She has been instrumental in the difficult task of maintaining consistency and accuracy in the preparation of the text, saved and sheltered the multiple drafts, and correlated the many steps to take in the completion of the work. But to those of us who know Carolyn best, it is her ever present enthusiasm, loads of encouragement and can do that shine through. Walker Mayo spent countless evenings and weekends, reading, editing, researching, and aiding the author to produce a book worthy of the individuals and the institutions herein enumerated. Whatever measure of success the book may attain, its value to the historical edifice so revered by the author, is in large measure because the author knew when to listen to his son.

I would also like to thank my family, especially my wife Pat, for their patience, encouragement and support.

The Medical Society has honored many a man and one woman on their election as president of the society. However, there is one instance when the process was reversed, when the society itself was not the donor but the recipient of such an honor; the occasion was the acceptance of the presidency in 1824 by Dr. Daniel Drake, foremost medical educator in America in the nineteenth century. His presidential address follows:

ADDRESS TO THE LEXINGTON MEDICAL SOCIETY

November 14, 1823

Gentlemen:

The animal body is an assemblage of organs, every one of which performs a function subservient to the general economy. But in relation to the whole they are not equal: some being of greater others of less importance. By a reference to this body, the structure composition, functions and diseases of which it is the object and will for several months be our object of most of you to study, I propose to illustrate the relation for the society of which I have had the honor of being elected the presiding officer to the university of which the greater part of you have become alumni and the remainder are trustees or friend professions. This society together with the private clubs of the pupils, the Kentucky Institute and all the facilities and contrivances which have been created or exist at present within the precincts of the town may be regarded as so many organs in the system of means, which have for their end or aggregate effect, the augmentation of literary scientifical and medical knowledge. The university is the principal; our society one of the subordinate or auxiliary organs, operating in concert, but in subserviency to the dominant or ruling department.

It is not, however, a lesser degree of the same, but differs from the medical college as specifically: as the sallivary glands differ from the liver, both of which, however remote in situation, different in size, and variant in function have the same object in view, the assimilation of foreign matter to our systems. It is not my design to express an opinion that this organ in the system of instruction is inferior in the dignity; but in the magnitude of its effects. When we contemplate it in reference to these we perceive at once, that it cannot afford the same advantages as the college but that the quality of what it affords and the nobleness of its operations as far as they go, may be regarded as equal to the institution to which it is auxiliary.

To render the society prolific in useful results, it must be conducted by the rules of sound common sense, and well regulated decorum. It must direct its attention to useful objects & conduct its operations with order and judgment. In the first place, it should adopt measures calculated to elicit from its members a regular succession of well written papers, on the various subjects which fall within the purview of the society; and these papers should if possible possess at least one of the three following excellencies.

1. Original facts or facts & speculation.
2. New speculations upon old facts.
3. In the absence of these an arrangement of existing facts & speculations, in such manner as to raise useful questions for

discusion. If measures should be adopted to secure an uninterrup ed succession of such papers, the meetings of the society ca not but prove highly interesting and beneficial.

Gentlemen, these benefits will be two fold 1st to ourselves & 2dly to the profession at large. To ourselves may come, if we choose the improvement in thinking & speaking that always results from debate, from the juxtaposition of inquisitive minds and the collisions that are the natural result of such a situation. The influence of occasions on the mind is so great, as to have given rise to the apothegm, that man is the creature of circumstances, which understood with proper limitations is undoubtedly true. Of the scenes in which it is possible for us, as students of medicine to place ourselves, I know of none, can indeed conceive of none, more eminently calculated to animate our intellectual faculties and desicate our stagnant pools of thought than debate; and I cannot believe it possible, that we shall even discuss the simplest questions in the science, without quicking our associations so as to send them into some new or untried region; nor examine the most difficult, without making some approximation toward the truths which it enveloped.

The second species of benefit which our society can be made to confer is on the profession at large and thro it upon mankind in general. This consists in promoting inquiries, and collecting and disseminating information, upon medical & scientific subjects. Such a society as ours may be made among the profession throughout our country what the voluntary or active powers of man are to his intellectual. Observation teaches us, that man requires to be stimulated; before he will act. When insulated & left to himself, his powers of mind too often remain passive his body quiescent. In this manner, hundreds of the profession vegetate to threescore then when sinking into the grave, the black waves of oblivion close over them & the world is as if they had not been. It is for association like ours, to disseminate the appropriate stimuli and rouse the slumbering lyons of literature & science to active effort. And this we may do in two different modes, 1. By resolving to engage ourselves in experimental researches; and at our various places of residence to prosecute such inquiries and make such original observations in the session or during the recess of the society or after our departure from it as may prove an example to other members of the profession, & serve to excite them to action. Secondly, we may accomplish much for the interests of the profession and of the manity by directing the attention of our professional confreres throughout the Western Country, to the countless number of interesting and important objects of investigation in which it abounds.

Among these I may refer to a variety of curious & beautiful atmospheric phenomena which daily pass before & seem to invite us to scrutinize them. The useful minerals of the Western Country, especially those employed in the processes of pharmacy. The investigation of our medicinal plants, many of which are doubtless entitled to great attention while very few of them have been thoroughly studied. The books which have been lately published on this subject indeed leave many desiderata. They are complete and worthy of great praise, in the botanical descriptions of the vegetables of which they treat but in the pharmacuetic and clinical histories of those substances they are so deficient, that I do not hesitate to say that such substantial advantage to medicine might be made to accrue by our society, would it undertake to exhort and advise the medical gentlemen of the West on this subject. It is necessary to direct their attention to specific objects if we would fix it.

The most important subjects, however, to which this society could point, those in which the community which we labor have the most deep & lively interests, are our diseases, particularly those of an endemic & epidemic character. Not a summer passes that does not give us an epidemic cholera which in certain places carries off many persons both adult & infantile; not an autumn which does not bring forth widespreading & fatal fevers which too often rage with such mortality as to spread over our social atmosphere as dark a gloom as that which in the same seasons shrouds our natural horizon. To ascertain all the physical & moral circumstances under which these maladies appear is the first step towards a discovery of their causes and a prevention of the effects of those causes. As, however, when discovered it may happen that that they are not of a kind that can be removed by human power, or avoided by human prudence it is of much importance that the diseases produced by them should be diligently & thoroughly studied: that the modifications which they exhibit in successive years, & in different situations should be compared with each other as well as the various means of cure which have been found most successful. For this to be done the profession throughout the country in which it is proposed to make observations should have a point of concentration-a sensorium commune where all intelligence should be received, compared, digested & again radiated to the profession and society at large to increase the powers of one & the blessings of the other, like the beams of heat & light which emanate from the sun to warm the earth make it prolific. To such objects might we direct our attention and it could scarcely be directed in vain.

Gentlemen, I hope to see our society active, & persevering, choosing good & great objects & prosecuting them with appropriate means, which is what constitutes wisdom; persevering in its ends and methodical functional & dignified in its proceedings. To assist in devoting it to such purposes & in conducting it in this manner are objects upon which I will cheerfully bestow every remnant of time and abilities that may be left after discharging my permanent duties to the University. I will conclude, Gentlemen, by offering you my unfeigned thanks for the honor you have bestowed upon me, in raising me to this responsible station. If I shall not be able to tread in the elevated footsteps of my learned & philosophical predecessor, I shall claim at least to equal him in my prayers for the prosperity & fame of the institution. [Daniel Drake]

W. Porter Mayo, M.D., Ph.D.

Chapter I

THE LEXINGTON MEDICAL SOCIETY

There are men and classes of men that stand above the common herd: the soldier, the sailor, and the shepherd not infrequently: the artist rarely, rarelier still the clergyman: the physician almost as a rule. He is the flower (such as it is) of our civilization: and when that stage of man is done with, he will be thought to have shared as little as any in the defects of the period, and most notably in the virtues of the race. Generosity he has, such as is possible to those who practice an art, never to those who drive a trade: discretion, tested by a hundred secrets: tact, tried in a thousand embarrassments: and what are more important, Herculean cheerfulness and courage. So it is that he brings air and cheer into the sick room, and often enough, though not as often as he wishes, brings healing.

Robert Louis Stevenson
Preface to *Underwoods.*

Of Progress and Of Medicine

The history of medicine in Lexington parallels the pattern set in earlier lands where the fates of medicine and of the economy were inextricably linked.[1] The pioneers of early Lexington conquered the wilderness, built a flourishing economy, and shared in the bounty of the early Republic. In their wake, medicine followed and flourished in its turn.

During Lexington's golden age, circa 1783 to 1820, the pioneers and their children turned Lexington into the *Athens of the West.*[2] Manufacturing, commerce, art, law, and politics flourished, and progress appeared to have no bounds.[3] The late 1790s welcomed the founding of the Lexington Medical Society and of the medical department of Transylvania University. By 1819, medicine had securely taken its place in the march of progress, with the medical department's possession of a faculty second only to that of America's oldest medical college, the University of Pennsylvania.[4] The people of Lexington played a decisive role in the formation of the medical department of Transylvania and were well rewarded for their generosity by the respect and admiration accorded *their* faculty, *their* students, and *their* Lexington. But the long shadow of history darkened the economic future of the *Athens of the West* and, inevitably, its prominent role in medicine.

Initially, geography smiled upon Lexington: "Lying as it did astride the major overland routes of the trans-Appalachian frontier, Lexington quickly became an important stopping place for new immigrants, a thriving mercantile entrepot, and a developing social and cultural center."[5] Within a generation of Lexington's founding, however, westward bound pioneers found travel on the rivers superior in terms of time, ease, and economy to the primitive overland trails leading to and from Lexington. Lexington's future troubles were foreshadowed in the comments of Joseph Espy of Philadelphia, who remarked in 1805, "The country around Lexington, for many miles in every direction, is equal in beauty and fertility to any thing the imagination can paint, and is already in a high state of cultivation....It has, however, one fault—to a Pennsylvanian an intolerable one—it is very badly watered."[6]

With the introduction of the steamboat in 1812, Lexington entered a long and humiliating decline that eventually culminated in the loss of its medical supremacy to the river cities of Cincinnati, Louisville, and St. Louis.[7] [8] Between 1814 and 1820, the population of Lexington dwindled from 8,000 to slightly over 4,000.[9] Its rivals, Cincinnati and Louisville, both of which were mere villages when Lexington became a budding city, rapidly surpassed Lexington in population. By 1830, Cincinnati had a population of 24,000, compared to 10,000 for Louisville and only 5,000 for Lexington.[10] Without river transportation, Lexington became just another inland town, without the prospect for prosperity. Even so, Lexington remained the center of medicine in the American West well into the latter 1830s. By then, however, Cincinnati and Louisville were burgeoning cities, each with several medical schools, while the medical faculty of Transylvania University declined in number and standing with the desertion in 1837 of several professors to the more prosperous and more promising medical schools in Louisville. Before its decline, however, Lexington made its mark on the world of medicine and preserved the seeds of a tradition that would come to fruition in the mid-twentieth century.

The Lexington Medical Society, a society including several members of national repute, but laboring under the same economic burden, closed its doors in 1834-35. Although the Transylvania Medical Department and the medical community plodded along into the mid 1850s, a state of dormancy prevailed in Lexington throughout the remainder of the nineteenth century and well into the mid-twentieth century. By the 1950s, however, the fortunes of Lexington revived with the arrival of newly crossing interstate highways and improved air traffic. Once again, some 130 years after the founding of Lexington's first medical school Transylvania University (1817-18), Lexington became home to a new medical school, led and fashioned by the shared ideas, courage, and tenacity of members of the Fayette County Medical Society and the

University of Kentucky.

First Society West of the Alleghenies

The enlightened ideas of the Revolutionary generation encouraged the founding of learned societies in the early Republic, including medical societies. In 1776, the Continental Congress urged the establishment in every colony of "A society for the improvement of agriculture, arts, manufactures, and commerce, and that a correspondence be maintained among them."[11] The usefulness of such a society was not lost on early Lexington. The December 7, 1787, issue of the *Kentucke Gazette* proudly announced the formation of "The Kentucke Society for promoting useful knowledge."[12]

The Kentucke Society literally put Lexington on the map (see endsheets). That map, a world map, depicts the full geographical extent of scientific societies in 1789. As related by the historian McClellan, "...at that date scientific societies extended from Philadelphia and Kentucky in the west to Saint Petersburg (or arguably Batavia, the East Indies) in the east, and from Trondheim (Norway) in the North to Sicily and Haiti in the south. If we include the *Academia Scientifica* which existed in Rio de Janeiro in the early 1770s, we can fairly say that eighteenth-century scientific societies extended worldwide. Scientific societies were scattered throughout Central Europe, the Low Countries, Scandinavia, and Great Britain. Two official scientific societies and four private ones represented North America [Boston, Hartford, New York, Philadelphia, Richmond, Virginia and Lexington]."[13]

For perspective, let us reflect on the nature of Lexington, Kentucky, in the year 1787: "Lexington, which stands on the head waters of Elkhorn River, is reckoned the capitol of Kentucky. Here, the courts are held, and business is regularly conducted. In 1786, it contained about 100 houses, and several stores, with a good assortment of dry goods."[14] A more earthy portrayal is given by Fielding Bradford, brother of the editor of the *Kentucke Gazette*, John Bradford: "In the summer of 1787 there was only a path where Main street now is, (up to) about where Masonic Lodge and Short street (now Short and Walnut). Gimson weeds grew so thick there you couldn't have seen a hog on either side 10 feet from the path."[15] Why then the recognition by a twentieth century historian of these Kentuckians, mud-deep in the forest, and for Lexington itself? How did they put Lexington on the map? No innovation, invention, publication or other attainments by the Kentucke Society explains such recognition. This seeming paradox is best answered by the following statement in Collins *History of Kentucky.*[16]

> Kentucky owed most of her remarkable intellectual development, at an early day in her history, to the fact that at the close of the Revolutionary war in 1781 many of the most intellectual and cultivated of the officers and soldiers in that war from the states of Virginia, New Jersey, Pennsylvania, and Maryland-being unsettled in their homes and business by its great duration, privations and calamities-sought new homes in the then richest land in the known world. Thus the times and the country itself, the very life of hardship, self-denial, and self-dependence, combined to make a race seldom equaled in the world for strength of intellect and will, physical and moral courage, personal prowess and personal endurance. Never did a population so small in numbers embrace so many who were giants in intellect, giants in daring, and all but giants in physical proportion.

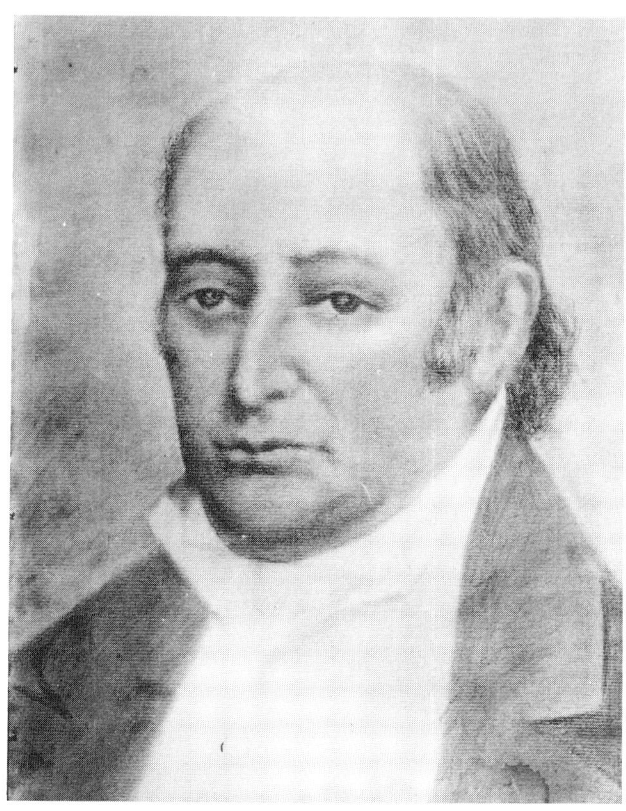

John Bradford
(1749-1830)
Courtesy of The Filson Club Historical Society, Louisville, Kentucky

That such a society could exist in the wilderness was, in itself, testimony to the realization of an important goal of the scientific societies, namely the diffusion of knowledge. What may have been most influential in their recognition is the settlers' awareness of themselves, simply the knowledge of who they were, where they were, and more important, *why*. As stated by John Bradford, editor of the *Kentucke Gazette*, in his first issue, August 18, 1787: "*...a Spirit prevails among my countrymen superior to their present circumstances.*"[17] That such an assertion was warranted can be found in the list of Kentucke Society's members: some became judges, governors, and United States senators, whereas others became famous and prominent in law, education, and politics. Although no physicians were among the original members of the

Kentucke Society, within a generation Lexington would have a medical society animated by the same spirit.

Medical Societies in America

A generation before the founding of the Lexington Medical Society in 1799, medical societies were active in the older American settlements.[18] The distinguished Medical Society of New Jersey, founded at New Brunswick on June 23, 1766, was the first important medical society in the American Colonies.[19] Its existence, however, was interrupted by the Revolutionary War from 1775 to 1781. The Massachusetts Medical Society has the honor of being the oldest medical society in the United States with a history of uninterrupted meetings, beginning in 1781 and continuing through the present.[20] Throughout the remainder of the eighteenth century, other medical societies sporadically dotted the Atlantic Seaboard. Continuity of existence was not a characteristic of American medical societies throughout the eighteenth century and the early nineteenth century.[21] Even so, those medical societies that languished and died led the way and gave impetus to those living societies to try ever harder. Although a given society might die, *the idea lived.*

Founding of the Transylvania Medical Department and the Lexington Medical Society

Early Lexington was preeminent in so many spheres that it is not unexpected to find it as one of the leaders of the medical profession, with the founding of the Lexington Medical Society. An advertisement (December 24, 1799) of Transylvania University in the *Kentucky Gazette* stated that "Law and Medicine societies meet each week in town...." This announcement was signed by William Morton, Chairman of the Standing Committee, Transylvania

University. The lead paragraph stated, "The trustees of the Transylvania University anxious to diffuse the benefits of the institution as extensively as possible, have resolved to inform the inhabitants of Kentucky and the Western country in general, of the arrangements which they have recently made for the promotion of academical and professional studies." The advertisement stated that Dr. Frederick Ridgely would teach "Materia Medica, Midwifery and the practice of Physick" and that the "important studies of Chemistry, Anatomy, and Surgery are confided to Dr. Samuel Brown."[22]

Samuel Brown

Samuel Brown (1769-1830), a native of Augusta (now Rockbridge County), Virginia, was the third son of John Brown, a Presbyterian minister, and Margaret Preston. Samuel began his schooling under the tutelage of his father. At the age of sixteen he continued his classical education at the seminary conducted by Dr. James Waddell in Louisa County, Virginia, preparatory to enrolling in Dickinson College in Carlisle, Pennsylvania. Subsequently, Samuel had the opportunity to serve an apprenticeship with his distinguished brother-in-law, Dr. Alexander Humphreys, of Staunton, Virginia. A young Kentuckian was also an apprentice with Dr. Humphreys at this time: Ephraim McDowell, of Danville, Kentucky.[23] After several months under the instruction of Dr. Humphreys, Brown transferred to the private tutelage of Dr. Benjamin Rush of Philadelphia, a signer of the Declaration of Independence and the most renowned American physician of the time.

Probably influenced by Drs. Humphreys and Rush, both graduates of the University of Edinburgh Medical School, in 1793 Brown set sail across the Atlantic to continue his studies at Edinburgh and once again found himself in the company of Ephraim McDowell. Two other fellow students, David Hosack

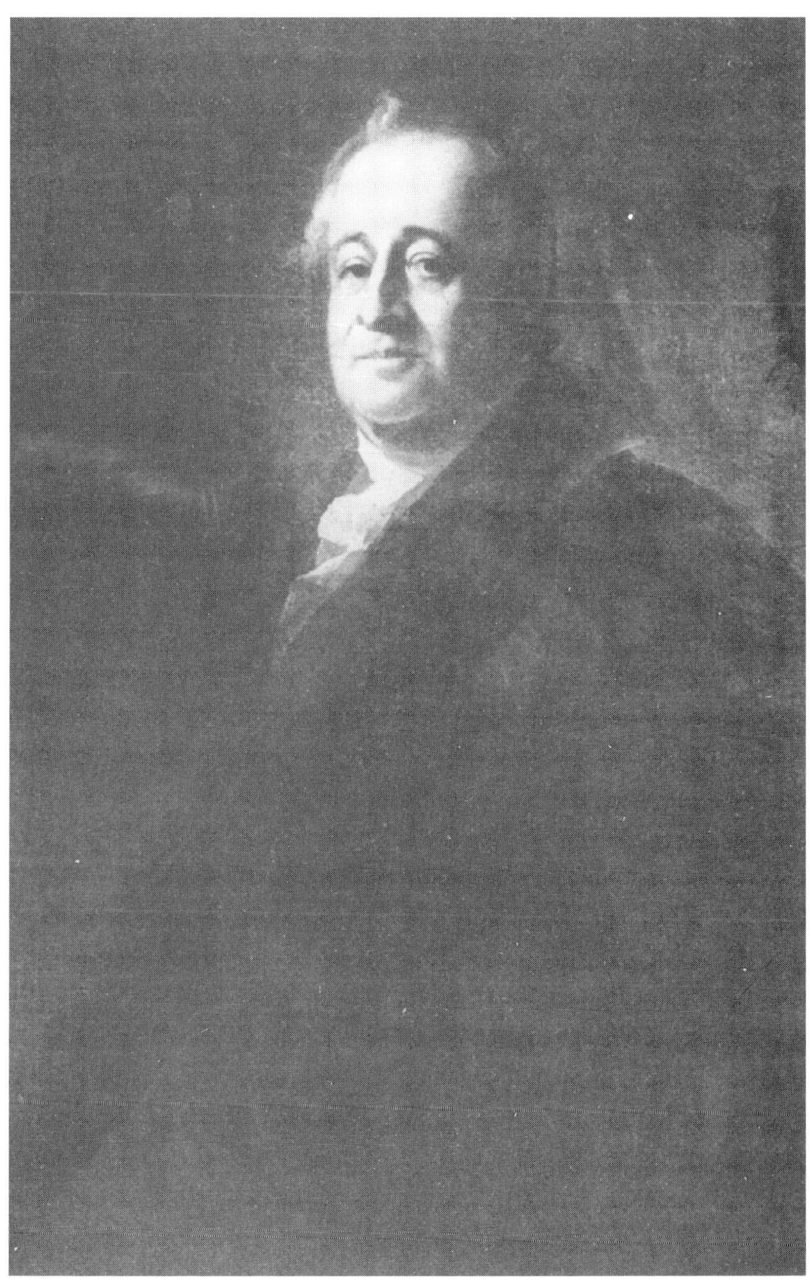

Samuel Brown, M.D.
(1769-1830)
Courtesy of Transylvania University Library

and John B. Davidge, later became famous American physicians.[24] At Edinburgh the young students attended lectures by the famous professors James Gregory, Joseph Black, Alexander Monro Secundus, and John Bell.[25] Although Brown did not receive his medical degree at Edinburgh, he did so at the University of Aberdeen before sailing for home. While in Scotland, Brown, Hosack, and Davidge each entertained the possibility of founding a medical school in America.[26] As Brown later recalled, the Scottish students ridiculed the Americans' ambition, but "we were not to be laughed out of our projects, and in a little while after his return Hosack was announced a professor in his native city [New York], and Davidge was at work laying the foundation of the University of Maryland. I was appointed a professor in this young University [Transylvania]…."[27]

In 1795, upon his return home, Brown began practicing medicine in Bladensburgh, Maryland, near Washington, D.C. Although he built an extensive practice, he longed for the companionship of his brothers, John, in Frankfort, Kentucky, and James, in Lexington.[28] [29] Brown's arrival in Lexington can be found in a short announcement in the *Kentucky Gazette* of September 6, 1797.

> Dr. Samuel Brown begs leave to inform the public that he will practice MEDICINE and SURGERY in Lexington and its vicinity-He occupies the house in which Mr. Love lately lived, opposite Mr. Stewart's printing office. He will undertake, on reasonable terms, to Instruct one or two pupils, who can bring Good recommendations (September 5, 1795).[30]

The prominence of the Brown brothers and the rapidly acquired reputation of Dr. Samuel Brown quickly led to his selection as one of two medical professors in the newly organized Transylvania College. Brown was the first professor of medicine west of the Alleghenies; his appointment was as professor of Medicine, Chemistry, and Surgery. The selection of Brown and Frederick Ridgely was first made by the Transylvania Board of Trustees on January 8, 1799. On the same date the Board "Resolved that a professorship of Medicine and Law and Politic be established; and that the committee hereafter named be empowered to make such rules for their regulations and provisions for the carrying them into effect, as to them shall seem proper; the rules so to be made, to continue in force until the mo[nth] of the next stated meeting of the Board and no longer." Notice of the appointments of Dr. Brown and Dr. Ridgely was dated December 24, 1799, and printed in the *Kentucky Gazette* of March 6, 1800.

> The reasons for introducing the study of Medicine and surgery were not less urgent...[than the study of law.] [James Brown, Samuel's older brother, was made professor of Law at Transylvania at this same meeting]....The important studies of Chemistry, Anatomy and surgery are confided to Dr. Samuel Brown.-His great application, and uncommon opportunities of acquiring an accurate and comprehensive knowledge of those subjects; his easy and perspicuous mode of conveying information have already gained him a considerable class; and from his perseverance and attention the trustees expect the happiest effects...
>
> Lexington Kentucky
> December 24, 1799

Brown was a man of many interests, anchored in medicine yet easily moving from medicine to science, particularly botany, agriculture, and archaeology, and other areas of study, all of which were one in his search for truth.[31] Dr. Robert Peter, in his *History of the Medical Department of Transylvania University,* gives this assessment of Brown:[32]

> Dr. Brown was a man of fine personal appearance and manners; an accomplished scholar, gifted with natural eloquence and humor that made him one of the most fascinating lecturers of his day. Learned in many branches, he was enthusiastic in his own profession, scrupulous in regard to etiquette and exceedingly benevolent and liberal of his time and services to the poor.

Dr. Brown's brilliant contribution to medicine did not stop here. He founded a national medical society, Kappa Lambda, and its companion journal *The North American Medical and Surgical Journal.* In 1819, he introduced Thomas Percival's "Code of Ethics" into the body of Kappa Lambda.[33] By 1800, Brown was a member of the renowned American Philosophical Society of Philadelphia, Pennsylvania, having been recommended by his friends Benjamin Rush and Thomas Jefferson.[34] He was the first American west of the Alleghenies to be so honored.

Frederick Ridgely

Frederick Ridgely (1757-1824), a native of Maryland, arrived in Lexington in 1790. Like almost all practicing physicians of the time, his medical training came by the apprentice system (Delaware), a process long in use in England. Dr. Ridgely also took advantage of medical lectures in Philadelphia preparatory to practice. He was said to be "a favorite pupil of Dr. [Benjamin] Rush."[35] At the age of 19, Ridgely was appointed surgeon to a rifle corps in Virginia. In early 1779, he was assigned duties "as surgeon to a vessel sailing with letters of marque and reprisal off the coast

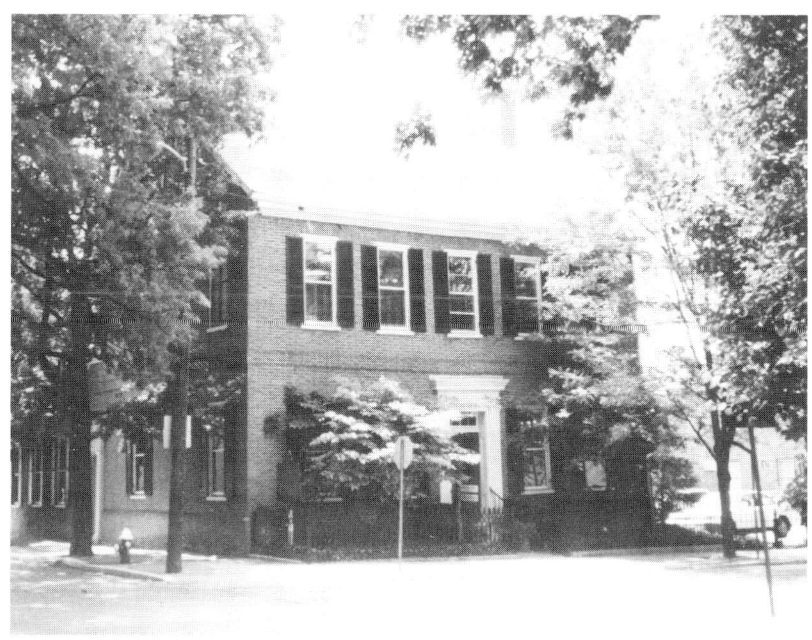

Ridgely-Brown House
Courtesy of Fayette County Medical Society

of Virginia. The vessel was chased into the Chesapeake bay by a British man of war. As the ship's colors were struck to the enemy, Dr. Ridgely leaped overboard, and narrowly escaped capture by swimming two miles to the shore."[36] He continued to be active in the military while in Lexington, accompanying the militia on its expeditions against the Indians, and he later served as surgeon-general in General "Mad Anthony" Wayne's army in 1794. While living in Lexington, Dr. Ridgely became close friends with Henry Clay. A highly successful practitioner, attracting patients not only from Lexington but also from remote settlements, he played an important role in medical education. Two of his apprentices became internationally famous, namely Walter Brashear (1776-1860) and Benjamin Dudley (1785-1870).

Dr. Ridgely was also active in the formation of the Medical Department of Transylvania University, being named as Professor of Physick in 1799, and, together with his friend and colleague, Dr.

Samuel Brown, delivering a course of lectures that same year to a small class of medical students.[37] He moved to Richmond, Kentucky, in 1806 and died in Dayton, Ohio, on December 21, 1824.

Records

Lexington, January 8th 1799.
Being the second Tuesday in the month.

Which day, was appointed by Law for the meeting of the Board of Trustees of the Transylvania University; In pursuance whereof the following Trustees met and took the Oaths prescribed by Law and their seats, to wit: Cornelius Beatty, Frederick Ridgely, George Nicholas, Andrew McCalla, William Morton, Robert Steele, John McDowell, Alexander Parker, Caleb Wallace, James Trotter, Levi Todd, James Blythe, Thomas Lewis, John Bradford, Bartlet Collins, and Buckner Thruston

The Board being thus met, proceeded to the appointment of a Chairman pro tem

Resolution of the Board of Trustees of Transylvania University appointing Drs. Brown and Ridgely as professors of medicine.
1st and 2nd pages – January 8, 1799
Both Courtesy of Transylvania University Library

2

tempore and John Bradford was unanimously elected.

After some consideration of the business before the Board it came to the following resolutions:

Resolved that a professorship of Medicine, and another of Law and Politics be established; and that the committee hereafter named be impowered to make such rules for their regulation, and provision for the carrying them into effect as to them shall seem proper: the rules so to be made, ~~the rules so to be made~~ to continue in force until the end of the next stated meeting of the Board and no longer.

Resolved, That the late President, assistant, Treasurer, and Clerk of the Transylvania Seminary, be continued in office with the emoluments now appertaining to their respective offices until the first day of January next and no longer.

Resolution of the Board of Trustees of Transylvania University appointing Drs. Brown and Ridgely as professors of medicine.
3rd page – January 8, 1799
Courtesy of Transylvania University Library

3

Resolved That Messrs. Cornelius Beatty, Andrew McCalla, William Morton, John McDowell, Alexander Parker, James Trotter, Levi Todd, James Blythe and Buckner Thruston, or any five of them, be a committee with full power until the next stated meeting of the Board, to do such acts and things, as by Law a committee may do.

Resolved, That there be two stated meetings of this Board in each year, to wit: On the first Mondays in April & October.

Resolved That Doctors Frederick Ridgely and Samuel Brown be appointed Professors of Medicine.

Resolved, That George Nicholas be appointed Professor of Law and Politics.

Resolved That Messrs. George Nicholas Caleb Wallace and Joseph Crockett or any two

Why a Medical Society?

We know that a medical society met weekly in Lexington in 1799 and that the members included practicing Lexington physicians, their student apprentices, and other selected physicians and citizens.[38 39] But in such a place and at such a time, why a medical society? The answer would be obvious by turning to the preamble of its constitution, and we would do so if one were available. But the 1799 constitution is lost along with almost all of the minutes.

Although we do not have the constitution and bylaws of 1799, the preserved constitution of 1821 is likely identical.[40] The 1821 preamble to the Act incorporating the Lexington Medical Society states in part: "there is a number of individuals, connected with the School of Medicine in Transylvania University, who are desirous of being incorporated as a society…for the purpose of cultivating to more advantage the science of medicine, and of awakening in these western states, a more lively zeal for greater attainment and improvements in that important branch of knowledge…."[41] Such minutes of the original society that survive (1803-04)[42] are invaluable and are consistent with the 1821 documents. The preamble of the 1821 Act affords an insight as to how the Lexington medical community, within but a relatively few years, came into national prominence.

Samuel Brown and the other members of the Lexington Medical Society were devoted to "the science of medicine." As "reputable" physicians, they sought to separate themselves in the public mind from medical practitioners who were not men of learning. In an era before licensing laws, medical societies helped to differentiate those who were reputable and scientific from those who were not. Membership in a medical society, together with a certificate from a preceptor, and, more rarely, a medical degree, were the insignia of the respected physician.

From the Colonial period in America, most physicians were trained by the apprenticeship method, serving for a given period of time, customarily five to seven years, and often living with the physician's family. The MD degree was so unusual that of the 3,500 practicing physicians in the colonies during the period of the Revolutionary War, less than 300 had received a medical degree. Of the 300 physicians with degrees, most had earned those degrees in Europe, because the Philadelphia Medical College (later the University of Pennsylvania) and King's College (later Columbia University) were the only medical schools available to Americans in their homeland.[43] Upon completion of the apprenticeship, the preceptor would give his student a signed certificate testifying to the readiness of the holder to practice medicine. The value placed on the certificate bearer, the new physician, was no more or less than that placed on the preceptor. If signed by Benjamin Rush of Philadelphia, William Goforth of Cincinnati, or Samuel Brown or Frederick Ridgely of Lexington, then the certificate had great value—the bearer would be recognized as a *reputable* physician.

In many instances, however, especially in the more rural areas, the preceptor had few if any books, and often little or questionable training; in such cases, the same incapacity, the same errors, would be passed on again and again. Charles Caldwell, the talented and contentious Professor of Medicine and Clinical Practice of the Transylvania Medical Department (1819-37) relates his apprenticeship experience:[44]

> I ... placed myself under the tuition of a gentleman of reputation and standing, who had not long previously graduated in medicine from the University of Pennsylvania. But, in relation to the advantages for improvement which I had anticipated, I encountered a sad and mortifying disappointment. Though my preceptor was a man of respectable talents, and no inconsiderable stock of knowledge, and though he was exceedingly attentive and communicative to me, in conversation, that was almost the only source of which I could avail myself. He had no library, no

> apparatus, no provision for improvement in practical anatomy, nor any other efficient means of instruction in medicine.

And too, there were others who practiced medicine without benefit of even the most rudimentary training. Writing in 1757, William Smith in his history of New York wrote, "Any man at his Pleasure sets up for Physician, Apothecary, and Chiurgeon. No Candidates are either examined or licensed, or even sworn to fair practice."[45]

And then there were quacks.[46] A partial list of the daily offerings of these quacks appeared in the *Kentucky Gazette* of April 27,1802:

- Hamilton's Grand Restorative; Is recommended as an invaluable medicine for the speedy relief and permanent cure of the various complaints which result from dissipated pleasures, juvenile indiscretions, residence in a climate unfavorable to the constitution, the immoderate use of mercury, the diseases peculiar to females at a certain period of life, bad lyings in, etc.

- Price 2 dollars, Indian Vegetable Specific, For the cure of a Certain Disease.

- The Genuine Persian Lotion, For cleansing and cleaning the FACE and SKIN, of all Scorbutic and other Eruptions—-particularly Freckles, Pimples, Pits after the Small Pox, Inflammatory Redness, Scurfs, Tetters, Ring Worms, Sun-Burns, Prickly Heat, Premature wrinkles, &c. Rendering the skin delicately clear and soft, improving the complexion, restoring and preserving the bloom of youth. Price 1 dollar and 50 cents, per bottle.

Others included Hamilton's Worm Destroying Lozenges; Tooth-Ache Drops; and the Genuine Extract of Mustard for the Cure of Rheumatism.

The obvious question, then, was how the competent physicians, those trained by reputable preceptors alone or by both preceptors and medical schools, at home or abroad, could identify themselves to their colleagues, to their patients, and to the public. For themselves and for the public good, they perceived a need for distinguishing their credentials from those of persons masquerading as physicians. The preceptor's certificate, letters of recommendation, published works, and word of mouth were the only means of proof.

Both Drs. Brown and Ridgely were familiar with the medical societies in Philadelphia, and Dr. Brown was also familiar with those of Europe, especially those of Edinburgh. Had he chosen to do so, Dr. Brown, in particular, could have had a lucrative practice in any of the larger cities along the Atlantic Seaboard. In fact, he left a prosperous practice in Maryland to come to Lexington. Such medical embellishments as societies were expected by men such as these as part of the medical tradition. The need of frontier physicians to fraternize, to share experiences, to exchange ideas, to diffuse knowledge, to investigate, and to abide by a universal ethical standard was a concept still in its infancy. For Brown, who was a frequent correspondent with President Thomas Jefferson and Dr. David Hosack of New York, among others, the society was a natural choice. This fraternal and intellectual thirst on the part of Brown, together with the desire of other Lexington physicians (ten to twelve physicians were in Lexington in 1799) to be distinguished as *reputable* physicians probably drew the members together. From what we know of other medical societies at this time, there were benefits to be derived and problems to be faced by those willing to commit themselves to membership.

These doctors often were many miles apart. The need to exchange ideas and knowledge, to present and discuss medical cases, new procedures, and experience likely prompted these frontier doctors to unite. The Society and its members had to be of such stature that the public would be impressed by their credentials. They were trained physicians. They craved respect. Members of such a society also had in mind the sharing of social and fraternal pleasures, but they did not, would not, care to do so with the quacks and the cunning.

We can summarize the extensive list of desirable traits given above in one word-**Respect**. **Respect** was the reason for the Lexington Medical Society; **Respect** is what later held the American Medical Association together during its tenuous and turbulent beginning; **Respect** came to physicians, but it took a century, the nineteenth, and it did not come easily.

The Founder of the Lexington Medical Society

The Lexington Medical Society is a self-portrait of its founder, Samuel Brown. Samuel Brown's role as the founder of the Society may be inferred from several facts. There is no record of a medical society existing in Lexington before 1799. Dr. Brown announced the opening of his office in Lexington in September 1797.[47] Samuel Brown quickly "became part of the civic life of Lexington," for within two months of his arrival in Lexington in 1797, he became a member of the "Immigration Society," together with George Nicholas and John Bradford, editor of the *Kentucky Gazette.*[48] [49] Although the Immigration Society had no connection with medicine, it was characteristic of Brown to act without delay. One of Brown's biographers states that "Dr. Brown was not long in acquiring at Lexington, a reputation equal to that he had enjoyed elsewhere, and in securing the confidence of a large number of the most respectable part of the population of the town and surrounding country. His reputation, indeed, soon spread over the whole State, and he was consulted far and wide."[50]

All who knew Brown were aware of his insatiable desire to be involved with the diffusion of knowledge and education. That is why he was the first person west of the Alleghenies to have published a medical paper, and why he was well ahead of physicians in New York City and other eastern cities in the introduction of vaccination for smallpox in 1801-02.[51] Equally convincing is Brown's gift for founding societies. Shortly after his return to Lexington in 1819 to join the Transylvania Medical Department, he started a new society, the first national medical society, Kappa Lambda of Hippocrates. A biographer of Brown states "He was active in the organization of societies for the discussion of questions of science and literature."[52] There is no record of a medical society existing in Lexington or elsewhere in Kentucky before the arrival of Brown in 1797, and during the years of his absence from Lexington (years spent in Mississippi, Louisiana, and Alabama, 1806-19), no other medical society was founded in Lexington.

The close associations of both Brown and the Lexington Medical Society with Transylvania University also point to Brown as the founder of the Society. The minutes of the Transylvania University Board of Trustees meeting of December 1799 announced the establishment of a medical department as part of the University. Drs. Samuel Brown and Frederick Ridgely were named professors. On December 24, 1799, the Chairman of the Board reported that "law and medical societies meet each week." And, further, the minutes of the Society note that medical students and professors met together, the hallmark of the Lexington Medical Society, "the mixed membership of students and physicians patterned on the medical societies clustering about Edinburgh University."[53] In 1799, Samuel Brown was the only Lexington physician to have studied medicine at Edinburgh University.

Of the physicians practicing in Lexington in 1799, there were but two whose names are undeniably tied to the Lexington Medical Society, Samuel Brown and Frederick Ridgely. Brown's name appears three times in the preserved 1803-1804 minutes, and Ridgely's name appears twice. Dr. James Fishback's name appears three times in the minutes, but he, however, probably did not arrive in Lexington until 1802.[54] Brown's penchant for founding and participating in societies, his experience in Edinburgh, and his general reputation and leadership all point to him as the founder of the Lexington Medical Society, the parent of the Fayette County Medical Society. Brown should be honored as the titular father of *all* medical societies west of the Alleghenies.

The Date of the Lexington Medical Society's Founding

The exact date of the origin of the Lexington Medical Society is unknown. One author categorically states that the Society was formed in 1799, and another in the winter of 1799-1800.[55] Unfortunately, these authors do not give a reference in support of these dates. Dr. Waller Bullock stated that the first meeting of the Society took place in 1802, but he, too, did not give a reference.[56] The noted Kentucky historian Dr. Emmet Horine states that "the earliest association of physicians in Kentucky was doubtless formed in Lexington sometime during the last decade of the eighteenth century."[57] The Society undoubtedly existed in 1799, while the possibility of an earlier date cannot be confirmed or denied.

An old *Kentucky Gazette* records the existence of the Lexington Medical Society as far back as 1803.[58] However, an attendance sheet dated February 2, 1803, confirms that society meetings had taken place in 1802 and lists the names of the members of the society.[59] The second extant entry by the Secretary of the Society was dated Wednesday Evening, October 5, 1803: "The Society met pursuant to adjournment last spring. Ordinary members [students] present, James L. Armstrong, Philip Barbour, William Wilmott, Robert McNitt, James M. Hamilton, Samuel M. Venable, & Rich Davison. Absent James Thompson, Bernard Farrar, Benjamin W. Dudley, Andrew Steele, Tho' C. Davis & Coleman Rogers."[60] The Secretary pro tempore was a bit put out by the absence of the Secretary and made this entry: "The Secretary finding it more his interest to attend a Ball, than the meeting of the

Society got leave of absence." The extant minutes of the meetings begin with that of October 5, 1803, and continue through twenty-one pages, ending on January 25, 1804. The roster, dated October 1803, discloses that there were fifteen "ordinary" members. Those members designated as "ordinary members" were medical students apprenticed to various Lexington physicians, especially Drs. Brown, Fishback, and Ridgely. There were also honorary members, physicians and laymen in Lexington, and Drs. Charles Caldwell and James Woodhouse of Philadelphia.

A reading of the minutes of the Society provides many interesting items of information. At the meeting of October 12, 1803, the Society resolved that "each ordinary member previous to his becoming an honorary member of this Society and after his having commenced the practice of medicine, shall write a dissertation on some practical subject and transmit it to the Society." The meeting of December 28, 1803, was highlighted by an assessment of James Armstrong, Secretary, who was fined 25 cents for absenting himself without leave. It was also resolved that "the skeletons are no longer considered as the property of the Society. But that one belongs to the student of Dr. Brown and the other to those of Dr. Fishback, and therefore, not subject to the collection of the curator." Drs. Brown, Fishback, and Ridgely were frequently mentioned in the 1803-04 minutes of the society.

Items such as the following, noting the continued existence of the Society, appeared from time to time in the Lexington newspaper, the *Kentucky Gazette and General Advertiser*. On September 20, 1803, we read that "The Lexington Medical Society will meet on the first Wednesday in October next in the Transylvania University at 6 o'clock. The members are requested to be punctual in their attendance. By order of the President, James L. Armstrong, Secretary."[61] The *Kentucky Gazette* of December 20, 1803, contains the following announcement: "Medical Society. Those who write to the Lexington Medical Society are requested to pay the postage of all communications so made. By order of the Society. (Signed) R. Davidson, Secretary, December 17, 1803."

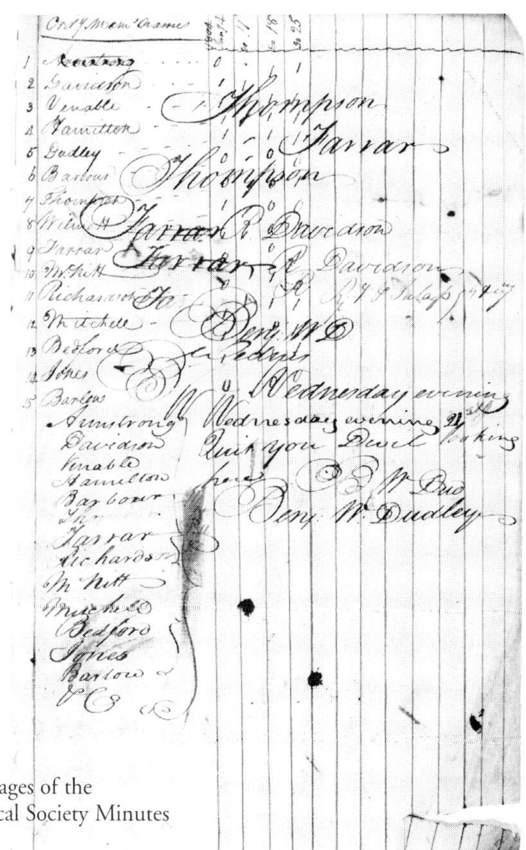

Representative pages of the Lexington Medical Society Minutes (1803-1804)

Courtesy of Transylvania University Library

The following announcement of June 5, 1804 is also of interest:[62]

> For the promotion of medical and Natural Science, there will be an intermediate meeting of the Lexington Medical Society on Saturday the 16th inst. half past two o'clock, at the Transylvania University Hall, where the following subject will be discussed: Is heat material, and the cause of the elasticity of the gases?

Student-Physician Society

Indeed, the Lexington Medical Society was not only the first medical society west of the Alleghenies, it was the first student-physician medical society in America in which both medical students and physicians held elected office.[63] The first student-faculty medical society in America was organized in Philadelphia during the latter part of the eighteenth century, a merger of a *Hospital Medical Society* of students and the *American Medical Society.* The Lexington Medical Society, therefore, was the second physician-student medical society in America. To our knowledge, however, students of the Philadelphia Society did not share in elected offices. The primacy of the Lexington Medical Society in this respect is recognized both by the delineation of students as ordinary members and of physicians as honorary members, and by the actual election of students as officers of the society along with physicians. The first known president of the Society was a student (ordinary member), S. L. Mitchell.[64] The second validated president of the society, Samuel M. Venable (elected November 5, 1803), was also a student.[65] A third student, John R. Bedford, was elected president; however, the date of the minutes is uncertain.

Another Transylvania University medical student, Henry Miller,[66] later the thirteenth president of the American Medical Society, was elected President of the Lexington Medical Society in 1822, the year of his graduation from Transylvania University.

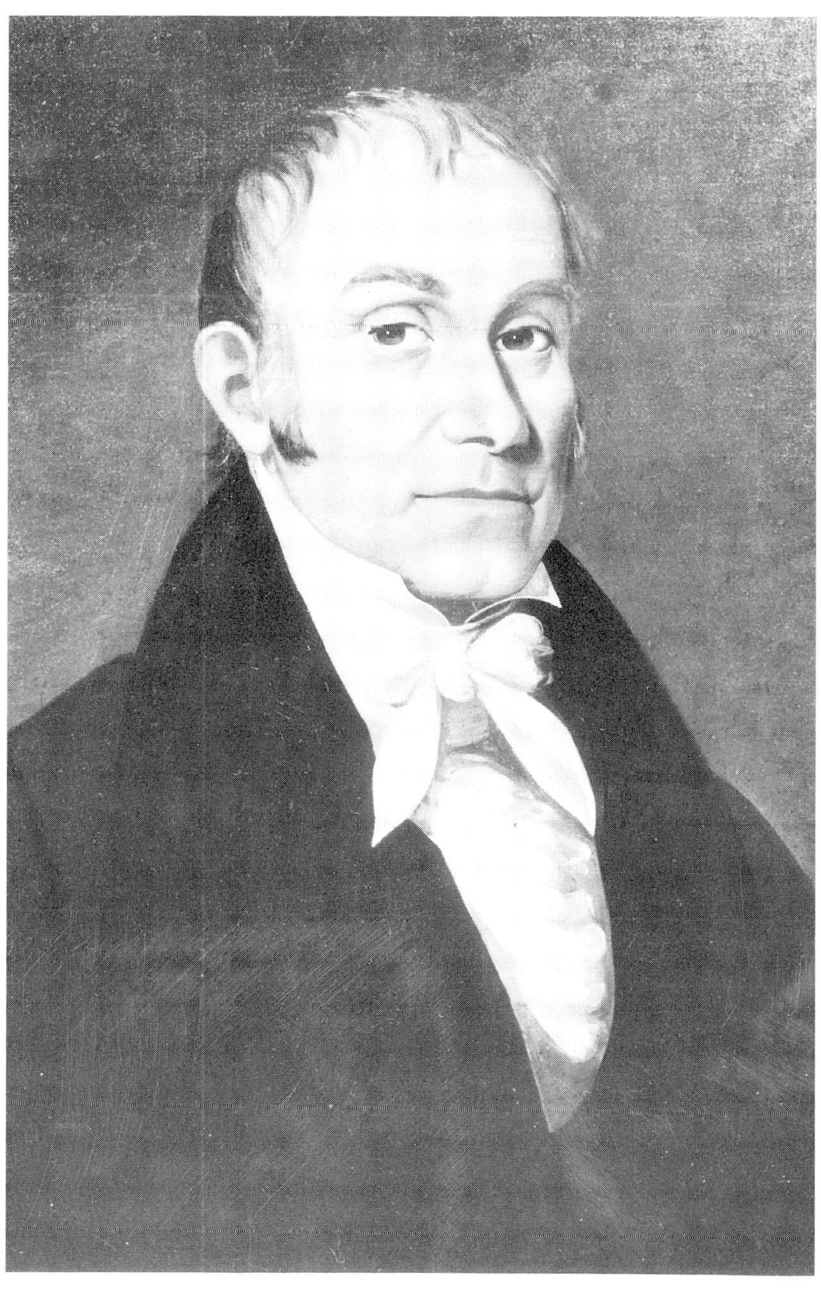

Ephraim McDowell, M.D.
(1771-1830)
Courtesy of McDowell House

(Miller was the last confirmed student to hold office). Doctors Benjamin Dudley (1818) and Daniel Drake (1824) were the first and second recorded physicians to hold the office of president of the Society.[67]

In the 1803-04 minutes of the Lexington Medical Society, the meeting date unidentified,[68] "John Pope, Esq., proposed honorary members—-Also Dr. McDowell." This was Dr. Ephraim McDowell of Danville, Kentucky, later to become the Father of Abdominal Surgery. His appointment would be in keeping with the knowledge that Ephraim McDowell and Samuel Brown had been apprentices together in Virginia and had continued their friendship as students while at Edinburgh (1793-95). Another student (ordinary) member of the society (1803) was Coleman Rogers[69] (1781-1855), an apprentice of Dr. Brown, who later completed his medical training at the University of Pennsylvania Medical School. For a period of four to five years (c. 1805-10) Rogers was a partner in the medical practice of Dr. McDowell in Danville, Kentucky, and assisted McDowell when, in 1809, he performed the favous ovariotomy on Jane Todd. He later became a professor of surgery at the Medical College of Ohio and subsequently moved to Louisville to form the Louisville Medical Institute (University of Louisville Medical School) in conjunction with Doctors Alban G. Smith and Harrison Powell.[70]

Student Officers

When contemplating officers of a medical society today, we customarily think in terms of members aged thirty to forty years or older. That the Lexington Medical Society's first extant officers, presidents and secretaries, were young men, even boys, represents quite a shocking contrast to our present system. Even so, these students were apprentices, customarily entering into contracts with their preceptors at the age of fifteen to seventeen, and sometimes younger. Benjamin W. Dudley (1785-1870), later to be the renowned surgeon of the West, was one of the early apprentice secretaries of the Lexington Medical Society (1804). William Richardson (c. 1785-1845), a fellow apprentice and member of the Lexington Medical Society (later a professor in the Medical Department of Transylvania University) was born in the same year as Dudley (1785) and probably began his training by age fifteen.

The age of fifteen, however young it may seem in today's society, was looked upon entirely differently during the eighteenth and nineteenth centuries. America was a nation young in every imaginable way, including the ages of its citizens. The median age of American white males in the year 1800 was fifteen years and seven months; in 1850, nineteen years and five months; in 1900, twenty-three years and eight months; and in 1950, thirty years and four months.[71] The further west one moved, the younger the average age.[72] As late as 1850, the Kentucky Census faithfully recorded the occupation of white males *fifteen* and over.[73]

The realization that the preserved early minutes of the society (1803-04) were recorded by boys fifteen to nineteen years of age helps explain the fact that portions of the minutes were crafted in beautiful penmanship whereas other pages were written in a decidedly "boyish" hand. Also, the numerous abortive penning in of capital letters, names, and drawings unrelated to the text and wherever convenient, is but a youthful doodling. These youths served as officers of the Lexington Medical Society, and did so intermittently with physicians, for a known period of twenty-four years, 1797-1821. To our knowledge, no other American medical society has ever had students play such a vital and salutary role in its affairs as did the Lexington Medical Society. In large measure, this unity between physicians and students was a reflection of the alliance of the Transylvania medical faculty and the members of the Lexington Medical Society for a period of approximately thirty-seven years.

The Lexington Medical Society played a central role in the education of the student members. As William Morton noted in

1799: "Law and Medical Societies meet every week in town, in which the fundamental principles of those professions are discussed with a freedom, which cannot fail of affording to every student the most permanent advantages. At these societies the professors attend, and placing themselves on a level with the students, encourage them to that free exercise of reason, which is so well calculated to elicit the dormant powers of the human mind."[74]

Lottery for the Medical Society

In 1803, the Kentucky General Assembly authorized a lottery for the building of "a house for the Kentucky [sic] Medical Society" in the town of Lexington.[75] The lottery was scheduled to begin in May 1804; however, "The drawing of the Medical Society Lottery is postponed until the 15th of September next. Those who purchased tickets before the first of August may have a credit until the commencement of the drawing."[76]

The Incorporation Statute

An act to incorporate the Lexington Medical Society was passed at the October session of 1821 by the General Assembly of Kentucky.[77] Henry B. Miller was the president of the Society when it was declared "a body corporate and politic, by the name and style of the Lexington Medical Society; and by that name shall have perpetual succession of officers and members, and a common seal, with full power to change, alter and make new the same as often as they shall judge expedient....All the officers of this Society shall be elected annually, by ballot, and each election shall require a majority of the members present.... It shall consist of honorary and junior members (students)." Meetings were scheduled to take place on "the first Friday succeeding the commencement of lectures in the Transylvania Medical School...." It is obvious that even after twenty-three years the association between the Lexington Medical Society and the Transylvania Medical Department remained intact and complementary.

The Lexington Medical Society Ends

A reference in the *Transylvania Journal of Medicine and the Associate Sciences* (1828) indicates that the existence of the Lexington Medical Society was long established and prosperous; it sets forth, under the date 1828, that "The Lexington Medical Society holds regular meetings every week throughout the winter and monthly during the summer. At these, communications are read by different members on subjects pertaining to Medical Science and free discussions are elicited by them. Medical professors occasionally attend, read papers, and partake in the debate."[78] There is further documentation of meetings of the Lexington Medical Society as late as 1834.[79]

The Lexington Medical Society came to an end in 1834. The demise of the Society and the apparently precipitous manner of its closing is puzzling. Many of the eighteenth and nineteenth century medical societies began, sputtered, and died, whereas others began and then died, only to be reborn. Daniel Drake (1837), the noted medical educator, makes this observation about the Tennessee Medical Society: "...notwithstanding a considerable array of names, as officers and committee heads, its meetings, on the whole, like those of other western state societies, are but thinly attended."[80]

The last extant evidence of the activities of the Lexington Medical Society was published in the *Transylvania Journal of Medicine and the Associate Sciences* in 1834.[81] At the last meeting, a resolution was unanimously adopted to establish a library to be known as the "Medical Library of the Lexington Medical Society." Honorary members were requested to give money or books. And further, an additional resolution was made to fund a museum to

THE

TRANSYLVANIA JOURNAL

OF

MEDICINE

AND THE ASSOCIATE SCIENCES.

EDITED BY
JOHN ESTEN COOKE, M. D.
Professor of the Theory and Practice of Medicine in Transylvania University,
AND
CHARLES WILKINS SHORT, M. D.
Professor of Materia Medica and Medical Botany in the same Institution.

VOL. I.

LEXINGTON, KENTUCKY.
PRINTED QUARTERLY, BY JOSEPH G. NORWO

1828.

The Transylvania Journal of
Medicine and the Associate Sciences
Vol. I., No. I – February, 1828
Courtesy of Transylvania University Library

THE

TRANSYLVANIA JOURNAL

OF

MEDICINE

AND THE ASSOCIATE SCIENCES

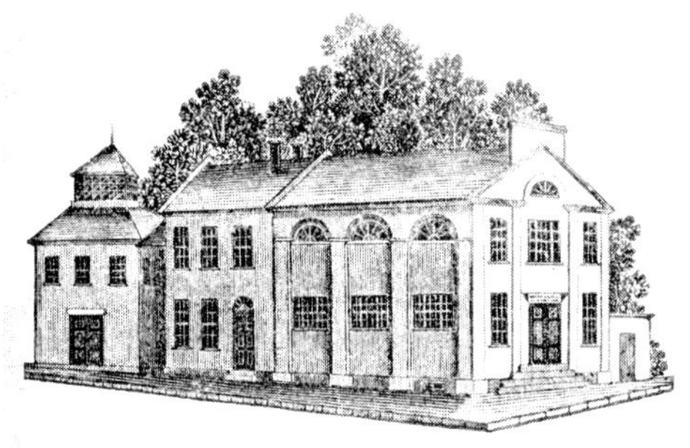

VOL. 2. NO. 2.—MAY, 1829.

LEXINGTON, KENTUCKY
Printed at the Transylvania Press,
BY JOSEPH G. NORWOOD

The Transylvania Journal of
Medicine and the Associate Sciences
Vol. 2, No. 2 – May, 1829
Courtesy of Transylvania University Library

collect the "mass of information respecting the extensive Mississippi Valley, of which so little is known." Lunsford P. Yandell, editor of the *Transylvania Journal of Medicine and the Associate Sciences*, remarked: "If medicine is destined ever to be erected into an exact science it can only be after all its isolated facts are collected, and impartially compared and arranged. Many attempts have been made to effect this object, but it is universally acknowledged that they have all failed, and failed for a want of a sufficient number of facts."[82] Such lofty ideals and plans do not mesh with the sudden collapse of the Society. We say sudden, for within a year the Lexington Medical Society was defunct. Writing from Cincinnati in 1837, Daniel Drake had this to say about the plight of the old and the new medical societies: "The Lexington Medical Society was incorporated many years ago, and has been the seat of numerous animated debates; but we Americans, get tired of our play things, and seek for new ones. Use and age, generate no endearments; and hence the physicians of Lexington, embracing several or all of the medical professors of the University, have lately had themselves incorporated, under a new charter, which styles them The College of Physicians and Surgeons."[83]

The College of Physicians and Surgeons

An entry in the *Directory of the City of Lexington* (1838-39) states that the College of Physicians and Surgeons was organized in 1835 and chartered by the Legislature of Kentucky on the 25th of February, 1836. Twenty-three Lexington physicians signed the charter.[84] Charles Caldwell, Dean of the Medical Department of Transylvania University, served as the first president of the society; Benjamin Dudley held the position from 1838 to 1839. Daniel Drake offers this further observation: "I had the opportunity of attending one of the meetings of this society...and found that a part of their exercises, consists in monthly reports of prevalent diseases of the city, and another part, in the report of individual cases, with speculations on their pathology and treatment."[85] The fact that a quorum of five members was seldom present was symptomatic of most of the medical societies, especially those in the West, and was probably the reason for their short life span. Records indicate that this society continued to exist until 1850. From that date and throughout the period of the Civil War, there is no known evidence validating the presence of a medical society in Lexington.

The 1838 *Directory of the City of Lexington* also lists The Transylvania Medical Society.[86] The existence of two medical societies following the ending of the Lexington Medical Society suggest that the original society may have voluntarily divided into separate societies, one for students (The Transylvania Medical Society) and one for physicians (The College of Physicians and Surgeons). The fact that Dr. Caldwell served as president of the College of Physicians while he was dean of the Medical Department of Transylvania suggests that there was an amicable split and not a rupture between Transylvania and the physicians of Lexington.

1 Philip Rhodes, *An Outline History of Medicine* (London: Butterworths, 1985), 17. According to Rhodes, "medicine tends to follow in the wake of progress in other fields, particularly those of conquest and flourishing economics and safe, sound politics."

2 Lewis Collins, *History of Kentucky* (2 vols.), rev. Richard H. Collins (Louisville: Richard H. Collins, 1877), II, 176. *"Lexington Manufactures* in 1817—At this date the manufactures, and capital employed in Lexington, as estimated by judicious men, were as follows: 12 cotton manufactories, employing a capital of £67,500; 3 woolen ditto, £32,600; 3 paper ditto, £20,250; 3 steam grist mills, £16,875; gunpowder mills, £9,000; lead factory, £14,800; foundries for casting irons and brass, connected with a silver-plating establishment, £9,000; 4 hat factories, £15,000; 4 coach ditto, £12,600, 5 tanners and curriers, £20,000; 12 factories for cotton bagging and hempen yarns, £100,400; 6 cabinet-makers, £5,600; 4 soap and candle factories, £12,150; 3 tobacco factories, £11,540; sundry others, £120,000; total amount of capital employed in the manufactories of Lexington, £467,225."

3 Robert Peter, *A Brief Sketch of the History of Lexington, Kentucky and of Transylvania University* (Lexington, Ky.: D.C. Wickliffe, Printer, 1854), 9. By 1802, ..."In short the town was flourishing to the highest degree, its merchants making rapid fortunes for an extensive and lucrative commerce, and its manufacturers complaining only of the scarcity of workmen."

4 Lewis Rogers, President, *Facts and Reminiscences of the Medical History of Kentucky,* address before the Kentucky State Medical Society (Louisville: John P. Morton & Co., Publishers, 1873), 6. In 1818, John Lawson McCullough, of Lexington, was the first graduate in medicine (Transylvania University) in the valley of the Mississippi.

5 Lee Shai Weissbach, "Growth and Mobility in a Frontier Town," *The Register of the Kentucky Historical Society* (Spring 1983) : 115-123. "Lexington was at the crossroads of the two principal ingress routes to the West: The Wilderness Trail, from Virginia through Cumberland Gap, to the Southeast; and the Buffalo Trace, from Limestone (Maysville), the point of debarkation for flatboats descending the Ohio River from Fort Pitt (Pittsburgh), to the northeast." Clay Lancaster, *Vestiges of the Venerable City, A Chronicle of Lexington, Kentucky* (Lexington, Ky.: Lexington-Fayette County Historic Commission, 1978), 11.

6 Collins, *History of Kentucky,* vol. II, 176.

7 Robert Peter, *The History of the Medical Department of Transylvania University* (Louisville: John P. Morton & Company, 1905), 57.

8 Willard Rouse Jillson, "Flamma Clara Maturae Medicinae Kentuckiensis, 1750-1850," *Transactions of the Kentucky Academy of Science, 1965* 25, no. 3-4 (1965), 97-98. "The rapid development of cheap long-distance transportation of passengers and freight on the Ohio River by steamboat marked this era and brought about a pronounced shift of merchandising, manufacturing, and business generally from the limestone uplands of central Kentucky in and about Lexington to the Ohio River flood plains and adjacent lowlands of Louisville."

9 Peter, *The History of the Medical Department of Transylvania University,* 57.

10 Ibid., 57-58; and Collins, *History of Kentucky,* vol. II, 262-264.

11 Lewis Cecil Gray, *History of Agriculture in the Southern United States to 1860,* vol. II (Washington, D.C.: Carnegie Institution of Washington, 1933), 783.

12 The announcement includes the following list of subscribers:

George Muter	John Jouett	Jno. Coburn
Sam M'Dowell	Tho. Allin	Geo. Gordon
Harry Innes	Robt. Todd	Alex D. Orr
James Speed	Jos. Crockett	Robt. Barr
Will M'Dowell	Ebenzr. Brooks	Hor. Turpin
Willis Green	T. Hall	Robt. Johnson
Thomas Todd	Caleb Wallace	John Craig
Thomas Speed	Will. Irvine	James Garrard
Gabriel J. Johnston	Chas. Scott	Isaac Shelby
Joshua Barbee	Levi Todd	David Leitch
Step. Ormsby	James Parker	H. Marshall
J. Overton, junr	Alex. Parker	Christo. Greenup
J. Brown	John Fowler	

"*The First Newspaper* ever published west of the Allegheny mountains (excepting the Pittsburgh *Gazette,* which preceded it only a few weeks) was the *Kentucke Gazette,* at Lexington—its first number having been issued on the 11th day of August, 1787. The matter intended for that number was set in type on board of a flat-boat while descending the Ohio river to Limestone (Maysville) or else at Limestone while waiting for pack-horses to transport it over the great buffalo 'Middle Trace,' which led over the 'sugar loaf' hill just back of that point, and *via* the Lower Blue Lick spring to Lexington....in that terrible carriage on pack-horses from Limestone to Lexington, 'a great part of the types fell into pi.'" Collins, *History of Kentucky,* vol. II, 180.

13 James E. McClellan III, *Science Reorganized, Scientific Societies in the Eighteenth Century* (New York: Columbia University Press, 1985), 4-5. (Reference Ribeiro, *Historia dos estabelecimentos sci-enfificas,* listing, vol. I.).

14 Thomas D. Clark, ed., *A Description of Kentucky in North America: to which are Prefixed Miscellaneous Observations Respecting the United States* (Lexington, Ky.: University of Kentucky Press, 1945), 90.

15 Charles R. Staples, *The History of Pioneer Lexington 1779-1806* (Lexington, Ky.: University of Kentucky Press, 1939), 47.

16 Collins, *History of Kentucky,* vol. I, 5.

17 "Kentucke" was changed to "Kentucky" in the 7 March 1789 issue.

18 Eric H. Christianson, "Medicine in New England," *Medicine in the New World,* ed. Ronald L. Numbers (Knoxville: The University of Tennessee Press, 1987), 101-153. Christianson states that "At least seventeen medical societies were either proposed or created in Massachusetts during the eighteenth century, fourteen appearing after 1750."

19 Walter L. Burrage, *A History of the Massachusetts Medical Society* (Mass.: privately printed, 1923), 8.

20 Ibid., 1.

21 Sherwin B. Nuland, guest ed., "A Matter of Great Importance to Mankind: The Origins of the New Haven County Medical Association," *Connecticut Medicine* 48, no. 9 (September 1984) : 559-561. Nuland claims that the New Haven County Medical Association (Conn.) is the second oldest in the United States, and "If continuous existence is the criterion, we are the *first!*"

22 *The Kentucky Gazette* (Lexington), 23 January 1800.

23 A. Scott Earle, ed., *Surgery in America*, 2d ed. (New York: Praeger Publishers, 1983), 92-103; and Laman A. Gray, Sr., *The Life & Times of Ephraim McDowell,* ed. Oscar Bryant (reprint, Louisville, Ky.: V.G. Reed and Sons, Printers, 1987), 20-27. **Ephraim McDowell** (1771-1830) was born in Rockbridge County, Virginia, and moved to Kentucky with his family while he was still a youngster (1783). He returned to his native state in 1791 to study under Dr. Alexander Humphreys of Staunton, Virginia. He then went abroad to further his medical education, spending two years at Edinburgh. He did not receive a medical degree, probably because of lack of funds. In December 1809, he performed the first ovariotomy, on Mrs. Jane Todd Crawford, and subsequently added a series of such cases with minimal mortality. He is known as the *Father of Ovariotomy and Founder of Abdominal Surgery.* He married the daughter of Governor Isaac Shelby and lived in Danville, where he died in 1830.

24 A native of the city of New York, **David Hosack** (1769-1835) attended medical lectures at Edinburgh; 1793-94. He formed a partnership in New York with his old friend and teacher, Samuel Bard, which continued for four years. In 1800, Dr. Bard retired, leaving the flourishing practice to Dr. Hosack. He served in several capacities as professor at Columbia College, the College of Physicians and Surgeons, and Rutgers Medical College. A founder of the latter two colleges, he was an outstanding teacher, an internationally known botanist, and an authority on yellow fever. Instrumental in the founding of Bellevue Hospital, he favored botanical treatment, opposing bleeding with the scalpel and purging with calomel.

Martin Kaufman, Stuart Galishoff, Todd L. Savitt, eds., *Dictionary of American Medical Biography,* vol. I (Westport, Conn.: Greenwood Press, 1984), 306-307.

John Beale Davidge (1768-1829), a native of Annapolis, Md., attended medical lectures at Edinburgh and graduated from the University of Glasgow with an MD in 1793. With associates, he chartered a medical school in 1807 that subsequently became the medical department of the University of Maryland. At the university he served as chair of anatomy and surgery and later as dean, College of Medicine of Maryland. In surgery he was noted for his amputation at the shoulder joint (1792). He is also credited as being first to ligate the gluteal artery, which he did for aneurysm. He is considered the inventor of the "American method" of amputation.

Kaufman, et. al., *Dictionary of American Medical Biography,* 182-183.

25 Gray, *The Life and Times of Ephraim McDowell,* 27.

26 August Schachner, *Ephraim McDowell, Father of Ovariotomy and Founder of Abdominal Surgery* (Philadelphia: J.B. Lippincott Co., 1921), 50-57; and Lunsford P. Yandell, "The Medical Literature of Kentucky," *Some of the Medical Pioneers of Kentucky,* ed. J. N. McCormack (Bowling Green, Ky.: Kentucky State Medical Association, date unknown), 134-137.

27 Ibid., 135.

28 "John Brown (1757-1837), the oldest of the four Brown brothers, entered Princeton College at the time of the Revolutionary War. When the American troops made their memorable retreat from the Jerseys, Brown joined the troops and remained with the army under Washington as a vol-

unteer. He later was under the command of the Marquis de Lafayette. After the war, Brown completed his education at William & Mary College, read law in the office of Thomas Jefferson, and in 1782 headed west to Kentucky. He was the first member of the Congress of the United States ever sent from the great valley of the Mississippi. In 1789 and 1791 he was elected by the people of Kentucky to serve in the first and second Congress. When Kentucky became a state in 1792, Brown served three consecutive terms as United States Senator. He enjoyed the personal friendship of Jefferson, Washington, Madison, and Monroe. He died at the age of 80 at his residence (Liberty Hall) in Frankfort."

Collins, *History of Kentucky*, vol. II, 252-253.

29 Ibid. "James Brown, the second brother, was a distinguished lawyer in Kentucky, and a contemporary at the bar of the Honorable Henry Clay (both of whom married daughters of Colonel Hart), and also of George Nicholas, Mr. Murray, John Breckinridge, and others, and was distinguished, even in such competition. He was appointed as first secretary of state of Governor Isaac Shelby. Upon the purchase of Louisiana, he removed to New Orleans, was several times elected to the senate of the United States and subsequently received the appointment of Minister to France. He died in Philadelphia in 1836."

30 The above printer's error in the *Kentucky Gazette* of 6 September 1797 gave the date of Brown's announcement as 5 September 1795; it should have read 5 September 1797. This error was repeated weekly for the next several months. The "corrected" notice appeared in the *Kentucky Gazette* of May 1798 and for several months thereafter.

31 One of Brown's biographers described him as "a dilettante in medicine as in his other interests. Though he introduced vaccination for smallpox at Lexington as early as 1802, its interest for him lay in its novelty." James M. Phalan, *Dictionary of American Biography*, vol. II (New York: Harper & Row Publishers, 1974), 153. Phalan drew his selected conclusions about Samuel Brown from a report by L. P. Yandell in his "Dr. Samuel Brown as an Author," *Western Journal of Medicine and Surgery*, vol. II, Louisville, 1854, 175-182. A far greater appreciation of Brown and his times can be found in the interpretation by Goddard:

"During the 18th and indeed much of the 19th century, particularly in England and America, distinguished scientists started their professional lives as physicians, but their interests were not limited to problems of disease and related questions. Because they were also interested in theories and ideas, to them is due much of the groundwork of modern science. Botany, for example, had its origins in the work of two Greek physicians, Theophrastus and Dioscorides. The disciplinary framework of the university, the haven for known facts and ideas and continued speculation, was the proper place for men such as these, and those who followed through by centuries to pursue their studies." David R. Goddard, "Medicine and the Universities," *J.A.M.A.* 194, no. 7 (November 15, 1965) : 133.

32 Peter, *The History of the Medical Department of Transylvania University*, 8.

33 Kappa Lambda and Percival's Code of Ethics are treated at length in Chapter II.

34 *Early Proceedings of the American Philosophical Society*, 18 April 1800, vol. II, comp. by one of the secretaries (Philadelphia: Press of McCalla & Stavely, 1884), 299.

35 Zachariah Frederick Smith, *School History of Kentucky, From the Earliest Discoveries and Settlements to the Year 1891* (Louisville, Ky.: *Courier-Journal*, 1891), 746.

36 Ibid. Dr. Ridgely devoted much time to teaching apprentices, such as Benjamin W. Dudley

and Walter Brashear. The former was the most successful lithotomist in the American West and the latter performed the first successful hip joint amputation in the world. Dudley, a surgeon, was the centerpiece of the Transylvania Medical Department throughout its days of renown. Brashear also practiced medicine for several years in Lexington before moving on to Louisiana, where later he became a United States senator.

37 Peter, *The Medical Department of Transylvania University*, 11.

38 *The Kentucky Gazette* (Lexington), 23 January 1800.

39 The following "Medicine Men" were listed as physicians in Lexington during the 1780s and 90s, although not all of them practiced medicine: James Wilkinson (1784); Richard W. Downing (c. 1787-1791); Andrew McKinley (1789); Hugh Sheil (1785); ——Beatty (1788); Thomas Lloyd ((1789); P. Rootes (1791); James Welch (1795); Basil Duke (1791); John Hole (1792); Daniel Preston (1791); Frederick Ridgely (1792); James Watkins (1795); John Watkins (1997); Thomas Huff (1796); John W. Scott (1796); Samuel Brown (1797); Walter Warfield (1797); Peter Trisler (1791); Walter Brashear (date uncertain—an apprentice of Dr. Ridgely); C. Freeman (1798); and Joseph Boswell (1786).

Staples, *The History of Pioneer Lexington*, 1799-1806, 320-321.

40 In a pamphlet published in 1818, Dr. Daniel Drake refers to the revision of the Medical Society's Constitution in 1817. Daniel Drake, *An Appeal to the Justice of the Intelligent and Respectable People of Lexington* (Cincinnati: Looker, Reynolds & Co., 1818), 21.

41 "An Act to incorporate the Lexington Medical Society," *Acts Passed at the First Session of the Thirtieth General Assembly for the Commonwealth of Kentucky* (Frankfort, Ky.: Kendall and Russell, 1821), 420. The Society's constitution is annexed to the Act.

42 Minutes of the Lexington Medical Society, 1803-04, Special Collections, Transylvania University, Lexington, Ky.

43 C. Keith Wilbur, *Revolutionary Medicine;* 1700-1800 (Old Saybrook, Conn.: The Globe Pequot Press, 1980), 1.

44 Charles Caldwell, *Autobiography of Charles Caldwell*, with a preface, notes, and appendix by Harriot W. Warner (Philadelphia: Lippincott, Grambo, and Co., 1855), 77.

45 Whitfield J. Bell, Jr., *The College of Physicians of Philadelphia; A Bicentennial History* (Canton, Mass.: Science History Publications, USA, 1987), 5.

46 *Kentucky Gazette* (Lexington), 27 April 1801.

47 *Kentucky Gazette,* 5 September 1797.

48 V.F. Payne, Signal Corps Engineering Laboratories, "Dr. Samuel Brown in Lexington, Kentucky from 1797 to 1806," (Atlantic City, N.J.: Division of the History of Chemistry of the American Chemical Society, 16 September 1952), Special Collections, Transylvania University, Lexington, Ky.

49 *Kentucky Gazette*, 9 September 1797.

50 René de la Roche, "Samuel Brown, 1769-1830," in *Lives of Eminent American Physicians and Surgeons of the Nineteenth Century*, ed. Samuel D. Gross (Philadelphia: Lindsay & Balkiston, 1861), 235.

51 Peter, *The Medical Department of Transylvania University*, 9.

52 Howard A. Kelly, *A Cyclopedia of American Medical Biography from 1610 to 1910*, vol. I (Philadelphia: W.B. Saunders Company, 1912), 118-19.

53 Bell, *The College of Physicians of Philadelphia, A Bicentennial History*, 4.

54 Staples, *The History of Pioneer Lexington*, 321.

55 John H. Ellis, *Medicine in Kentucky* (Lexington, Ky.: The University Press of Kentucky, 1977), 44; and George W. Ranck, *History of Lexington Kentucky: Its Early Annals and Recent Progress* (Cincinnati: Robert Clarke & Co., 1872), 223.

56 Minutes of the Fayette County Medical Society, 12 April 1938.

57 Emmet Field Horine, "Sketch of the Kentucky State Medical Society," presented at The Ephraim McDowell Memorial Meeting, Centennial of the Kentucky State Medical Association, Bowling Green, Ky., *KMA Journal 90* (June 1992) : ix.

58 *Kentucky Gazette*, 27 September 1803.

*Even though, as stated, the exact date of origin of the Society is not known, the minutes of the society meeting of Wednesday, January 3, although undated as to year, are found in the collection of minutes of the Lexington Medical Society from 1803 and 1804, thus raising the possibility of a date of origin earlier than 1799. Otherwise, all entry dates in the 1803-04 minutes have been confirmed and are correct. By agreement, all meetings of the society were held on Wednesday evenings. From the date of January 3rd, certain assumptions could be deduced that would date the existence of this society in 1797-98. Wednesday, January 3, coincided only with 1798 from the period of 1796 through 1809. Other facts, however, suggest that the date Wednesday, January 3 was incorrect and should have read Wednesday, January 4, thus corresponding to the year 1804. The short entry begins with two abortive 'inking ins' of the word Wednesday and followed by "Wednesday [sic] the 3rd of January the Society met according to appointment. Members present at that meeting: Ordinary members; Davidson, Mitchell, Dudley, Barbour, Thompson, Bedford, Mitchell [the names of two members could not be interpreted- Author]. Honorary members present; James Fishback, Samuel Brown, and James More. Fortunately, one of the attendance records includes the dates of January 1804; the fact that the names of members present or absent match those listed above strongly suggests that the date Wednesday, January 3rd, should have been Wednesday, January 4th (1804). Another point of concern is the fact that Benjamin Dudley, whose name appears in the list of members attending, was as of January 3, 1798, only twelve years of age (he was born April 12, 1785). Even though two writers state that Dudley entered the service of Dr. Ridgely at a very young age, they fail to give a date or Dudley's age. Another writer gives Dudley's initial apprentice age as fifteen (corresponds to 1800), a beginning age that, although consistent with the age at which many apprentices at that time entered their service, would not be in keeping with the very young age assigned by other writers [by WPM].

59 Minutes of Lexington Medical Society, 1803-04. Nine columns are marked with a 1 (for presence) or 0 (for absence). Because each of the nine columns had been appropriately marked, the dates would have had to reflect prior attendance dates extending back into the year 1802.

60 Minutes of the Lexington Medical Society, 1803, Special Collections, Transylvania University, Lexington, Ky.

61 *Kentucky Gazette and General Advertiser,* 20 September 1803.

62 Ibid., 5 June 1804.

63 One author cites the Lexington Medical Society as being the first student-faculty medical society in America. Eugene H. Connor, "Kentucky's Bicentennial and a Brief Overview of 200 Years of Medical Practice and the Physician," *KMA Journal 90* (June 1992) : 285-288.

However, our research indicates that this honor belongs rather to a joint student-physician medical society existing in Philadelphia in the last quarter of the eighteenth century. Whitfield J. Bell states that a student medical society, the Hospital Medical Society, existed in Philadelphia under the patronage of Dr. Thomas Bond in the latter part of the eighteenth century and that it merged with the American Medical Society of Philadelphia (founded in 1770), forming a "mixed membership of students and physicians, patterned on the medical societies clustering about Edinburgh University." Dr. William Shippen was president of the combined society in 1790. Such a society would, therefore, be distinguished as the first student-physician society in America. The author (WPM) believes that the Lexington Medical Society was the second such student-physician society in America, as stated above, and the first student-physician society in which elected offices were held by both students and physicians.

Whitfield J. Bell, Jr., "For Mutual Improvement in the Healing Art, Philadelphia Medical Societies of the 18th Century," *JA.M.A.* 216, no. 1, (5 April 1971) : 125-129.

64 This information comes from the minutes of Wednesday evening, October 12, 1803, which contain the following statement: "By order of the President S. L. Mitchell." Minutes of the Lexington Medical Society, 1803, Special Collections, Transylvania University, Lexington, Ky.

65 Ibid.

66 Henry Miller, "The Relation Between the San Guiferous and Nervous Systems" (M.D. diss., Transylvania University, 1822).

67 *Kentucky Reporter,* 12 January 1824. A circular requests that replies to an "Autumnal fever" survey be submitted to the President of the Lexington Medical Society, Dr. Daniel Drake.

68 Minutes of the Lexington Medical Society, 1803-1804, Special Collections, Transylvania University, Lexington, Ky.

69 *Kentucky Gazette* (Lexington), 7 November 1805. "Married on Sunday evening last, by the Reverend Jas. Moore, Dr. Coleman Rogers of Danville, to Miss Jane Farrar, of this county."

70 Otto Juettner, *Daniel Drake and His Followers* (Cincinnati: Harvey Publishing Company, 1909), 46-47. "He [Coleman Rogers] rode to Philadelphia on horseback in twenty-three days...He attended lectures at the University of Pennsylvania, and remained in Philadelphia for eighteen

months. He was too poor to be able to pay the expenses incidental to graduation, and left for his Kentucky home without the coveted diploma." In 1816 he returned to Philadelphia and took his degree. Rogers practiced with Dr. Ephraim McDowell, Danville, Kentucky, in the intervening years, 1810-1816.

71 Department of Commerce, *Historical Statistics of the United States: Colonial Times to 1970,* pt. I (Washington, D.C., 1976), 19 and 28.

72 Mark C. Carnes and John A. Garraty with Patrick Williams, *Mapping America's Past* (New York: Henry Holt and Company, 1996).

73 "Kentucky Census," a loose-leaf document in the census files of The Kentucky Room, Lexington Public Library (Main), Lexington, Ky.

74 *Kentucky Gazette,* 23 January 1800.

75 "An Act authorizing a Lottery for the benefit of the Kentucky Medical Society," *The Statute Law of Kentucky* (5 vols., Frankfort, 1809-1819) III (25 May 1803) : 159. The Act should have referred to the "Lexington Medical Society."

76 *Kentucky Gazette and General Advertiser*, 22 May 1804.

77 An Act to incorporate the Lexington Medical Society," 420-24.

78 *Medicine and its Development in Kentucky,* Sponsored by the State Department of Health of Kentucky and the Kentucky State Medical Association (Louisville, Ky.: The Standard Printing Company, 1940), 67-68. Reference is to the *Transylvania Medical Journal and The Associate Sciences I* (Lexington, 1828) : 300.

79 *The Transylvania Medical Journal and The Associate Sciences* 7, no. 2 (1834) : 291. The *Transylvania Journal of Medicine and The Associate Sciences* was published from 1828-1839 (vol. 1-12). With the departure of a portion of the medical faculty to Louisville the newly assembled medical faculty of Transylvania initiated the *Transylvania Medical Journal,* which was published for two years, June 1849-June 1850 (vol. 1-2).

80 Daniel Drake and Wm. Wood, eds., *The Western Journal of the Medical and Physical Sciences* IX, Second Hexade—vol. III, Cincinnati, 1836), 470-480. (Note that the year of publication of the Journal was given as 1836; the dateline of Drake's article was 1837. WPM)

81 *The Transylvania Medical Journal and Associate Sciences* (1834).

82 *The Transylvania Medical Journal and Associate Sciences* 7, no. 2, 291.

83 Drake and Wood, eds., *The Western Journal of the Medical and Physical Sciences,* 470-480.

84 "An Act to establish the College of Physicians of the city of Lexington," *Acts Passed at the First Session of the Forty-Fourth General Assembly of the Commonwealth of Kentucky* (Frankfort, Ky.: J. H. Holeman, 1836), 333-34.

85 Drake and Wood, eds., *The Western Journal of the Medical and Physical Sciences,* 475.

86 Julius P. Bolivar Mac Cabe, *Directory of the City of Lexington and County of Fayette, for 1838 & '39* (Lexington: Printed by J. C. Noble, 1838), 19 and 87. The constitution of the College of Physicians and Surgeons was adopted on 18 December 1835 and was chartered by the Legislature of Kentucky on 25 February 1836.

Chapter II

KAPPA LAMBDA SOCIETY

One of the most pressing goals of the American medical profession in the early part of the nineteenth century was to bring about civility among physicians. During the first forty years of the nineteenth century, in particular, infighting, fist-fights, duels, and confrontations of every variety plagued the doctors. James Thomas Flexner, in his classic *Doctors on Horseback,* describes conditions in Lexington in 1823-24 as follows: "Yet, despite their fame and prosperity, the [Transylvania] professors were continually warring with each other, while the doctors of Lexington had not a good word to say for the institution that was bringing their obscure settlement international fame."[87] He also comments that there was not a spot in the whole nation where the doctors were not at each other's throats.[88] Skirmishes were not limited to the frontier West but also affected the more cultivated East, especially urbane Philadelphia, which saw a feud between the partisans of the University of Pennsylvania and those of Jefferson Medical College.

That the forces of change in medical fraternity would be conceived and implemented on the American frontier rather than in the medical pinnacle of Philadelphia begs an explanation. First, it might be said that bickering and mistrust among physicians were so prevalent and so vicious in Philadelphia that the probability of the city's doctors rallying around one side or another in the search for harmony was remote. If not Philadelphia, then where would physicians look for guidance? Perhaps Baltimore or New York? But no one came forth, and there was no let up in the chaos. Even so, reform of the tarnished relationships between physicians weighed heavily on the mind of one physician, Samuel Brown, Founder and Honorary Member of the Lexington Medical Society and professor in the Transylvania University Medical Department. At the request of the Trustees of Transylvania University, Brown accepted a professorship of Theory and Practice in 1819. Being acquainted with or the friend of many of the leading physicians in Philadelphia and New York, Brown may have been prompted to act solely on their behalf, yet there was enough discord between members of his own faculty in Lexington to acquaint him with the need for reform.

Dr. Charles Caldwell of Philadelphia had also received an appointment to the Transylvania Medical Faculty in 1819, as Dean and Professor of the Institutes of Medicine and Materia Medica. His feisty nature fed on dissent. And just two years earlier, two members of the medical faculty, Drs. Benjamin W. Dudley and William H. Richardson, fought a duel. Amid this turbulence, the imaginative faculties of Brown charted a course by which social, ethical, and professional harmony could be restored. He envisioned a national medical society made up of reputable and enlightened physicians who could through their common interests promote honor, harmony, and the advancement of medical knowledge throughout the land.[89] The society, Kappa Lambda of Hippocrates (KΛ), was begun in Lexington in 1819. Chauncey Leake expressed the spirit and substance of the Kappa Lambda Society in articles published in 1922 and 1962.[90 91] In the later article, Leake wrote:

> Taking his cue both from the efforts of Thomas Percival [medical ethicist] (1740-1804) in trying to develop some intra-professional courtesy and decorum in the English medical groups and from the example set by the Phi Beta Kappa Honorary Society of William and Mary College in Virginia, Dr. Samuel Brown (1769-1830) thought he might improve the standards and ideals of medical education and medical practice in the burgeoning frontiers of the United States by organizing a secret society of intellectual medical leaders who might set an example to the rest of the profession.

Before the vision and action of Samuel Brown in the founding of the Kappa Lambda Society in 1819, there was no national medical society, no single code of medical ethics to guide all American physicians, no national medical journal, no cry for harmonious relations among physicians, and no call to address professional ills on a national scale. The Kappa Lambda Society was born out of the need to rectify what were known to be serious defects in medical education, licensing, practice, and ethics. The society was the first serious effort to correct the many professional wrongs, and in doing so it attracted many of the elite physicians of the day.

The formation of Kappa Lambda Society, the first national medical society in America, had an immediate and favorable impact, especially on the physicians of Philadelphia, as described by Dr. René de la Roche:[92]

> Before the reforming power was made to bear on the medical men of that city [Philadelphia] these, although inferior to none elsewhere, in point of

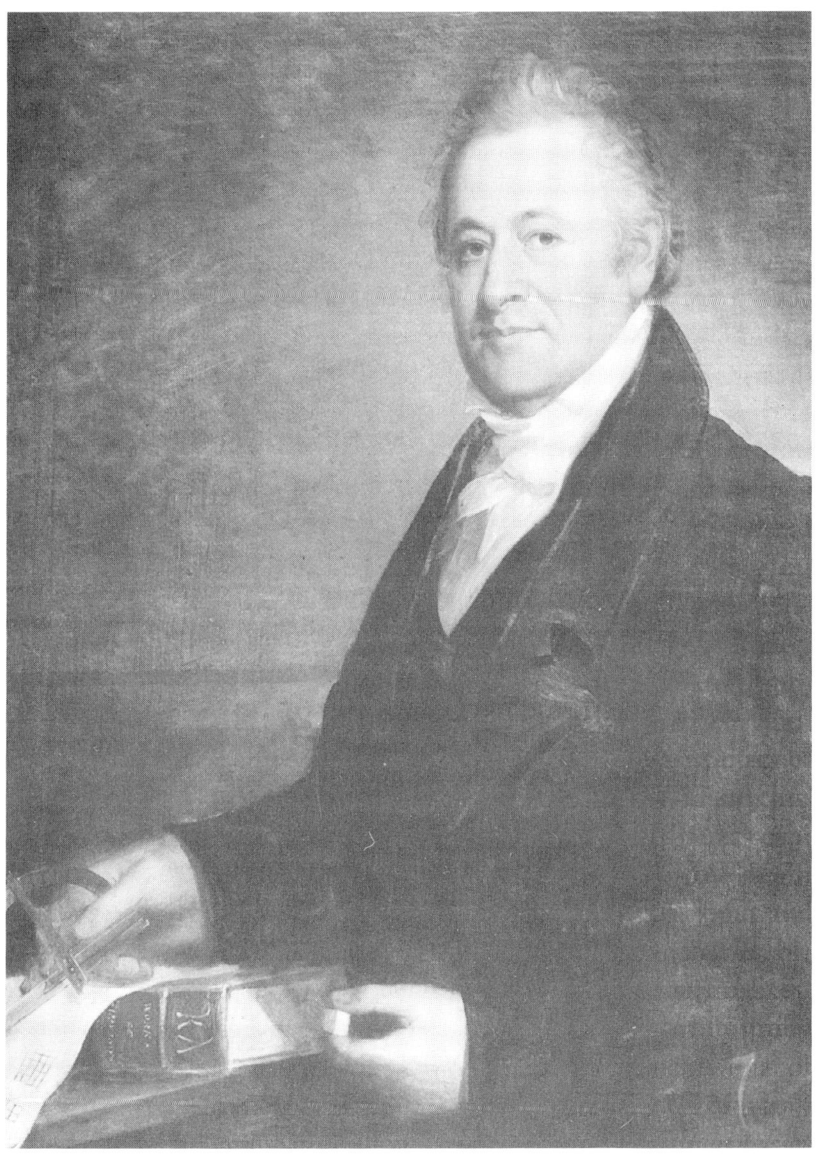

Samuel Brown, M.D.–holding book with
Kappa Lambda insignia (1769-1830)
Courtesy of Transylvania University Library

> intelligence, scientific attainment, or practical skill, so far from fraternizing together, lived in an almost constant state of warfare,-quarrelling, and even worse, was not uncommon among them, and now and then street fights occurred. Soon after its establishment, harmony, comparative harmony, at least, was restored among its members, and before long, through their influence, among other medical men around them.

Spurious Link to the Lexington Medical Society

Some writers have linked the Lexington Medical Society with the legendary Kappa Lambda Society (1819), both of which were founded by Dr. Samuel Brown. These writers based their conclusion on (1) the presence of what appear to be drawings of Kappa Lambda insignia on one page of the 1803 minutes of the Lexington Medical Society and (2) a letter directed to the Lexington Medical Society and published in the *Lexington Gazette* of August 16, 1803. Whether the scribbling in the minutes represents a group of carelessly drawn Lambdas is apt to remain unknown. Likewise, the letters presumed to be ΚΛ are not sufficiently interpretable to warrant their acceptance as such.

The first paragraph of the 1803 letter states the motive of the writer:

> Gentlemen,
>
> I beg leave to suggest to your society, the propriety of petitioning our next Legislature, to enact a law for the regulation of the practice of medicine, in this state, as there is no doubt, but that the number and respectability of the gentlemen, who form your society, will entitle such a petition to the serious attention of our Legislature. I also take the liberty of offering a few observations on the necessity of such a law, which I submit to the consideration of the society.[93]

CONSTITUTION

OF THE

K. Λ. SOCIETY

OF

HIPPOCRATES,

ADOPTED NOVEMBER 27, 1821.

LEXINGTON, KY.

PRINTED BY WM. G. HUNT.

1821.

Title page of the Constitution of the Kappa Lambda Society of Hippocrates, Adopted November 27, 1821
Courtesy of the Library of the College of Physicians of Philadelphia

The "few" observations extend several hundred words in length, and at the end of the letter the signature is that of "MEDICUS." Neither the words Kappa Lambda nor the letters ΚΛ appear in the salutation, the body, or the closing of the letter. In a 1941 letter in the Samuel Brown papers in the Transylvania University Library, the librarian wrote that the "...letter from a Kappa Lambda (1803)...reasonably must have been the beginning of Dr. Brown's Kappa Lambda."[94] Why the librarian assumed a Kappa Lambda member wrote the letter is not explained by the librarian nor is there any mention in her letter of the pseudonym Medicus. In a very thorough review of the Kappa Lambda Society in 1922, Chauncey Leake made no mention of this letter. Leake gave the date of the establishment of the Kappa Lambda Society in Lexington as 1819.[95]

The name of the person who wrote the letter to the Lexington Medical Society and signed it MEDICUS remains a mystery.[96] That the letter was written by a physician well acquainted with the English tongue and with the knowledge and necessity of laws for medical licensing is certain. The letter also was of sufficient interest to the Lexington Medical Society members to cause them to call a special meeting on August 13, 1803, to deal with a letter "from some gent. who subscribes himself Medicus." The eight members present for the special meeting recommended that the secretary "wait upon the printer of the K. Gazette and request him to give the letter a place in his paper in the name of the Society." That Dr. Samuel Brown nursed serious misgivings about the means by which *any impostor* could feign the practice of medicine, and that Brown was the only Lexington physician at that time to have written and published a medical paper *suggests* that he may have written the letter and adds interest and intrigue *but not certainty* of authorship.[97]

The First Code of Medical Ethics

Why the importance of Kappa Lambda? What meaning did it have for its members and for the public in the 1820s? Before Kappa Lambda, the vision of a national medical society had not yet materialized; medical societies were either local or regional. Because the society was first conceived by Dr. Brown, *he, then, is the originator of the first national medical society in the United States.* Of the various components of the Kappa Lambda charter none was more crucial than that of a single code of ethics. To this end Brown modified the works (1803) of Thomas Percival of Lancashire, England.[98] As pointed out by Leake: "The term 'medical ethics,' introduced by Percival, is really a misnomer. Based on Greek traditions of good taste, and on Thomas Percival's 'Code,' it refers chiefly to the rules of etiquette developed in the profession to regulate the professional contacts of its members *with each other.*"[99]

Later in the century (1846-47) the American Medical Association members adopted a further modification of Percival's Medical Ethics, as did most of the state medical societies. A single code of ethics was one of the main goals of the American Medical Association (A.M.A.) convention delegates in 1847. Brown's adoption of Percival's Medical Ethics into Kappa Lambda became the model. Leake states that Nathan Smith Davis was "impelled" by the need to upgrade the standards of medical practice, now (1847) recognized as essential even by the local medical societies.[100] Whether acknowledged or not, all such societies were directly influenced by Percival's work, and whether knowingly or not, by the vision and the guidance of Brown.

At the preliminary American Medical Association convention held in New York City in 1846, one resolution designed specifically to address medical ethics read, in part, as follows: "that it is expedient that the medical profession in the United States should be governed by the same code of medical ethics."[101] The report was presented to the Association in 1847 by Dr. Isaac Hays, but not before he made some explanatory remarks. Dr. Hays and other committee members had conducted extensive reviews of "a great number of codes of ethics adopted by different societies in the United States and found that they were all based on that of Dr. Thomas Percival and that, moreover, the phrases of this writer were preserved to a considerable extent in them." In fact, the code of ethics adopted by the New York State Medical Society was "almost wholly similar to the code prepared by Thomas Percival....Isaac Hays stated clearly that the code had been derived from that of Percival and thus neatly reprimanded the New York and Baltimore Societies, which adopted these codes without giving credit to Percival."[102]

It is evident then that the inclusion of Percival's Medical Ethics into a national medical society by Brown in his Kappa Lambda Society of Hippocrates (1819-20) preceded by four years its incorporation into the New York State Medical Society Articles (1823), by thirteen years its incorporation by the Medico-Surgical Society of Baltimore (1832), and by some twenty-seven years its adoption by the American Medical Association (1847).[103]

Demise of the Kappa Lambda Society of Hippocrates

The historical veil shadowing Dr. Samuel Brown is, in all likelihood, a manifestation of the demise of the Kappa Lambda Society. What led to the downfall of this august society? In a large measure, the seed of its fall was planted from the very beginning when Brown decided that Kappa Lambda, in conformity with almost all previous societies, would be secret.

Brown desired to bring into Kappa Lambda the most eminent physicians of the day, and he believed that this could best be accomplished under secrecy. In particular, he did not wish to embrace any "irregulars," pretenders, or other persons believed to be unfit for the practice of medicine.[104] The concept of an exclusive organization was not original with Brown. Members of the Massachusetts Medical Society in 1781 did not shy away in their declaration "that a just discrimination should be made between such as are duly educated, and properly qualified for the duties of their profession, and those who may ignorantly and wickedly administer medicine whereby the health and lives of many valuable individuals may be endangered, or perhaps lost to the community." That the Kappa Lambda Society was selective in its membership was quite consistent with the times. Indeed, because of the lack of licensing in most states—identifying those with credible credentials—there was more need for exclusivity in 1820 than in 1781.[105]

As René de la Roche relates, "The society [Kappa Lambda], which was originally planted in Lexington, where Dr. Brown was then attending to his professorial duties, and the existence of which was some years, for various reasons fully appreciated at the time, concealed from the public, was soon established in other places,-Philadelphia, New York, Baltimore, and other cities. Laws and regulations framed by Dr. Brown, for the government of the entire association, were there adopted....A promise, modelled in great measure on the celebrated oath of the Father of Medicine, was exacted of each member at the moment of his admission; to obtain which a unanimous vote of those present was necessary."[106] However valid the reasons for the secrecy, it proved to be a yoke that the society could not afford and could not shed.

The New York Massacre

The dissolution of Kappa Lambda began in Philadelphia and climaxed in New York City.[107] In 1826, Dr. George McClellan succeeded in establishing a new school of medicine in Philadelphia, the Jefferson Medical College, and a very short time later engaged in a dispute with Dr. Francis S. Beattie, a fellow-member of the Jefferson faculty and a member of Kappa Lambda.[108] McClellan sued Beattie for libel. The trial ended in McClellan's favor. On appeal, Beattie received the support of the editors of Kappa

Lambda's publication, *The North American Medical and Surgical Journal.* The public reports of the trial reached much further than desired by the Philadelphia medical community, especially further than desired by the members of Kappa Lambda. By October 1829, the publicity of the trial had led to an anonymous article captioned "Secret Medical Associations," published in the *New York Medical and Physical Journal.* The article not only lambasted the "secret organization" but also distanced itself from the Philadelphia scene with this bit of sarcasm: "the expression of a sincere opinion that the medical atmosphere of New York is untainted by the exhalations of any branch from such a parent stem."[109] This unwelcome intrusion into the affairs of the Philadelphia medical community was answered by the editors of Kappa Lambda's publication, who asserted that Kappa Lambda did have a "very excellent branch in New York City."[110] The revelation of the New York chapter proved to be unfortunate. The rebuttal helped to rekindle the underlying ferment in New York medical circles, and in 1830 a denunciation of the secret society was published by "Medicus," together with a list of known members of Kappa Lambda, which included "most of the new faculty (1826) of the college of Physicians and Surgeons."[111] Another blow to the New York chapter of Kappa Lambda came with the publication in 1839 of a vitriolic tirade against Kappa Lambda, *History of the New York Kappa Lambda Conspiracy*, signed by Dr. Valentine Mott and "made up of anonymous essays taken from the *[Medical Examiner]*, a department of the *New York Weekly Whig.*"[112]

Kappa Lambda Secrecy and the Antimasonic Crusade

When one reads the history of the development of medical societies before and after colonial days, it is striking how short a time often existed between their beginning and their end. In comparison to many of the medical societies of the day, the Kappa Lambda Society had an extended run (from 1819-20 to the

1860s).[113] [114] As Schafer, in his *The American Medical Profession 1783 to 1850*, relates:[115]

> Medical societies often passed out of existence soon after their organization. For example, the Medical Society of North Carolina of 1800 and that of Georgia of 1804 seem to have had few, if any, meetings. Other groups, such as the Wisconsin State Medical Society of 1842, are known to us only through the researches of medical scholars. Many of the state societies like the Massachusetts Medical Society were dying at their roots....In both Maine and Tennessee the state society had a most irregular existence, to say nothing of the situation in Illinois and Indiana, where organizations were alternatively sponsored and abolished by the state legislatures.

For the most part, the societies failed for a lack of interest, failure to attend meetings and failure to pay dues. This was not the case for Kappa Lambda. And yet, by the secrecy element, the society opened the door to those inclined to view any closed system as a power-driven conspiracy. Unfortunately for Kappa Lambda, the Antimasonic crusade began in 1826-27.[116] Although there was no relationship between the Masons and Kappa Lambda, the times were not conducive to secret rituals, whatever their constituency. A nationwide revulsion toward secret organizations came with the disappearance of William Morgan, "an obscure and derelict stonemason," in 1829, a disappearance presumably brought about by the Masonic Order.[117] "The popular belief that he had been murdered by Masons of northern New York because of his threat to reveal the secrets of Masonry resulted in the strongest feeling against all ritualistic fraternities of the day, even resulting in the formation of a short-lived Anti-Masonic political party."[118] By 1831, the anti-secret-society movement stormed through the United States. In New York much was made by Kappa Lambda's accusers of a closed system of referrals within the Kappa Lambda group.[119]

Secrecy was not the driving force of Kappa Lambda. Indeed, early on, many members recognized the error of secrecy and sought to remove it. The minutes of the July 11, 1827, meeting of the Philadelphia Chapter of Kappa Lambda state: "Secrecy as to the name and existence of the society was removed from the members' obligation to take effect September 1, 1827, and Lexington and New York to be notified of the action."[120] Members stayed with and believed in Kappa Lambda for its espousal of harmony, a common code of ethics, the fostering of education, the advancement of knowledge, and elevation of the standards of medical practice, in all sections of the nation. That this devotion held true is best revealed by the numerous and celebrated members of the society, their admiration for Dr. Brown, and, even more so, the values by which members could conduct themselves, individually and collectively as physicians, through membership in Kappa Lambda. That they were so respected for their beliefs was amply evidenced in the actions of the A.M.A. delegates in the formative sessions of the society.

Whether some few members of Kappa Lambda engaged in acts designed for personal gain is irrelevant to the aims and actions of the founders and of most of the members of Kappa Lambda. The New York mishap was not experienced elsewhere. The debacle that played havoc with the Kappa Lambda Society of New York apparently did not dim the fortunes of at least two of its members, Edward Delafield, named vice-president at the 1846 preliminary A.M.A. Convention, and Alexander Stevens, who served as vice-president of the A.M.A. in 1848 and became the second president of the A.M.A. in 1849. The widespread knowledge of the jealousy and faction-ridden quarrels prevalent in New York City probably led the A.M.A. delegates to downplay, if not to dismiss, accusations from any source.[121]

The experience of what went right and what went wrong with Kappa Lambda would not have been lost on the A.M.A. delegates, and that experience may well have saved the struggling A.M.A. from a similar fate. With due respect to both men, Samuel Brown and Nathan Smith Davis (and the weight of evidence fully supports this contention), the American Medical Association is the public flowering of the Kappa Lambda Society. The building of the fortunes of one society on the dust of another is not to deny the merits of the latter.

Birth of The American Medical Association

It is not suggested or implied that Samuel Brown was the founder of the *American Medical Association*, for it was, as Leake observes, Dr. Nathan Smith Davis (1817-1904) who "succeeded in spite of much opposition in organizing the American Medical Association in New York City in 1846."[122]

Samuel Brown died in 1830, seventeen years before the founding of the American Medical Association. It is imperative for us today to explain and to perpetuate *how*, in his absence from the A.M.A. Convention of 1847, he left so many footprints. As stated by Chauncey Leake: "It is interesting to note…that the same forces were at work in the formation of Kappa Lambda that succeeded later in establishing the American Medical Association in 1847, and in passing its elaborate code of ethics."[123] This is a profound statement, even provocative, and calls for clarification. If the statement is true, a far greater recognition of Brown's contribution is well overdue; if not true, then the evidence to support Leake's contention is lacking and it should be laid to rest. Leake himself does not offer specifics; thus, we are left to ponder whether Samuel Brown has somehow been unjustifiably lost amid the decline of the Transylvania Medical Department, the dissolution of the Kappa Lambda Society and the founding of the American Medical Association.

What evidence would support Leake's assertion? Certainly, the chronology, the similarity of scope, and the purpose of each society would be factors, yet even more conclusive would be the identity of the leaders involved in Kappa Lambda and in the formative Conventions of 1846 and 1847 of the American Medical Association. How often did the same person or group belong to both Kappa Lambda and the A.M.A.? What importance and influence did these members have in establishing the similar principles and purposes of the American Medical Association and Kappa Lambda?

Similarities of the A.M.A. and Kappa Lambda

First, we need to identify the essential elements of the A.M.A., namely the establishment of a national society, with representatives from all counties and states, the publication of a journal of the society *(J.A.M.A.)*, the advancement of education, the diffusion of knowledge, the promotion of harmony among its members, and the inclusion of a single code of ethics for all physicians. These same elements were first set forth by Brown in 1819-20, in his Kappa Lambda of Hippocrates: the formation of a national medical society "to embrace all reputable practitioners;"[124] representation by members throughout the nation, North, South or East or West;[125] publication of a society journal *(The North American Medical and Surgical Journal)*;[126] a code of medical ethics applicable to all members, modeled after Percival's Medical Ethics; promotion of *"science, friendship, virtue, and honor;"* and diffusion of knowledge.[127]

The commonality of the two organizations, Kappa Lambda and the A.M.A., is again called to our attention by the words of the eminent René de la Roche, Philadelphia physician and member of that city's Kappa Lambda Society:[128]

> This Association [Kappa Lambda] he [Brown] proposed to be formed through means of local societies established in various sections of the

> country. Its object was to unite its scattered members - whether residing in the north or south, east or west, - into a single homogenous body, and by **fostering** among them reciprocity of kindly, fraternal and **honorable** feelings, insure the establishment and **cultivation** of harmony in their ranks; while at the same time, it would, through various means, be instrumental in **exciting emulation, and promoting the advancement of medical knowledge.**

The striking similarity in wording between the purpose of Kappa Lambda (1819), as expressed above by Dr. René de la Roche in his biography of Dr. Brown, and the preamble of the American Medical Association (1847), is obvious as shown by the bolding of words and phrases in both quotations. The A.M.A. Preamble follows:[129]

> for **cultivating** and **advancing medical knowledge;** for elevating the standard of the medical education; for **promoting** the usefulness, **honor**, and interests of the medical profession; for enlightening and directing public opinion in regard to the duties, responsibilities and requirements of medical men; for **exciting** and encouraging **emulation** and concert of action in the profession, and for facilitating and **fostering** friendly intercourse between those engaged in it.

Delegates to the National Conventions of 1846-1847

The historian Philip Van Ingen states that the New York chapter of Kappa Lambda sent delegates to the early and formative meetings of the American Medical Association, and the chapter continued to be active as late as 1862.[130] The New York delegation included Dr. Edward Delafield,[131] a Kappa Lambda member, who was in the chair when delegates first met in New York on May 5, 1846, and Dr. Alexander H. Stevens, also a Kappa Lambda member.[132]

Two other prominent delegates who were also members of Kappa Lambda were Drs. Isaac Hays[133] and John Bell[134] of Philadelphia.[135] Dr. Hays, one of the most active members at the 1846 Convention, presented the resolutions proposing a national medical association.[136] Dr. Bell was chairman of the Committee appointed to prepare a code of medical ethics (1846-1847). According to Dr. Davis, "The report on Medical Ethics, made by Drs. Bell and Hays, was very full and explicit and was unanimously adopted by the Convention."[137] Drs. Franklin Bache, George B. Wood, Hugh Hodge, Joseph Parrish, Charles Meigs, Joseph Pancoast, Samuel Jackson, and René de la Roche were additional members of Philadelphia's Kappa Lambda chapter who participated in the founding of the A.M.A. The Philadelphia group loomed large in the first A.M.A. conventions, and not the least of their representatives was Dr. Wood (ΚΛ), acknowledged by Dr. Davis in the Convention of 1848-49 and, together with Dr. Stevens (ΚΛ) and Dr. Jonathan Knight, named to the Special Committee on Education. They were described by Davis as "three of the ablest and most experienced professors in the country."[138]

The second president of the American Medical Association, Alexander H. Stevens of New York, was a member of Kappa Lambda as were the ninth, George B. Wood of Philadelphia; the thirteenth, Henry Miller of Louisville; and the twentieth, Samuel David Gross of Louisville and Philadelphia. In addition, vice presidents of the A.M.A. who were members of Kappa Lambda include Dr. Edward Delafield (1846), Dr. Stevens, Dr. Wood (1847), and Dr. Samuel Jackson (1849).[139] That these men were committed to and nurtured by the values of Samuel Brown's Kappa Lambda Society inexorably links the constituency, chronology, and goals of the two societies, Kappa Lambda and the A.M.A.

Dr. Davis describes the 1850 meeting of the American

AN

INAUGURAL THESIS

ON

THE RELATION BETWEEN

THE

SANGUIFEROUS AND NERVOUS

SYSTEMS,

SUBMITTED TO THE EXAMINATION

OF THE

Rev. HORACE HOLLEY, A. M; A. A. S. President,

THE

TRUSTEES AND MEDICAL PROFESSORS

OF

TRANSYLVANIA UNIVERSITY,

ON THE 12th DAY OF MARCH, 1822.

FOR THE DEGREE OF

DOCTOR OF MEDICINE.

BY HENRY MILLER,

President of the *Lexington Medical Society*, and member of the K. Λ *Society of Hippocrates*.

"Felix, qui potuit rerum cognoscere causas."—VIR.

LEXINGTON, KY.

PRINTED BY WILLIAM GIBBES HUNT.

1822.

Transylvania University Thesis submitted by Henry Miller
for the degree of Doctor of Medicine
Henry A. Miller, M.D. (1800-1874)
Courtesy of Transylvania University Library

Medical Association in Cincinnati as the "occasion of bringing many eminent members of the profession from the Atlantic cities into the great Valley of the Mississippi for the first time in their lives."[140] At this meeting, Daniel Drake,[141] a member of Kappa Lambda and former President of the Lexington Medical Society (1824), was defeated for the presidency of the A.M.A. by a fellow Cincinnatian, Reuben D. Mussey.

The Legacy of Samuel Brown and Kappa Lambda

That Samuel Brown of Transylvania University, Lexington, Kentucky, is the founder of the Lexington Medical Society and of the first national medical society in America, Kappa Lambda of Hippocrates, the prototype for **all** subsequent national medical societies, and, as such, is the **Father of all National American Medical Societies** cannot be denied. To fail to fully recognize him as such would be shameful.

With the founding of Kappa Lambda in Kentucky, the diffusion of knowledge, the education of the new nation's citizens so sought by the Revolutionary generation, had now come full circle. No longer was the diffusion of knowledge simply one-sided, East to West, for Professor Samuel Brown, through his wit and fortitude, had materially and spiritually reversed both the direction of its diffusion from West to East, and its substance, not merely the diffusion of knowledge but rather the advancement of knowledge. He was first in so many ways: in forming and implementing the first medical school West of the Alleghenies, the Transylvania University Department of Medicine; in the founding of a medical society West of the Alleghenies, the Lexington Medical Society; and in founding a national medical society in America, Kappa Lambda, and its affiliated medical journal, *The North American Medical and Surgical Journal.* Altogether, it was the educational and scientific endeavors of Samuel Brown,[142] a man of virtue and of vision, which, together with the successful hip amputation

(1806) by Walter Brashear (1776-1860), the ovariotomy (1809) by Ephraim McDowell (1771-1830), and the first successful excision of the clavicle (1813) by Charles McCreery (1785-1826), all of Kentucky, that brought to fruition the prophecy by Thomas Jefferson:[143]

> **Indeed, I have such an opinion of the talents of the professors in the other branches which constitute the school of medicine...that it is from this side of the Atlantic, that Europe, which has taught us so many other things, will at length be led into the sound principles in this branch of science, the most important of all others, being that to which we commit the care of health & life.**

87 James Thomas Flexner, *Doctors on Horseback: Pioneers of American Medicine* (New York: The Viking Press, 1937), 210.

88 Ibid., 221. "The two Cincinnati institutions [the Medical College of Ohio and the Medical Department of Cincinnati College] engaged in a free-style battle with no holds barred; even the students had fist fights. One day [Daniel] Drake met an Ohio College professor on the street. They both walked straight ahead until they faced each other chest to chest. 'I do not propose to step aside for a fool,' said the Ohio professor. 'I will,' replied Drake and stepped aside."

89 L.P. Yandell in his 1854 publication, "Dr. Samuel Brown as an Author," *The Western Journal of Medicine and Surgery,* Volume II, leaves no doubt as to Brown's contributions. He attributes to Brown the idealistic belief in universal harmony among physicians and does not hesitate to credit him as "the founder of the *'Kappa Lambda Society of Hippocrates,'* an institution framed by his benovolent mind to bring harmony to the profession. He hoped to *see every worthy physician in America enrolled among the members of the society* and thus, by becoming brethren in a double sense, be made to exhibit a fraternal spirit in their intercourse with each other." [Italics added.]

90 Chauncey Leake, "What was Kappa Lambda?" *Annals of Medical History,* 4 (1922) : 192-196.

91 Chauncey D. Leake, *"Some answers to* What was Kappa Lambda?" *Journal of History of Medicine* 17 (1962), 525. Leake remarks, "It would seem sentimentally appropriate to revive the Kappa Lambda Society of Hippocrates as some kind of honor society for the purpose of preserving and expanding the high standards and ideals of medical education and medical practice. This might be an appropriate undertaking in the splendid new College of Medicine at the University of Kentucky, which has now been established in Lexington."

92 R. de la Roche, "Samuel Brown, 1769-1830," in *Lives of Eminent American Physicians and Surgeons of the Nineteenth Century,* ed., Samuel D. Gross (Philadelphia: Lindsay & Balkiston, 1861), 231 and 245. Dr. René de la Roche, a leading practitioner of medical journalism and professor of medicine, added that this state of things gave way under the influence of the *Kappa Lambda Society.* "He [la Roche] was a prolific contributor to medical journals of the first order elsewhere and was one of the chief powers in the editorial staff of the Kappa Lambda Society's journal, *The North America Medical and Surgical Journal,* Philadelphia. He is probably best known for his great work on Yellow Fever, which is a classic on that subject. He was a member of nearly all the leading medical and scientific societies of the city [Philadelphia] and was one of the strong influences of this period."

Burton A. Konkle, *Standard History of the Medical Profession of Philadelphia,* ed. Frederick P. Henry, 2d ed. (New York: AMS Press, 1977), 209.

93 In *The Kentucky Gazette,* 16 August 1803. A note was printed immediately above the letter addressed to Mr. Bradford (Editor) stating "The enclosed letter was directed to the Lexington Medical Society—you will very much oblige the Society, by giving it a place in your paper. By order of the President, James L. Armstrong, Secretary."

94 Mrs. Charles F. Norton, Librarian, Transylvania Library, Lexington, Ky., to Dr. Philip Van Ingen, New York City, 9 December 1941, Special Collections, Transylvania University, Lexington, Ky. The same misinformation is also contained in Benjamin Hobson Frayser, "Kappa Lambda, the First Professional Fraternity," *Banta's Greek Exchange* 23, no. 4 (October 1935), 335.

95 Leake, "What was Kappa Lambda?" 192-196.

96 Ibid., 200. A letter published in 1830, also bearing the pseudonym MEDICUS, and written

by Dr. John Stearns of New York, strongly opposed the Kappa Lambda Society, thus effectively eliminating the possibility that the pseudonym generally served to disguise a Kappa Lambda member.

97 One author, Zachariah Frederick Smith has stated that Dr. Frederick Ridgely published several articles in the *American Medical Repository*, published in Philadelphia. Zachariah Frederick Smith, *School History of Kentucky* (Louisville: *Courier Journal*, 1891), 746. (Konkle and Henry in their *Standard History of the Medical Profession of Philadelphia* do not include the *American Medical Repository* in the list of Medical Journals of Philadelphia). Smith cites no reference. I am unable to confirm or deny his statement; however, in Yandell's review of the medical literature of Kentucky, and in his discussion of Dr. Ridgely, there is no mention of a publication. Dr. Brown's works were published in June 1799 in the *American Medical Repository* (New York), founded in 1797, the only journal of medicine published in the United States at that time. Dr. Yandell states that it was "the first medical paper from the pen of a Kentucky physician." Lunsford P. Yandell, "The Medical Literature of Kentucky," read at a meeting of the State Medical Society at Henderson, April, 1875, *Kentucky Medical Journal*, Historical Number, no. 11 (November 1917) : 134-137.

98 Born September 29, 1740, in Warrington, Lancashire, Thomas Percival began to study at Edinburgh in 1761 and there enjoyed the same exhilarating medical tutoring as did the Americans Benjamin Rush, Samuel Brown, Ephraim McDowell, and David Hosack. Graduating with his medical degree from Leyden in 1765, he was made a fellow of the Royal Society of England that same year at the age of 25. Two years later, Percival published a series of general medical and philosophical essays and commentaries on medical life. It was an argument initiated by the medical staff of the Manchester Infirmary that led to his long-delayed publication on medical ethics. The difficulties arose when, after an outbreak of typhoid that "taxed the capacity of the Infirmary," the hospital board decided to double the size of the medical staff. Two of the most prominent members of the staff took this action as an affront and resigned. In 1791 as a close friend of many members of the "old" and "new" staff, "Percival was asked by the trustees of the Infirmary to draw up a *scheme of professional conduct relative to hospital and other medical charities.*" His much deliberated and delayed work unquestionably led to the codification of the principles that were the first formal code of ethics submitted to the English medical profession. Drafts of the manuscripts were circulated for many years among his friends for their criticism. The completed work was finally published in 1803. Chauncey D. Leake, ed., *Percival's Medical Ethics* (Baltimore: The Williams & Wilkins Company, 1927), 25-32.

99 Ibid., 1.

100 Ibid., 49.

101 Morris Fishbein, *A History of The American Medical Association, 1847-1947* (Philadelphia and London: W. B. Saunders Co., 1947), 36.

102 Ibid., 37.

103 Konkle relates the presentation of the report on medical ethics by Isaac Hays and John Bell of Philadelphia and its adoption in May 1847. He states, "...higher educational standards were recommended to the colleges, and the constitution was so framed as to invariably secure a majority of the delegates from permanent state and county societies. The latter provision was intended to animate and encourage state and county organization, and ultimately to limit the membership to such bodies. These were features that at once showed Philadelphia's leadership of the conservative element." Konkle, *Standard History*, 184.

In February 1823, the New York State Medical Society unanimously adopted a code of ethics submitted by a committee of members. In his *History of Medicine in New York*, James Walsh states: "The reading of the two codes (code of Medical Ethics of the Medical Society of the State of New York and that of the American Medical Association) makes it clear that of the National Association was founded to a considerable extent on the system of ethics of the New York State Society. This is not surprising if we recall that the American Medical Association originated from the efforts of the State Society of New York." Chauncey Leake disputes the conclusions drawn by Dr. Walsh: "Dr. J.J. Walsh has tried to show that this important document (A.M.A. Code of Ethics) was taken directly from the New York State 'Code,' but there is little evidence, aside from chapter headings, to support this view."

104 Regular physicians were those who had received medical degrees from the European or American Medical Schools. Also, included were those physicians trained by the apprentice method by a "reputable" physician. Often the regular physician's training included a given number of years as an apprentice together with one to two years of lectures in a medical school. Other so-called "physicians" were those with little training or training by an unqualified physician. The irregulars were rounded out with quacks, herb doctors, Indian doctors, et. cetera. The distinction between regular and irregular physicians was often murky. This fault was one of the driving forces to establish medical societies. It also fostered the need for exclusivity in the earlier societies.

Medicine and Its Development in Kentucky, comp. and written by Medical Historical Research Projects Administration for the Commonwealth of Kentucky (Louisville: The Standard Printing Company, 1940), 79. "The legal position of medical men claming to be regular remained in great measure undefined at least up to the outbreak of the Civil War. That is pretty much the same thing as saying that it was under no restrictions imposed by the Legislature at Frankfort. Regulation was a matter of membership in and loyalty to some association, through what one may call 'a gentlemen's agreement.' A rebel might be boycotted, left outside of consultation, whispering campaigns might be resorted to and were in cases where something like a feud developed, but it was well not to go too far. Always the law of libel was there as remedy. In extreme cases there might be a challenge and a duel. The non-regulars were prosperous just the same, much as, in more recent days, the advertising dentist; they were not only feathering their nests, but making friends who told of cures and conspired against the regulars. Real control did not exist in Kentucky, not through legislation at all events."

William G. Rothstein, *American Physicians in the Nineteenth Century* (Baltimore and London: The Johns Hopkins University Press, 1972), Appendix II, 335. "No licensing law in Kentucky before 1860."

105 Rothstein, *American Physicians in the Nineteenth Century*, 65.

106 René de la Roche, "Samuel Brown, 1769-1830," 244.

107 The following description of the happenings related to Kappa Lambda Society in Philadelphia and New York is liberally taken from the essay of Leake, "What was Kappa Lambda?" 192-206.

108 George McClellan (1796-1847), Chairman of the Department of Surgery and founder of Jefferson Medical College (organized in 1824), Philadelphia, Pennsylvania. (Dr. McClellan was the father of Civil War General George McClellan.)

Ibid., 199.

109 Ibid., 200.

110 Ibid.

111 "Medicus" was said to be Dr. John Stearns.

112 Leake, "What was Kappa Lambda?" 201.

Some of the members of the New York Kappa Lambda Society were John Watts, President of the College of Physicians and Surgeons; John Augustine Smith, Professor of Anatomy; Joseph M. Smith, Professor of Theory and Practice of Medicine; Alexander H. Stevens, Professor of Surgery; Edward D. Delafield, Professor of Obstetrics.

Valentine Mott (1785-1865), a distinguished American surgeon who took his MD degree from Columbia University (1806) and completed his training both in London under the famed Sir Ashley Cooper, and in Edinburgh. His fame rests foremost on his triumphs in vascular surgery.

113 Leake, "What Was Kappa Lambda," 196; and Benjamin Hobson Frayser, "Kappa Lambda, the First Professional Fraternity," *Banta's Greek Exchange,* Vol. 23, No. 4, (October, 1935) : 334, 337.

114 Van Ingen, "Remarks on Kappa Lambda. Elf or Ogre? And a Little More Concerning the Society," 513-538.

115 Henry Burnell Shafer, *The American Medical Profession* 1783 to 1850 (New York: Columbia University Press, 1936), 134-135.

116 William Preston Vaughn, *The Antimasonic Party in the United States 1826-1843* (Lexington: The University of Kentucky Press, 1993), 10-14.

117 Ibid., 1.

118 Lee D. van Antwerp, "Kappa Lambda, Elf or Ogre?" *Bulletin of the History of Medicine* xvii, no 4 (1945) : 327-350, 331.

119 Ibid., 330-331. "There is probably some basis in fact in the contention that the New York branch of the Society used the secrecy of the organization for the mutual profit of the members, but considering the Society as a whole, there is little or no evidence that it was the hydraheaded monster sometimes pictured."

120 Ibid., 338.

121 "In New York City, where the factions never were reconciled throughout the period [1783-1850], jealousy alone seems to explain the deplorable situation....Again ill-will prompted some physicians to charge the members of the Kappa Lambda Society of New York...with aiding each other." Shafer, *The American Medical Profession*, 1783 to 1850, 36.

122 Leake, "What Was Kappa Lambda?" 192-206.

123 Ibid., 196.

124 A. H. Barkley, "Dr. Samuel Brown, The First Professor of Medicine West of the Alleghenies," *Annals of Medical History* III, no. 4 (1931) : 367, quoting Brown.

125 Ibid.

126 In 1826 when the *Kappa Lambda Society* of the United States founded the *North American Medical And Surgical Journal,* editors of the journal included Hugh L. Hodge, Franklin Bache, Chas. D. Meigs, B. H. Coates, and R. de la Roche; later George Wood, David Francis Condie and John Bell, all of whom were nationally known and highly respected members of the Philadelphia Medical profession. The journal, according to de la Roche, "[was] placed under the guidance of a committee of the [Philadelphia] society by Dr. Brown, established and continued to appear quarterly during six consecutive years." de la Roche, "Samuel Brown," 245. *It was the first such journal to be published by a national medical society as a constituent arm of the society.* As the journal title indicates, Dr. Brown's vision was national, even continental, and the *journal* itself has since become the standard organ by which a medical society, national or otherwise, conveys its scientific and literary philosophy, diffuses knowledge, and exhorts its members to a higher standard of excellence. *Indeed, the medical journal is among the most important discoveries of all times.* [Author]

The editors of this timely and influential journal knew precisely the intent of Kappa Lambda's founder, as evidenced in their preface to the fourth volume of the journal issued in 1827: "Several years ago, an Association of American Physicians was founded by the zealous and philanthropic exertions of Dr. Samuel Brown, late Professor of Medicine in Transylvania University. This institution, under the title of the KAPPA LAMBDA ASSOCIATION of the United States, was intended to be co-extensive with the Union, and accordingly, its branches, which, in the progress of this design, have been established in various parts of the country, acknowledge a mutual connexion....the objects of the Institution are to elevate the character of the Medical Vocation, by inculcating a higher standard of excellence, not merely in the professional or ministrative, but also in the ethical relations and duties of physicians."

127 Horine, "Sketch of the Kentucky State Medical Society," 290-303; and Henry Miller, "Resolutions of 11 December 1822 Meeting of the Kappa Lambda Society of Hippocrates," Special Collections, Transylvania University, Lexington, Ky.

128 de la Roche, "Samuel Brown, 1769-1830," 244.

129 *Proceedings of the National Medical Conventions Held in New York, May, 1846 and In Philadelphia, May, 1847* (Philadelphia: T.K. & P.G. Collins, Printers, 1847), 401.

130 Philip Van Ingen, "Remarks on 'Kappa Lambda, Elf or Ogre?' and a Little More Concerning the Society," eds. Henry R. Sigerist and Genevieve Miller, *Bulletin of the History of Medicine* XVIII (December 1945) : 513-538.

131 Edward Delafield, of New York, chairman of the National Convention in New York, 1846. He, along with John Bell, was elected Vice-President at this organizational meeting.

Fishbein, *A History of the American Medical Association,* 24.

132 Fielding H. Garrison, *An Introduction to the History of Medicine,* 3d ed. (Philadelphia and London: W. B. Saunders Co., 1922), 806-807; Leake, "What was Kappa Lambda?" 192-206.

133 Isaac Hays (1796-1879), a distinguished Philadelphia physician and Editor of the *American Journal of Medical Sciences* for forty-two years.

Fishbein, *A History of the American Medical Association* 1847 to 1947, 37.

134 John Bell (1796-1872), a graduate of the University of Pennsylvania (MD degree), an editor of several books including *Stokes Lectures on the Theory and Practice of Physics.* He was one of two vice-presidents of the organizational meeting of the A.M.A. at the National Convention, New York City, 1846.

Davis, *History of the American Medical Association*, 42.

135 Konkle, *Standard History of the Medical Profession of Philadelphia,* 210-211. Dr. Hays was a member of the Committee on Ethics and Chairman of the Committee on Arrangements at the Philadelphia Convention of 1847, one of three members appointed "...for the promotion of our national medical literature..." and, beginning in 1847, a five-term Treasurer of the American Medical Association.

136 Ibid., 210.

137 N. S. Davis, *History of the American Medical Association,* ed. S. W. Butler (Philadelphia: Lippincott, Grambo & Co., 1855), 45.

138 Ibid., 41 and 77.

139 Some historians have asserted that the officers at the 1847 meeting in Philadelphia, Dr. Knight, President, Dr. Alexander Stevens and Dr. George B. Wood, (two of four) vice-presidents, should be accorded the title of first president and first vice-president(s) of the A.M.A. Sherwin B. Nuland in his manuscript "A Matter of Great Importance to Mankind: Origins of the New Haven County Medical Association" declares, "When the American Medical Association was founded in 1847, it was a member of our society, Jonathan Knight, who was the first President." *Connecticut Medicine* (September 1984) : 559-561. He also was the seventh president of the A.M.A.

140 Davis, *History of American Medical Association*, 87.

141 Emmet Field Horine, *Daniel Drake (1785-1852), Pioneer Physician of the Midwest* (Philadelphia: University of Pennsylvania Press, 1961), 393.

142 Dr. Samuel Brown and Dr. Ephraim McDowell (Danville, Kentucky) were members of the Lexington Medical Society. Minutes of the Lexington Medical Society, 1803-1804. Dr. Brashear took his apprenticeship in Lexington under the tutelage of Dr. Ridgely and practiced in Lexington during the second decade of the eighteen hundreds. He, too, probably was a member of the Society.

143 Thomas Jefferson, "Letter to Dr. Caspar Wistar," June 21, 1807, *Thomas Jefferson Writings* (New York: Library Classics of the United States, Inc., 1984), 1185.

Chapter III

DISEASE AND THERAPY IN ANTEBELLUM LEXINGTON

Late Eighteenth- and Early Nineteenth-Century Medicine

What was it like to practice medicine in the latter part of the eighteenth century and in the early nineteenth century? What differences were there between the practice and the care given in Lexington and that given in Philadelphia, Paris, or London? In the two centuries following the founding of Jamestown (1607), what was known and what was done by the medical practitioner of any standing had little changed; recovery from the smallpox, the "bloody" flux, the fevers, and other ailments were still at the whim of nature. Indeed, the number of colonists prematurely ushered to their graves by well-meaning practitioners can more easily be conceived than counted. Were we to assume that the medical care afforded most men, women, and children of America during the seventeenth, eighteenth, and nineteenth centuries was significantly inferior to that available to their counterparts in Europe, we would err, "for much of what passed as medicine, both in Europe and America, was delivered by neighbors, clergy and self-proclaimed doctors....It was also a time when any enlightened person could read, understand, and apply medical care in a manner equal to that of many so-called physicians."[144]

The First American Physicians

Rarely did the English physician choose to leave his homeland for the uncertainty of America. The first physicians in America were clergymen and a few peripatetic ship surgeons. The Puritan clergy were not empirics; they had prepared themselves for the dual professions of medicine and religion, echoing the ancient practice of the priests of Egypt. Cotton Mather of Boston, perhaps the best known of this highly respected group, called the duo "the angelic conjunction."[145] Although this paired profession was especially prevalent in New England for nearly a century, the clergy-physician practice was similarly combined in other colonies, but seldom with the idealism and the command of the Puritans.[146]

It was not unusual for the physician to wear many hats, perhaps physician, cleric, and farmer. The added hats worn also added to the physician's income, a necessity in the smaller communities. A few of the early Lexington physicians, such as the infamous General James Wilkinson, never practiced medicine in Lexington; the eminent Dr. Walter Brashear eventually found the United States Senate (Louisiana) more to his liking; Dr. Basil Duke favored business; Dr. Joseph Buchanan, professor of the Institute of Medicine, Transylvania University, abandoned medicine to serve as editor of the Louisville Focus in 1812; and Dr. James Fishback served as both a physician and a clergyman.[147]

The British tripartite system of clinician, surgeon, and apothecary was alien to the American scene.[148] American physicians from the beginning integrated these three roles into one, not by design but by necessity. For Americans, the term "Doctor"

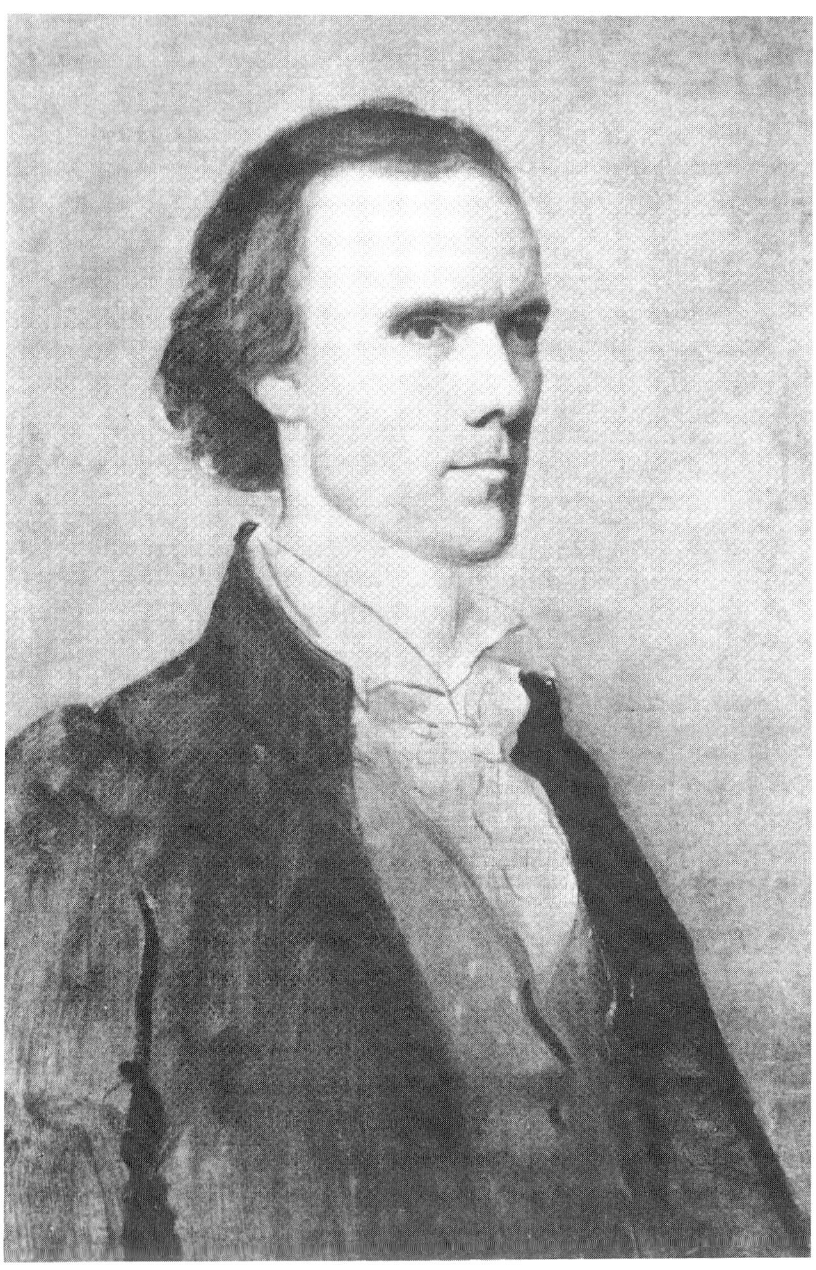

Joseph Buchanan, M.D.
(1785-1829)
Courtesy of Transylvania University Library

described a practitioner who treated, for better and often worse, all that could ail a person. The American doctor, in contradistinction to his British counterpart, did what he found necessary to do: concoct medicine, bleed and purge, pull teeth, prescribe herbs, set fractures, amputate limbs, practice midwifery, and nurse.

The doctors in London, Philadelphia and Lexington practiced with basically the same knowledge, the same drugs, the same instruments, and the same results. Because Americans could detect no particular difference between their medical care and that of their European counterparts, there was no hue and cry to establish medical schools. Why pay handsome sums to the physician with formal training when the care and outcome delivered by him offered no additional protection to the patient's well-being? Even though Philadelphia was the medical center of the Colonies, there was no demand by Philadelphians for the medical school founded there in 1765. "The city fathers had to be persuaded by a local boy (John Morgan,1735-1789) returning from Edinburgh that they really needed one."[149]

The West

As American colonists moved farther and farther westward from the eastern seaboard, they, out of necessity, faced the wilderness with the same fortitude as the original settlers, but often with even less knowledge of medicine and with less education in general than their forebears. By the turn of the eighteenth century, clergymen of various denominations traversed the wilds of Virginia and the neighboring colonies. Like their scholarly Puritan predecessors, they were customarily the leaders in their frontier settlements; and though not always men of exceptional learning, they were, even so, knowledgeable in comparison to the remainder of their congregations. And they knew their flocks, their patients, far better than did any other person, and so attended simultaneously to their physical and their spiritual needs. Settlers made do with what was at hand, placing their faith in God and their trust in the cleric-physician.

During these early years in the backwoods of Lexington, the pioneers had one primary aim-to *survive.* Indian raids took a heavy toll on the settlers, and if that alone was not misery enough, cold, starvation, and disease added to their plight. But these pioneers stood their ground, and, with the ending of the Revolutionary War in 1783, the danger of the savage Indian attacks was less pressing. For the first time, the settlers were able to build outside the forts. Even so, frequent and deadly encounters with small bands of Indians continued to plague the settlers. In the *Kentucky Gazette* of July 18, 1789, an extract signed by Levi Todd, county lieutenant, reads as follows: "That each of the militia in the several counties on the western waters, shall keep always ready a good musket or rifle, half a pound of lead, to be produced whenever called for by the commanding officer, or be fined at the discretion of a court martial, in any sum not exceeding ten shillings, for each musket, unless he be too poor as to be unable to furnish the same."[150] Throughout the balance of the 1780s and 1790s, the newspaper published numerous accounts of slayings and horse raids by bands of Indians.[151]

In a tale told by an old lady to the Lexington physician Dr. Samuel Brown (1769-1830),[152] we are momentarily whisked back into this wilderness, back into a time when violence raged:

> …that during the first two years of her residence in Kentucky, the most comely sight she beheld, was seeing a young man dying in his bed a natural death. She had been familiar with blood and carnage and death, but in all those cases the sufferers were the victims of the Indian tomahawk and scalping knife; and that, on an occasion when a young man was taken sick and died, after the usual manner of nature, she and the rest of the women sat up all night, gazing upon him, as an object of beauty.

Early Lexington Physicians

We have previously acknowledged the personal background and the works of Drs. Frederick Ridgely and Samuel Brown, the first two professors of the Transylvania Medical Department.[153] Of the other physicians practicing in Lexington during this period (1784-1800) we know considerably less. James Wilkinson is believed to have been the first physician to settle in Lexington (1784); however, his interest was principally in the selling and transporting of goods down the Mississippi River. His employee, Dr. Hugh Sheil (1784), managed Wilkinson's store. Neither physician is thought to have practiced medicine in Lexington other than for their personal needs. Among the practicing physicians were Dr. Joseph Boswell (1787); Dr. Richard W. Downing (arrival 1787 or 1791); a Dr. Beatty (left his practice in Lexington on November 14, 1788); Dr. Andrew McKinley (opened his office August 8, 1789); Dr. Thomas Lloyd (1789); Dr. P. Rootes (1791); Dr. Basil Duke (1791); Dr. Daniel Preston (1791); Dr. John Hole (1792); Dr. James Welch (1795); Dr. James Collins (1795); Dr. Thomas Huff (1796); and Dr. John W. Scott (1796).[154]

Early Migration to Lexington

What brought about this migration of physicians to Lexington? The rapid growth of the population and the increasing notoriety given Lexington by the presence of schools and men of prominence in the law, the clergy, and other fields probably played their part. Another distinct possibility is that "after the Revolution colonial army officers, including surgeons and surgeons-mates, received sizable Kentucky land warrants as bounties for military service."[155] Although several of the pioneer physicians stayed on in Lexington, others sought their fortunes elsewhere, for Lexington was a point of departure for the vast reaches of the west.

Early Lexington physicians were less than shy in announcing their virtues. In 1798, a Dr. C. Freeman, physician and surgeon, wrote in detail of his qualifications, occupying almost one-half of a front-page column: "Late of the Indian towns; from the North-Western Territory of the United States, now at Lexington, Kentucky...attended Dr. William Shippen, Jr.'s [1736-1808] lectures on anatomy, surgery and midwifery.... Since which times, he has traveled through twenty-two different tribes, among whom he has resided nearly four years, and made it his constant study to investigate all kinds of herbs, roots plants...."[156 157]

We are likewise given a lengthy list of "Fresh and Genuine Medicines" just received from Philadelphia by Dr. J. M. Schawg of Lexington in 1806. A partial list includes "rhubarb, root and powder; laudanum; venereal pills; rose water; gum opium; quill bark; orange peal; lemon peal; gum Arabic; sugar candy; camphor; oil of vitriol; ipecacuanha powder; Red precipitate mercury...." He added this footnote: "I will sell the whole furniture with the medicine, to any person inclining to purchase."[158]

To more fully grasp the vagaries of medicine as practiced in Lexington during the period 1790 to 1850 we look not only to physicians but to the homes of settlers and their descendants, to the women, to their neighbors, to the ever-ready "irregulars": quacks; herbalists, "Indian doctors," and physician pretenders. Self-reliance was to the forefront of those far removed from the physician "where everyone is disposed, from his earliest childhood, to think and to act for himself."[159] Medicinal drugs (calomel, jalap, ipecac et cetera) were as readily available to the public as to the physician, but when home remedies failed it was time to call on a neighbor or perhaps a nearby herbalist.

The Theorists

For the regular physicians, i.e., those having acceptable credentials by apprenticeship or the few with medical school diplomas, the practice of medicine in Lexington and essentially the entire United States was first framed by a philosophical system fashioned by the medical theorists of the University of Edinburgh Medical School in Scotland. Although several young physicians returned to America from Edinburgh during the eighteenth century, the most celebrated and influential graduate and purveyor of the Edinburgh system was Dr. Benjamin Rush of Philadelphia, professor of Medicine, University of Pennsylvania Medical School. He, in particular, brought home the Edinburgh medical systems of William Cullen (1710-1790) and John Brown (1735-1788). Cullen emphasized the role of the nervous system and nervous energy in bodily function, the qualities of sensibility and irritability (irritability was later transformed into excitability). John Brown had a somewhat different approach; by his system "all diseases were due either, to an excess or to a lack of nervous stimulation and thus indicated either "depleting" or "stimulation" remedies.[160] Rush initially embraced the two theorists in thought and in action but later developed a system of his own and with it a therapy wrapped in the trappings of "Old Glory." Rush had no tolerance for the modest blood-letting practices of the Europeans. Such practices, he insisted, could not be trusted to repulse the "particular harshness" of American disease. The greater mettle of the American called for a more rigorous therapy that could, in Rush's opinion, be both withstood by the gallant Americans and, in turn, tame if not defeat the disease. It was appropriately dubbed the "heroic treatment" consisting in the main of blood-letting, purgatives, emetics, and sweating.

Rush counseled his devoted Philadelphia medical students, "that there was but one fever in the world, be not startled Gentlemen, follow me and I will say that there is but one disease in the world." Central to his theory Rush assumed "an underlying pattern of bodily reaction in disease a pattern common to all types of illness regardless of the remote or external causes."[161] All disease, he concluded, was brought on by one "proximate" cause, a state of excitability ("vascular spasm," "vascular tension," "convulsive action") in the blood vessels which summoned the one treatment of "depletion" by bleeding and purging.[162] Several ounces to two- and a-half gallons of blood were taken from the adult over a period of hours or days. The greatest fear was in taking too little, not too much, blood. Even babies of three months of age were not exempt from the lancet.

Our interest in Dr. Benjamin Rush is through his national reputation and the fact that over two thousand of his medical students subsequently dotted the states and territories, their practice and their results being much as their master's. The practice of medicine as advised by Rush had numerous followers in Lexington. Several outstanding Lexington physicians while students in Philadelphia attended his lectures: Samuel Brown, Daniel Drake, Benjamin Dudley, William Richardson, John Esten Cooke, and Charles Caldwell. Drugs were given to treat symptoms not disease. Their purpose was to lessen the severity of fever and of loose bowels, etc. Writing in 1832 on the "diseases of the summer and fall," Dr. Lunsford P. Yandell, a Transylvania University professor, furnishes us with this insight into heroic medicine: "The remedies that succeeded best in the treatment of the disease [scarlet fever] were emetics and calomel, preceded by blood-letting when the arterial excitement was high. Ipecacuan, administered in such doses as excited vomiting, and repeated throughout the day produced the best effects. The calomel was repeated from day to day so as to keep up free purging."[163]

In the treatment of cholera, Dr. Benjamin Dudley was prone to give emetics to relieve spasms with the added benefit of "recalling the pulse to the wrists." Unlike most physicians of the time, Dudley opposed blood-letting, "and used to say that a man's life was shortened a year for every bleeding."[164] Daniel Drake, however, employed blood-letting in many entities including pneumonia when actual inflammation had developed. The initial bleeding, he advised, should "produce syncope…and the second, if the heart should recover its power, should be carried to the verge of fainting but not further."

Diagnosis and treatment climaxed when the patient and the doctor met: be it at home; in the field; on the roadway; or the doctor's shop. And there were times when the patient was brought into the home of the physician and cared for sometimes for days or weeks. One such instance is related by Dr. John Esten Cooke, professor of the theory and practice, Transylvania University. For a period of two months in 1824 Cooke treated a patient with huge doses of calomel, rhubarb, aloes, and jalap without apparent benefit. In an attempt to reverse the man's decline, Cooke took him to his own home for care. Here he remained for several months at which time he died.[165] Well-known for his prescribed doses of calomel varying only from large to huge, Cooke initially had a solid following; however, as his speculative theory of the common origin of all diseases increasingly fell into disrepute his credibility collapsed and he voluntarily resigned from the medical faculty of the University of Louisville in 1843.[166]

The "Pox"

At a time when even the concept of disease was still captive to speculative theories and to the tenets of ancient ritualism, what should come forth and take hold in the cities of America but the practice of preventive medicine for smallpox.[167] According to Rosen, the term "smallpox" appeared early in the sixteenth century as the counterpart of the French term *la petite verole.*[168] The latter was employed in contradistinction to *la grosse verole,* syphilis. The terms imply a recognition of some similarity between the two conditions. The common element is the eruption that occurs in both diseases.[169] Until the year 1721, in Europe and Colonial America, preventive measures for smallpox and other infectious diseases were limited to the ancient practice of quarantine. For centuries, it was common knowledge that persons who had had an attack of smallpox were not subject to further attacks; they were immune. When Europeans became aware of "inoculation" as a means of preventing smallpox, it was first put to the test in England.[170] The principle was simple: smallpox matter from a person having a light case of smallpox was inoculated into one who had never had smallpox, causing a mild attack and so protecting that person from any further smallpox infection. The procedure was relatively simple, carried out by the use of a lancet and a thread containing smallpox matter. Inoculation, the use of the serum from a pox pustule to confer immunity, was the only tried and proven measure for prevention of smallpox, but it was not without risk and thus remained highly controversial throughout the eighteenth century in Europe and America. The stage was set, therefore, for the implementation of a new form of immunity, one that was both safe and effective. Such a method was discovered by a physician, Edward Jenner (1749-1823), of Gloucestershire, England. Jenner observed that persons who had had cowpox were immune to smallpox.[171] Through human experimentation in 1796,[172] he confirmed that people could be inoculated against cowpox in the same manner as against smallpox.[173] Who would have dared to believe that at that time one physician, Samuel Brown, intellectually primed and placed in the wilderness of Lexington, would have the knowledge, the courage, and the audacity to perform mass vaccinations for smallpox well before such extensive vaccinations were performed in Philadelphia and New York City?

To inoculate a person for smallpox had its risks for physicians, and the risks were not limited to those of a medical nature, nor in just one section of the colonies. In 1768 a riot took place in Norfolk, Virginia, brought on by the desire of a physician, Dr. Campbell, and some of his friends to have their wives and children inoculated by Dr. Dalgleish.[174] The first site set for the inoculation, under threat by the anti-inoculators, had to be abandoned, so Dr. Campbell chose to have the vaccinations performed at his plantation. A concession was further made by Dr. Campbell to the anti-inoculators, namely to limit the number of those to be inoculated. The procedures were carried out by Dr. Dalgleish on June 25, 1768. Although both sides agreed to move the inoculated patients to the pesthouse, the mob attacked Dr. Campbell's house on June 27 and forced the patients to go to the pesthouse in foul weather, before it could be readied for them. Two days after the riot, Dr. Campbell's house was burned.[175]

To fully appreciate the enormity of the "pox"[176] as it was conceived in Kentucky in 1798, the main features of the Statute enacted by the Kentucky Legislature on January 30, 1798, is given:[177]

An ACT to reduce into one the several acts for regulating the Inoculation of the Small-Pox, within this Commonwealth.

> Sec.1. If any person or persons whatsoever, shall willfully or designedly presume to import or bring into this commonwealth, from any country or place whatever, the small-pox...with a purpose to inoculate any person or persons, whatsoever, or by any means to propagate the said distemper within this commonwealth, he or she so offending shall forfeit and pay the sum of one thousand pounds for every offense so committed;
>
> Sec.2. That if any person shall think him or herself, his or her family, exposed to the immediate danger of catching the said distemper, such person may give notice thereof to the sheriff of any county, or to the mayor or chief magistrate... (to) consider whether upon the whole circumstances of the case, inoculating may be prudent or necessary, or dangerous to the health and safety of the neighbors;
>
> Sec.3. Any person having first obtained in writing ...the consent of a majority of the housekeepers residing within three miles, and not sepa-

rated by a river, creek or marsh a quarter of a mile wide, and conforming to the following rules and regulations, may inoculate or be inoculated for the small-pox, either in his or her own house, or at any other place.

Sec.4. Every physician, doctor, or other person undertaking inoculation at any house, shall cause a written advertisement to be put up at the nearest public road or other most notorious adjacent place, giving information that the small-pox is at such house...

Sec.5. If any person who hath not had the small-pox other than those who have been or intended to be inoculated, shall go into any house, where the small-pox then is, or intermix with the patient, and return from thence, any justice of the peace for the county or corporation, on due proof thereof, may by warrant, cause such person to be conveyed to the next hospital

Sec.6. Be it enacted, That it shall and may be lawful for the justices of any county... to levy on the titheable persons... so much tobacco or money as will be sufficient to defray the expences [inoculation] necessarily incurred.

Sec.7. If any sheriff, mayor or chief magistrate...shall refuse or neglect to attend accordingly to such summons, every such sheriff... shall forfeit the sum of one hundred pounds upon his refusing or neglecting to give such notice.

Sec.8. If any person or persons shall inocu-

> late or procure inoculation for the small-pox... without obtaining a license or consent to inoculate...he, she or they, shall forfeit and pay respectively, for every such offense, the sum of one hundred pounds.
>
> Sec.9. Every person willfully endeavoring to spread or propagate the small-pox, without inoculation, or by inoculation in any other manner than is allowed by this act, in special cases, shall be subject to the penalty of five hundred pounds, or suffer six months imprisonment without bail or main prize.
>
> Sec. 10. All the penalties inflicted by this act, may be recovered with costs, by action of debt or information, in any court of record.

The severity of the punishment, i.e., a fine of several hundred pounds, for failure of citizens to obey the law is ample testimony to the fear of and concern about smallpox held by the members of the legislature.

Throughout the colonial period, smallpox had been confined principally to the cities and towns along the eastern seaboard. Isolation itself protected most of the rural populace from the ravages of this "terror" until the time of the Revolutionary War.[178] Lacking immunity, military recruits from the small villages and the backwoods were easy prey to this prince of death. Further outbreaks of smallpox were precipitated with the unannounced movement of troops into isolated and vulnerable villages. George Washington called smallpox "more destructive to an army in the natural way than the sword," and after 1777 he ordered the entire army to be inoculated.[179] Many of the settlers in and about Lexington had served in the Revolutionary War and so had had the "pox" or had witnessed it first-hand. Their sentiments for or against inoculation would have been dictated by their own experiences.

Smallpox Inoculation in Lexington

The historian Staples informs us that "Of all the diseases that human flesh is heir to none is mentioned in the pages of the (Kentucky) Gazette, before 1806 so frequently as the dreaded smallpox. The disease was very common among the early pioneers, and frequent reference to it is found in the tales of travelers passing through this country."[180] The first public notice of "inoculation for smallpox" in Lexington appeared January 4, 1794, in the *Kentucky Gazette:*

> On Thursday last the inhabitants of this place began the inoculation of smallpox and have agreed to continue until the fifteenth, after which they are determined to cease. They have appointed a committee to draw up a remonstrance to the court of Fayette County requesting that the order of that court granting liberty to the inhabitants of said county to inoculate may be rescinded, so far as respects the town of Lexington after that date.

The *Gazette* for the first of February following has this terse announcement, illustrating the great hazard of this primitive operation:

> That the smallpox had been very fatal within the three weeks past in the town [Lexington] and vicinity under inoculation, that at least one out of fifteen died who had been inoculated, and very few children had recovered. At present most of those who survived are out of danger, and it is thought

> that within ten days all those who have taken it will be entirely well and the town freed from this disorder.

Simply the fact that inoculation for smallpox was given would imply that an epidemic had already struck. The following quote from the journal of Robert McAfee confirms this as fact: "In 1794 when I visited Lexington, Mr. Breckinridge advised my father to take me back home on account of the smallpox which had been brought to Lexington by returning soldiers from Ft. Washington."[181]

Learning About the Jennerian Vaccine

By 1800 Dr. Samuel Brown was a member of the renowned American Philosophical Society of Philadelphia, having been recommended by his friends Benjamin Rush and Thomas Jefferson. Brown was the first American West of the Alleghenies to be so honored. We may surmise that it was through his correspondence with other members of this august society that he learned of the Jennerian mode of vaccination. Brown and David Hosack of New York, both members of the society, were frequent correspondents (Dr. Hosack, following the lead of Dr. Benjamin Waterhouse in Boston, was the first to perform vaccination in New York). Or perhaps the first news may have come through Dr. Waterhouse in the same manner by which Brown later received the cowpox thread. Other possibilities include the English journals that he received in Lexington, or the report of cowpox vaccination by Dr. Waterhouse in March 1799 in the *Columbian Sentinel*, a Boston publication.[182] [183] We know that Brown had vaccinated at least two patients by May 1801, according to the newspaper account found in the *Kentucky Gazette* of May 25, 1801. It is through the journal of the famous French naturalist F. A. Michaux that we learn that 500 Lexingtonians were vaccinated by Dr. Brown by the year 1802.[184]

It is likely that most of the patients, at least the initial patients, were vaccinated with material taken from the thread received by Dr. Brown in May-June, 1801. It should be noted that in his account of the vaccination, John Bradford, editor of the *Kentucky Gazette,* includes the name of Dr. Ridgely with that of Dr. Brown. The newspaper notice by the Lexington Physicians pertaining to the smallpox includes the names of Drs. Brown, Ridgely, Downing and Boswell. These accounts indicate that Dr. Brown probably was supported, if not assisted with the vaccinations, by these other physicians.

An article in the May 25, 1801, *Kentucky Gazette* suggests that some Lexingtonians were not well-informed about the immunization as practiced by Dr. Brown and Dr. Ridgely. "A report having been circulated that Doctors Brown and Ridgely have inoculated with the infection of the small-pox in this town, the Editor thinks it his duty to inform the public that the report is (in his opinion) absolutely false."[185]

> Two young men have been inoculated with the Vaccine or cow-pox infection; no medical facts are better established than, that the Cow-pox cannot be communicated by any other means than inoculation- and that the person who has once had it is forever after incapable of taking the small-pox in any other manner.

Evidently, the Editor's effort was less than convincing, for in the issue of the *Gazette* published but two weeks later, the following two notices appeared. The first was by Lexington physicians:[186]

> SMALL POX
> Lexington, June 8th, 1801
>
> IGNORANT, interested and malicious persons, having asserted on several occasions, that

> the SMALL POX now prevails in Lexington and the intercourse between the town and country, being considerably interrupted by belief in this unfounded report; we the undersigned practitioners of medicine in the town of Lexington, after the most diligent inquiries which we have been able to make, are authorized unequivocally to assert that not one case of SMALL POX (either by natural infection, or by inoculation) has occurred in Lexington or the vicinity, for several years, nor do we believe that any contagious disease at present exists among us. For the truth of the above facts we pledge our reputation and honor. Given under our hands,
>
> R.W. Downing
Joseph Boswell
Sam. Brown
F. Ridgely

Some citizens may have been terrified at the possibility of unleashing a deadly disease upon the populace. Many Lexingtonians were all too well acquainted with the "pox" and with the death, the misery, the blindness, and the disfigurement that accompanied it; many also were aware that the same ill-results could come about by smallpox inoculation. Such valid reasons may have fed rumors that inoculation by smallpox and not vaccination for cowpox had been used by the physicians. Likewise, since cowpox vaccination was so recent a medical innovation, it is unlikely that the townspeople knew about or understood its safety and reliability in affording immunity to smallpox.

That such rumors were not easily quelled and that a number of people were incensed by the introduction of the vaccine can be deduced from the following article that appeared in the same issue of the *Kentucky Gazette,* June 8, 1801, and immediately below the notice by the physicians.

> We, the subscribers, being prompted, in the consequence of a report, which has been propagated through the country that the SMALL-POX has been lately introduced into this Town; have made every possible inquiry respecting it, and are happy to have it in our power to say, that the report is not only unfounded, but neither that, nor any other infectious disease has existed here for several years.
>
> Being convinced, that this report, must derive its origin from malicious motives; The subscribers, as well as citizens of Lexington at large, will consider it an act of Justice in any person to inform them of the name or names of the propagators thereof.
>
> *James Morrison,*
> *Will. Morton,*
> *John Jordan, Jun.,*
> *Andrew. M'Calla,*
> *John Bradford,*
> *Henry Marshall,*
> *John McNair*
> *Henry Clay,*
> *George Poyzer,*
> *C. Coyle,*
> *John Postlethwait,*
> *Arch. McIlvain, sen.,*
> *Thos. Bodley,*
> *James Trotter,*
> *G.R. Tompkins,*
> *William Ross,*
> *James Maccoun,*
> *George Tegarden,*
> *Alex. Parker,*
> *Thomas Wallace,*
> *John A. Seitz,*
> *Benjamin Stout,*
> *Thomas Whitney,*
> *George Mansell,*

We have used the terms "inoculation" and "vaccination" as means by which immunity can be given to a person; however, the words have different implications both historically and medically. Smallpox inoculation was not without complications, e.g., in some instances, the pre-conceived mild case turned into a "full-blown" attack from which the patient may have suffered the ravages of a devastating disease, possibly scarred if not dead. And not the least of concern was the fact that such patients could infect others, if not start an epidemic. The fear of inoculation was not born of hysteria. The fear was justified, the relevant question being what risk is the greater, inoculation with its blessed immunity or possible complications versus the chance of not being infected or of having the full effects of the "pox"? The argument for or against inoculation was never settled, for with the advent of cowpox vaccination it had lost all relevance.

Two considerations strike the reader about the vaccinations given by Dr. Brown: first, the large number of vaccinations (500), and second, the source of his cowpox material.[187] The latter can be determined by letters stipulating the source and the manner in which it reached him. The first is open to conjecture in the absence of any written documentation by him. Of course, we have the number as given to Michaux, presumably by Dr. Brown, and we have no reason to doubt that Michaux is a reliable witness. As earlier stated, the populace at large did not customarily partake of inoculation until the disease had reached epidemic proportions. Although Brown was a man of remarkable persuasive skills, the author questions the likelihood of townspeople rushing to line up for vaccination in this relatively short time span without cause. In all probability, the threat of a smallpox epidemic in Lexington in 1802 created rapid converts to vaccination.

Passage of the Cowpox "Thread"

Although we know the date and source of the vaccination material supplied to Brown after June 1801, the identity of the person from whom cowpox matter was taken for the vaccinations of the two young men reported in the *Kentucky Gazette* of May 25, 1801, remains unknown. However, it is altogether possible that the cowpox matter was taken from the teats of a local cow and before Brown's access to the "thread." The June 1, 1801 edition of the *Kentucky Gazette* prints two letters drafted in May 1801, one from Basil Duke in Washington, DC, and the other from George Graham of Dumfries, Virginia, relating to the "thread infected with cowpox matter."

> Letter from Dr. Duke to Dr. Brown:
> Washington, May 19,1801
>
> I forward you by Mr. Bodley some matter which has lately been taken from the arm of a patient inoculated with the cowpox. I intend to inoculate some persons here immediately and will acquaint you with the results and shall be glad to hear as soon as you have made sufficient trial.
>
> I am Dear Sir Yours, &c B. Duke[188]

A second letter to Dr. Brown from George Graham of Dumfries, Virginia, of May 22, 1801, traces the passage of the "thread" through Dr. Waterhouse of Boston to Dr. Brown.

> Dear Sir:
>
> Mr. Tebbs takes out with him some thread infected with the vaccine matter, part of which is for you. This matter was obtained by Dr. Spencer of this place through the means of Doctor Post of New York, from Dr. Waterhouse of Boston,[189] and so far no experiments have been made here. We have no doubt that the matter is genuine, and that it produces the real disorder, as described by Dr. Jenner, but as we have had no opportunity of inoculating for the smallpox the experiment has not been made complete-but Doctor Hartford of Norfolk obtained some matter from this place and has inoculated very extensively; he is now preparing

inoculating with the variolous matter and as soon as we hear the result you shall be informed of it. The sooner you inoculate after receiving the thread the better-the heat and the length of time are apt to destroy its powers.

With very great respects, and esteem
I remain, Dear Sir, Yours &c
George Graham

Dumfries, May 2^{d}, 1801
Doct Samuel Brown
Lexington, Kentucky

That vaccination had been a marked success in Lexington is borne out by a letter from Dr. Brown to Mr. John Vaughn.

June 10, 1802.[190]

It will give you satisfaction to hear that the Jennerian inoculation has gone on here, [Lexington] with astonishing rapidity. Many thousands have passed through that disease. People of all descriptions communicate the infection and although it is to be apprehended that some spurious cases may have occurred, under the management of such untutored practitioners, yet it is believed that the genuine disease is pretty generally known and diffused. Not less than one hundred and fifty thousand of our inhabitants [Americans] have never had the smallpox. What obligations do we owe to Dr. Jenner for the discovery of so safe and easy a mode of escaping the ravages of that horrid distemper.

Although Brown, as did Waterhouse, Hosack, and others, showed the safety and effectiveness of the vaccination for smallpox, there continued to be pockets of resistance to vaccination throughout America in the nineteenth century. Dr. James Fishback, in an open letter to the editor of the *Kentucky Gazette* of February 12, 1805, made this dire comment: ".... it was much to be lamented that the mild disease of cowpox had not been encouraged in this state; as no doubt could remain that it would effectively prevent smallpox which had raged with violence on Licking and in lower parts of the state."

The "Pox" Returns

Smallpox recurred in Lexington in May and June 1837 and in October 1849. In 1837, the disease began in Louisville and was transmitted to a visitor from Lexington (brother to brother), after which several members of the Lexington family were likewise infected. An infant child, who had slept with the affected father until the time of eruptions, was vaccinated and, together with the other children who had previously been vaccinated, escaped the variola. Even though the household harboring smallpox was isolated, a family in the country that had been visited by the infected Lexingtonians also fell prey to the pox. Fourteen persons in this family were infected, "Three of them had, I suppose, five thousand pocks each."[191] The attending physician relates that two colleagues visited the latter family with him and agreed with his conclusion, "That in many instance, practitioners of medicine have done too much in the management of this disease; and that the better method is to watch and assist the efforts of nature, instead of burthening the patient with medicines."[192]

Thirty cases of smallpox were reported to be in the Lexington City Hospital in 1849, and an undetermined number of victims were lodged in their homes.[193] These cases were reported in the *Transylvania Medical Journal* because fourteen patients, all of whom had been previously vaccinated, sometimes repeatedly, developed moderate to clearly defined smallpox. One of the fourteen patients died. The author, Dr. J. M. Bruce, was not questioning the protective value of the vaccine when properly instituted but believed that not enough attention was given to the "acquisition, propagation and preservation of pure vaccine." He was unable to determine why there were so many exceptions, and why the disease should have become epidemic; however, suspicions were aroused by the possibility of contamination of the pure vaccine lymph from Cincinnati: "The greater portion of the lymph used in Lexington was procured from Cincinnati where small pox had been prevailing to a very great extent, and it becomes a question of grave interest to the profession and to society, whether we may not have imported the disease instead of the remedy, the poison in place of the antidote."[194]

The Cholera Years

Cholera was not the most common cause of death in the Pre-Revolutionary and early Post-Revolutionary period in America, but when it came, it did so with such a vengeance that it not only took lives but also changed even the socioeconomic well-being of many citizens, together with the cities and communities in which they lived.[195] Although a sporadic number of cholera cases occurred in 1817 and 1832, Lexingtonians, for the most part, felt rather smug in their "Athens of the West." And why not? Lexington was widely known for its salutary climate, the nearby healthful springs, the absence of severe epidemics, a plentiful supply of doctors, and the celebrated Medical Faculty of Transylvania University. And even if cholera came, they took heart in knowing that cholera victims were almost always limited to the poor, the filthy, the ignorant, and the sinful. Morality was believed to play an awesome role in those afflicted by disease. "It was fondly believed that this beautiful city would escape [cholera] entirely, on account of its elevated situation, freedom from large collections of water, and general salubrity."[196 197] And further, they believed that the hand of the Lord, even if not directly culling his cholera victims, nevertheless offered no haven for those guilty of transgressions. Unquestionably, the poor, the filthy, the drunks, the blacks, and the freshly immigrated Irish were the most gifted intemperates; they had little else of the world's goods.

For the unsuspecting citizens of Lexington an unbelievable new judgment was at hand. An article in the *Lexington Observer and Kentucky Reporter* of July 12, 1832, warned the citizens that cholera was apt to strike "every portion of the United States" and urged that they take immediate steps to protect themselves. The reader was referred to a recent and excellent report on cholera by Dr. Lunsford P. Yandell (1805-78) of Transylvania University. Other journalistic precautions included keeping the streets clean and dry and the houses white-washed. Exposure to the sun in the middle of the day should be avoided, and measures to prevent chilliness were especially urged, such as avoiding the night air and cold bathing if in a sweat. "Every species of ardent spirit" was viewed as poisonous. Water, coffee, and milk were encouraged, but acidic drinks were to be shunned. Easily digested foods were recommended: good beef, lamb, good white bread, peas and beans, "potatoes, if they are good." All fresh vegetables should be well cooked. Crowds and every species of excess should be avoided. If any symptom of diarrhea, "stomach" pain, or nausea should develop, "lose no time in sending for your doctor." And finally, the reporter entreated his readers to "preserve that tranquillity of mind that springs from confidence in Him who has the life of all beings in His hand."

A second newspaper entry on November 15, 1832, conveys a little more anxiety but falls short of alarming the public.[198] The deaths of three blacks and two whites were reported. The author of the article continues: "The disease, as it exists here, is, we believe, much milder in its attacks than it has been in other parts of the United States. It does not extend itself much, and has created but very little alarm or excitement among our citizens. The probability is that it soon will disappear altogether." A few more specifics were given by the writer to prevent or offset the pestilence. For the treatment of any watery and frequent intestinal discharge or uneasiness in the stomach, however mild, the afflicted should immediately take liberal doses of *Calomel*.[199] The limbs should be kept warm by the use of mustards, cayenne pepper, horse radish or any other article that might hasten the effect. For more urgent consideration, vomiting might be induced by taking "ten spoonfuls of *Ipecac*, frequently repeated, in large draughts of warm water or with liberal portions of warm salt water."

As the months passed, there was an increasing uneasiness in Lexington. Travelers and nearby families told of outbreaks of cholera in near and distant towns and on the rivers. Even so, Lexingtonians continued to cling to their belief that "it can't happen here." "Early in the year [1833], rumors of cases occurring on board the steamboats, both of the Mississippi and Ohio, reached our ears; and presently cases were reported in the towns between this and the Ohio River; of these, Paris and Millersburg suffered most severely; and about the commencement in June the work of death began in Lexington."[200] By June 5, 1833, there was no longer any question of the virulence and of the indiscriminate nature of cholera. Newspaper columns were now occupied by a list of the dead, and the numbers reported were usually far behind and far short of the actual fatalities. "In the short space of nine days, fifteen hundred persons were prostrated, and dying at the rate of fifty a day."[201]

Cholera was indiscriminate: all classes and all colors fell before it. People lay dying, and there was no one to comfort them. People lay dead in their beds, and there was no one to lift them. People lay dead in the streets, and there was no one to bury them. "The grave-yards were choked. Coffins were laid down at the gates by the score, in confused heaps; and among them, horrible to relate! corpses wrapped up only in the bed-clothes in which they had but an hour or two before expired. There they lay, each waiting their turn to be deposited in the long trenches...."[202] The high and the low were buried side by side, if at all. Religious rites were ignored. Wives, husbands, and children did what they could for one another, but often they were too sick and too weak to call for help. Many who were not ill stayed indoors, fearful that they might be the next cholera victims. The reassurance from certain members of the Transylvania Medical Faculty that cholera was not infectious fell on deaf ears. As Dr. C. W. Short, Dean of the Transylvania Medical Faculty, recalls, "And as to give the lie to the slanderous reports of its being confined in its visitations to unhealthy places; and of its selecting its victims from the poor, the profligate and the intemperate,- reports by which many, we have reason to believe, were lulled into a fatal security,- the pestilence continued longer; destroyed a larger number of sober, useful, and wealthy citizens;- and was perhaps more mortal in proportion to the population here, than in any other town or city of the union."[203] Clerics did their duty, day and night, but there were too few for too many.

Although the people of Frankfort felt the wrath of the cholera, the catastrophe existing in Lexington was such as to draw the sympathy of the publisher of the *Frankfort Commonwealth*, Orlando Brown: "But *yesterday* that City [Lexington] was the Eden of the western world—*there*, there was an union of all the comforts of life—of all its elegancies—a people hospitable in their homes, accomplished in their manners. That spot seemed, of all others in this favored land, more exempt from the visitations of disease and those sad occurrences which interrupt the enjoyment of life. *Look at her to-day*? Gloom, and sorrow, and mourning in every habitation—instead of being at Goshen, with lights in each dwelling, the sound of gladness is unheard, for the voice of grief has penetrated every abode."[204] And so, with both the streets and the dead deserted, what of the living? As reported in Philadelphia's *Niles Weekly Register*, those who had the means to do so fled to the countryside:

> We have never witnessed such anxiety, such alarm, such a panic....The proudest hearts seemed to quail before the relentless destroyer, that was striking among us unseen, giving scarcely an intimation to the persons whom it had selected for its victims, before prostrating them upon a dying bed. No one pretended to claim an immunity from its grasp, and no one knew what moment he, or some of his family, would be one of its victims. All seemed to be seized with an awful dread. We heard an old veteran say he had been in many a hard fought battle; he had heard the sound of cannon and musket balls passing through the air; he had seen the dead and dying strewed around him, and heard the groans and shrieks of the wounded; but never had he felt such an awful dread of impending danger, he felt during the four days ending yesterday...there are but few left in this place to have it [cholera], nearly all that could go to the country have been gone some days; many of whom have died. There are not enough well persons left to take care of the convalescent and inter the dead. I have been told that there were twelve or fourteen uninterred at one time this morning, at one of the graveyards. It is useless for any one to attempt to guess how many have fallen. Three hundred would probably be a reasonable computation. On yesterday and today it has been impossible to get coffins or rough boxes made sufficiently soon to put them away.[205]

That the physicians of Lexington stayed the course (in no instance was a single physician of Lexington accused of fleeing the city), took the risk alongside their patients, and in some instances gave their lives, is testimony to their courage and reflects honor on the medical family.[206] It is , however, as tragic as it is ironic that, as Rosenberg concludes, "The lesson of cholera was clear enough; those physicians who had not fled had merely hurried the passage of their patients from this world."[207]

Various accounts confirm that almost all of the physicians in Lexington came down with the cholera. Drs. Dudley, Bush and James Miller reportedly remained exempt, even though they were as intensely involved with the care of the sick as were other physicians.[208] Professor Dudley, nationally known for his mastery of surgery, was also well versed in the medical maladies, especially cholera.[209] He prepared a letter (June 22, 1833) published in the Philadelphia *National Gazette and Literary Register* on July 4, 1833, "...to answer the many inquiries of his professional correspondents." Speaking of the prevailing epidemic, he asserts: "The opinions of medical men upon this, as upon most other professional subjects, are not found to correspond." With respect to specific treatment, he recommends emetics: "But above all, I conceive them valuable, as possessing the faculty of arousing the stomach to the lively and active impression of calomel; a cathartic superior to all others, for the purpose of exciting bilious secretion, and of securing thick or consistent evacuations from the bowel." For patients experiencing collapse, he dashed buckets of cold water upon the patient's entire surface, without the "pleasing results...urged by the advocates of that practice." He rebuked the use of the lancet (bleeding) and favored cataplasms of mustard and pepper to the stomach, bowels, and limbs.[210]

The *Niles Weekly Register* of June 22, 1833 printed a letter from Lexington: "I do assure you we have seen and heard enough since I wrote you, two days since, to strike terror to the strongest nerve; even the physicians wore such awful countenances, that it was enough to confound and terrify the weak and the timid. Nearly all the physicians are completely prostrate, and many of them now in bed; surely there never has been such mortality in any place of the same number of inhabitants....There are not enough well persons left to take care of the convalescent and inter the dead....On yesterday and to-day, it has been impossible to get coffins or rough boxes made sufficiently soon to put them away."[211] Indeed, three physicians and three Transylvania medical students gave not only their time and their energy but also their lives to the people of Lexington: **Dr. Joseph Boswell; Dr. Joseph Challen; Dr. John Steele.** The three medical students, **Alexander McChord**, from Alabama, died June 12, 1833; **Milton W. Thurmond**, of South Carolina, died June 26, 1833; and **Alexander W. Dillon**, of Paris, Kentucky died June 30, 1833.[212]

In the long history of the human race, there are times when the actions of one man or one woman are so inscrutable, so at odds with all their past, that the feat is not only improbable but also inexplicable. Such an instance took place in Lexington in 1833 at the height of the cholera epidemic. The man involved was William Solomon, the town drunk. To be known at that time as the town drunk of Lexington was no small feat, for Solomon had numerous competitors. Solomon drifted to Lexington from Virginia in the late 1790s, and his low character was, in part, a reflection of the level of his workplace: the cellar and the graves. For nigh on forty years the people of Lexington had become familiar with this vagrant, never expecting him to rise above his rank and knowing full well he could sink no further. These years of indolence earned for Solomon the derisive title of "King." The "King" was a white man, when and if scrubbed, but he was judged to be lower than life, even lower than the slaves. Indeed, in June 1833, just before the outbreak of the cholera, "...his labor as an indentured servant for a twelve month period was sold at public auction." Aunt Charlotte, a black and an acquaintance of Solomon's during his boyhood days in Virginia, outbid two Transylvania students for his services.[213] Once the cholera began its deadly beat, Aunt Charlotte begged Solomon to leave town. He refused. Why? Solomon, like the other residents of Lexington, could see and could smell the corpses, piled up in makeshift coffins or less, left at the door or on the street or tossed in carts, all destined for the cemetery, for bur-

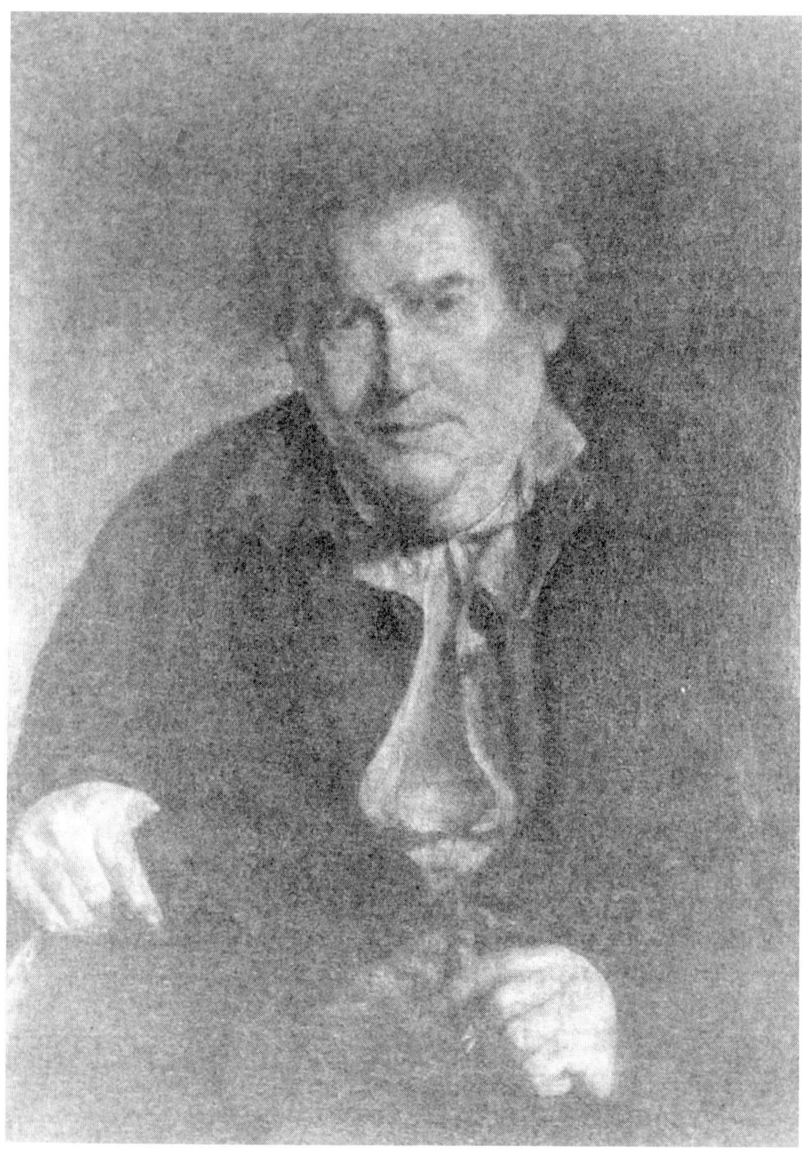

William "King" Solomon(1775-1854)

Courtesy of Special Collections and Archives Service Center, University of Kentucky Libraries ial without ceremony. It was at this moment that the "King" *ascended*, for he took on the task of grave digging without reservation and with little help. Why did he do so? One could speculate that Solomon, who had been in Lexington for almost forty years, knew many of the dead, and that perhaps some of those lying in the street had at some time befriended him by giving him a cigar or a slug of whiskey. But many other Lexingtonians knew the dead and yet had fled the city. I doubt that Solomon thought his act through and believed that he had a duty to perform. Had he given much thought to the situation he probably would have fled with the others. Solomon, without reflecting, and for perhaps the first time in his life, saw himself in better circumstances than all those about him, the sick and the dead. He, Solomon, now was the provider, the caretaker, the master of his world; it was he who could give when others could not or would not do so; it was the dead who gave him life. *Some would say that it was a miracle that he escaped the clutches of cholera, but the miracle was not that he escaped cholera, but that for one crowning moment he escaped himself.*

And so, this tragedy unfolded. Cholera took its toll. So, too, did pride. The proud people of Lexington had been reduced in number and in esteem by an invisible and remorseless foe. What once had seemed to be invincible, now smoldered in ruins. Dr. C.W. Short, Dean of the Transylvania Medical Department, assessed the situation: "...here in Lexington-the boasted seat of medical science, and heretofore so noted for its healthiness, that some of our physicians vainly affirmed that cholera could not come here- on one visitation were six hundred of our people swept off; being more than a decimation of its inhabitants."[214]

Why had this plague chosen the promising and gallant people of Lexington on whom to unload its fury? Lexingtonians had weathered the savagery of Indians, but Fortress Lexington was not equipped to repel the veiled violence of cholera. The promise of tomorrow lay buried. "At length it [cholera] has ceased and its departure is certain. Years will roll away before the memory of this visitation is forgotten....The cholera brought with it more terror than hords of savages, for it came on the 'viewless couriers of the air,' and bade defiance to human strength. *Why was it so fatal in Lexington*? There is truth in the answer, that the citizens did not believe that the cholera could come there."[215]

John S. Chambers tersely describes the change: "Lexington, formerly the 'Athens of the West' but now the less pretentious 'Heart of the Bluegrass…'"[216] An announcement by the Medical Department of Transylvania University, appeared in the *Kentucky Gazette* of August 14, 1833:

> The lectures in this institution will reconvene, as usual, on the first Monday of November, and terminate on the first Saturday in March....During the entire term, the Professor of Surgery lectures nine times each week, and the other professors daily, Sabbaths excluded;-The fee to the entire course, with matriculation and the use of the library, amount to $116.-The graduation fee is $20.
>
> The cholera having left it, Lexington now enjoys its ordinary health.

Chambers states that "poverty and want made their first appearance in the city as a result of its visitation [cholera]."[217] He further notes that the beginning of the present school system at that time resulted from the need to establish a free school in the city. The Lexington City Directory of 1838-39 documents the establishment of an orphan asylum in the aftermath of death.

> In the summer of 1833, the benevolent citizens of Lexington got up a meeting for the purpose of raising funds sufficient to establish an Asylum for the destitute and friendless Orphans (deprived of both parents) who were deprived of their parents by the Cholera, with which the City had just been severely visited. Between 4, and 5000 dollars were raised;

> a house and lot was purchased which cost $3000. The remaining funds were then placed in the hands of twenty four Ladies, who furnished the house, procured a Matron and Assistant, and received such children as they found destitute.[218]

Cholera-The Next Wave

By the latter part of the 1840s, Lexington had once again *regained its composure if not its pre-eminence. According to the Lexington Observer and Reporter,*[219] "fall business" was highly prosperous and the stores were crowded, not only by Lexingtonians but also by people from a distance. During the forties, capital had flowed into the city, and "business had increased in a very great ratio." The writer indicates that many buyers who had been accustomed to trading in Cincinnati and Louisville now found that in Lexington "...purchasers of all kinds can be accommodated with every thing they want" and as advantageously as anywhere in the West. In the same issue and speaking of Transylvania University, the writer asserts "There is now a much larger number of students attending preparatory courses of lectures in the Medical Department than have ever been at this time. And a larger class is expected to assemble this winter than has for several years sought instruction from the able faculty of the School....On the whole the prospects for Old Transylvania were never brighter." An occasional minor entry in the *Observer & Reporter* in 1848 spoke of multiple outbreaks of Cholera in Europe, but these did not raise any special concern for the people of Lexington.

On December 13, 1848, the *Observer & Reporter* copied an item from the New York correspondent of the *Philadelphia Ledger:* "The Cholera is here." He took to task the New York newspapers for discrediting the report. The cholera was brought over by a packet from France. Seven passengers had died of cholera en route, and many others were in the ship's hospital. At the end of the report, a telegraphic dispatch from New York stated that three deaths from cholera had occurred at Staten Island Hospital.[220] On December 20, 1848, a newspaper account referred to a letter from New Orleans detailing the deaths of 160 passengers of cholera on passage from Bremen (Germany) to New Orleans. From March through August 1849, news articles listing cases and deaths caused by cholera from Nashville, Louisville, Cincinnati, and Maysville became more common in the Lexington newspapers.

On May 23, 1849, the *Lexington Observer & Reporter* headlined a column, "THE CHOLERA." The cholera had struck Lexington, or had it? The first reported cases of cholera were from the Lunatic Asylum, "in the suburbs of the city." Fifteen inmates of the asylum had been stricken with cholera, and four of them were men, but the article offered no explanation for this sexual discrepancy other than that it is "singular." The writer is far less hesitant in expressing his belief that cholera "...may be truly said not to prevail at all in our city," a conclusion he reaches because "...The disease has confined its attacks exclusively to the unfortunate inmates......not a single case being reported in the city outside the walls of the hospital [Lunatic Asylum]." Even though the journalist recognized that the disease was active only in a public institution in the "suburbs," he cautioned his readers to take preventive measures. The writer's interpretation of the boundary lines between suburb and city may have comforted the citizens, but it failed to impress the cholera. Even so, for a time the disease remained content to reside at the Lunatic Asylum. A further report on Wednesday, June 8, 1849, a self-congratulatory exercise, states that upon the authority of the Board of Health and of "our most respected physicians.... the health of the city continues remarkably good." The writer once again emphasizes the necessity of prevention, "strict attention to diet, clothing and cleanliness..." He goes on to assure the many friends abroad that Lexington "never enjoyed more perfect exemption from disease of every description and that they cannot visit any city in the West with a certainty of being more entirely free from all liability to disease."

Lexington residents became a bit more humble on June 13,

1849, when the *Lexington Observer & Reporter*, under the headline "HEALTH OF OUR CITY" acknowledged the presence of cholera in the city; however, "the subject of the disease was a laboring, debilitated man...."[221] Once again the writer sought to reassure the public that "they [cases of cholera] were not in the slightest degree calculated to create alarm." The number of cholera deaths swelled to thirty-eight within two weeks (seventeen whites and twenty-one blacks). Deaths from the Lunatic Asylum, about sixty, were listed separately. During the course of the cholera, in particular the onslaught at the Lunatic Asylum, Dr. John R. Allen, superintendent, frequently reported to the newspaper the prevailing conditions of the inmates and staff. A comment by Dr. Allen on June 2, 1849, is most telling of the medical intellect of the day with respect to the concept of cholera in particular and disease in general:

> On Thursday [May 31] the cannon was used and as you perceive the abatement continued. I can form no opinion as to the influence of the concussion, etc., but think it is not unreasonable to suppose, that good may have resulted. I may state that we now have cases apparently relieved, of a character, which have heretofore proved altogether intractable.[222]

According to Dr. Allen, the firing of cannons strategically placed on the Asylum grounds resulted in "a sharp decline in the number of cases and deaths."[223] What had the firing of cannon to do with the decline in deaths? Nothing, for as previously noted the number of deaths at the Asylum in the latter part of June was sixty, and most of these occurred after the firing of the cannon. The use of the cannon testifies to the unflinching belief in the spread of disease by the miasma (poisoned atmospheric vapors), and that the air could be purified by the smoke escaping from the cannon fire. In 1793, Philadelphians had used a similar plan of action, including guns and cannon, to relieve the agony of the Yellow Fever, in the belief that the resulting heavy smoke would destroy the plague.[224] So many people were wounded by the gunfire that the mayor had to forbid it. The only relief obtained from either event was its ending.

The Ancient Greeks knew that the plague invariably attacked near and distant localities at the same time. What was the one common factor? The ambient air, of course; the cause was in the air. Did not everyone know that the change of seasons brought with it its own array of disease, the dysentery in summer, the fevers in autumn, the flu and pleurisy in winter?[225] Even more proof lay in the atmospheric properties of hotness, dryness, cold, and moisture, the same elementary and universal properties basic to the universe. Each of these properties accommodated one of the four basic humors; fire (yellow bile), earth (black bile), water (phlegm), and air (blood). As long as these four humors were in harmony, health flourished, but if one or more of them gained favor, the resulting imbalance led to disease. At the beginning of the nineteenth century, this ancient humoral theory still held sway in Lexington, as it did throughout most of the world.[226]

By the latter part of June and the first week of July 1849 the number of deaths per day ranged from six to fourteen. The faith of the people was now severely shaken, and, as one observer noted, "Our town [Lexington] looks deserted, scarcely any one from the country in. Quite a number affected-nearly every one has symptoms. It is supposed that 1500 white persons have left town."[227] By the time the scourge ended its rampage, 283 Lexingtonians had died from the cholera and 58 (other accounts list sixty) at the Asylum, for a total of 341 dead.[228]

Among the dead were three physicians, **Drs. James Jones, Lemuel Sanders, and W. W. Whitney.** The first two physicians were victims of cholera; Dr. Whitney died of an intestinal illness, "not cholera." The death of Dr. Whitney was reported by the *Lexington Observer & Reporter* on Saturday, July 7, 1849: "It is our painful duty this morning to announce the death of this amiable, accomplished and excellent man....He had been very unwell some three or four weeks ago....upon the breaking out of the epidemic, he entered at once upon a most extensive practice, and for two or three weeks enjoyed scarcely any repose from the arduous duties of his profession. About a week since he was compelled by recurring illness to take his room, but not satisfied to remain there when the cries of his friends were heard all around him for medical aid, he continued, at intervals of each day since, to his practice, when he no doubt needed the ministering hand of a physician as much as any one of his patients....He fell a noble martyr to his profession."

Bloody Flux

Dysentery, or the "bloody flux" as our forefathers called it, denotes a complex of symptoms including frequent passage of blood, pus, and mucus in the stools, abdominal pain, and straining. Known from the time of Hippocrates, dysentery was responsible for many of the ancient plagues.[229] In 1669, Thomas Sydenham (1624-89), the "English Hippocrates," provided a classic description of dysentery:[230]

> I observe this disease come in for the most part about the beginning of Autumns. It is sometimes accompanied with a feaver and sometimes without but always with great torment in the bowells upon goeing to stoole with frequent dejections and those for the most part not stercoros but mucous with which are mixt streaks of blood in the beginning, but in the farther progresse of the disease bloud in larger quantitys and unmixed often is evacuated....Upon the continuance of this disease, the intestines seeme to be affected successively downward until the whole mischeife be terminated upon the rectum....It is for the most part mortall to old persons, lesse fatall though very dangerous to youth

> but benigne enough to infants, who if let alone and not tamperd with may have it for some months without prejudice to their lives.

Dysentery, an illness most apt to occur in summer, and one most familiar to Southern physicians, can be transmitted from one person to another. It may occur in two forms, *endemic,* i.e., always present, or *epidemic,* i.e., occurring in intervals with appalling cruelty. Of the 1758 preserved theses of Transylvania medical graduates during the years from 1820 to 1859, fifty-five were on the topic of dysentery. Lunsford P. Yandell, editor of *The Transylvania Journal of Medicine and the Associate Sciences,* published an essay on dysentery in the *Journal* in 1836, reporting nine cases (case narratives) under his care. Yandell presents the cases of slaves, whites, children, and adults at length while always maintaining the physician's discipline, the distance between his heart and his mind. Excerpts from three cases have been selected:

> Case 7. The case next to be reported occurred this summer. W.Y . a boy age 6 years, of robust frame, subject to attacks of bowel complaint and fever since he suffered with cholera infantum, from which he was recovered slowly and with great difficulty, was taken with diarrhea and slight fever on the evening of the 9th of June. Next morning, his fever increasing and his bowels continuing to be disordered, he took 6 grains of calomel. When it operated, he rose from bed and was dressed, and that evening appeared well. During the night his bowels were repeatedly moved-passages not seen, but one observed next morning was bilious.
>
> [June] 11th. Up and dressed early-fever gone-surface pale-blood discovered in his stools, with mucus. Cal. 5 grs. and ip.1 gr. at once given-

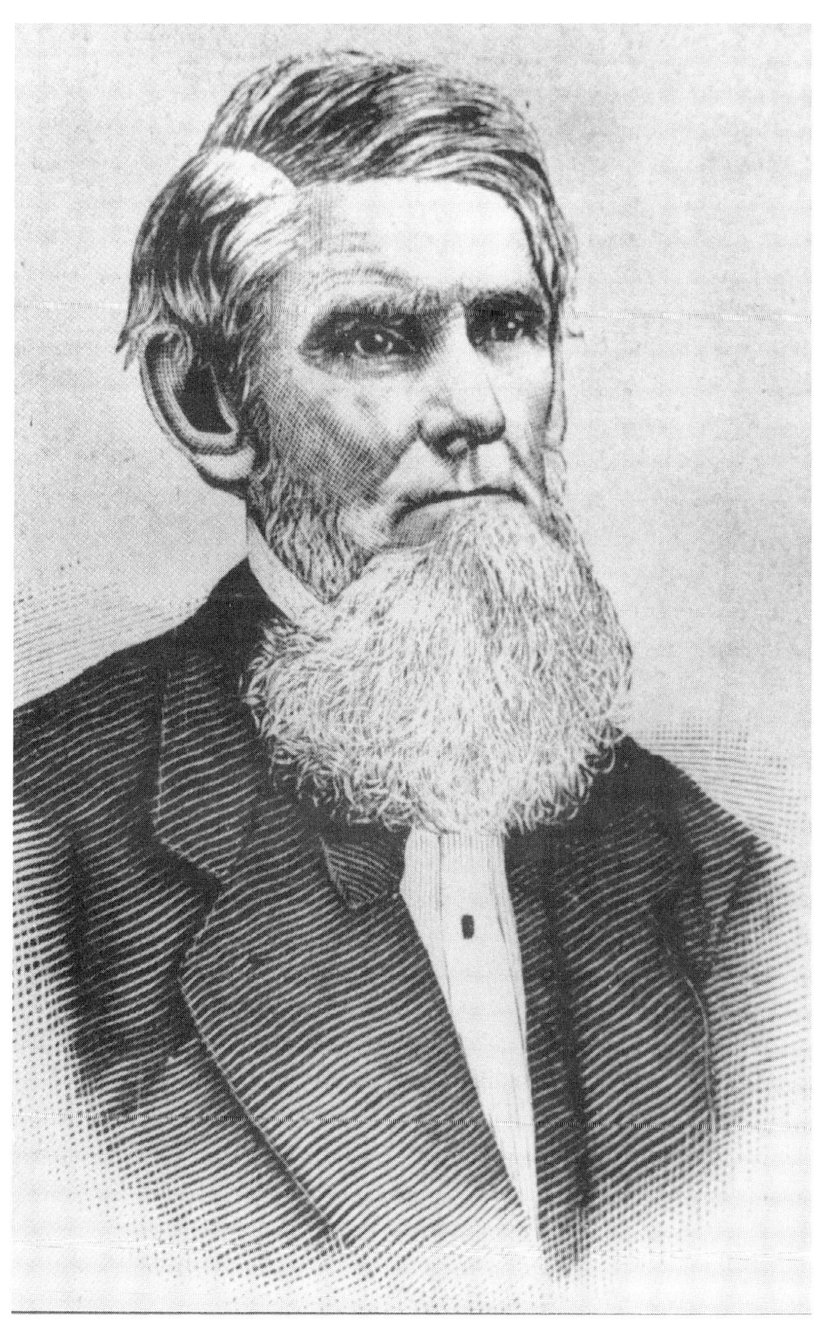

Lunsford P. Yandell, M.D. (1805-1878)
Courtesy of Transylvania University Library

> vomits him. Repeated at intervals of two hours through the day, in smaller doses. Frequency and character of discharges not affected by the remedies.
>
> [June] 12th. A bad night-bowels disturbed every hour, with tormina—appearance of exhaustion this morning—extremities cold and clammy. A bilious passage at 8 o'clock, but blood and mucus soon followed. Anodyne enema given, but cannot be retained. Flannels dipped in hot spirits, applied to extremities and abdomen, cal. And ip. continued through the day with the addition of 1 gr. opi. to each portion. Bile appears occasionally in stools. Thirst moderate, and drinks toast and slippery elm water, but asks for ice. In the evening, evacuations resemble the washings of raw beef. Tenesmus never very great-no tenderness of abdomen. Hands and feet cannot be kept warm. Great tossing-8 o'clock, P.M. took 10 grs. cal. Restlessness increasing. At 12, becomes delirious. At half past 8 in the morning, dead.[231]

Following this case report, Yandell made several observations: "This was an extraordinary case. The patient died in eight-and -forty hours after the first dysenteric symptoms appeared.…It is quite remarkable that these symptoms should have come on *while he was under the operation of calomel,* and that the discharge of green bile afforded no relief.…The appearance of the patient, thirty-six hours after his attack, was that of a person about failing into the collapse of cholera, which disease, in many of its symptoms, and especially the fearful rapidity of its progress, this case resembled more than dysentery." Case 8, on the 29 year old mother of the little boy, is narrated at considerable length, and followed for a period of twelve days, the last day being the 26th (June).

"Convalescent. Takes rhubarb and mag. calc. once daily. No untoward symptom presented from this time, and her recovery was rapid." Case 9, the last reported by Yandell, was a 19 year old girl "in the same family," whose illness lasted six days and with an "uninterrupted convalescence."[232]

Yandell closes the case report with certain observations and conclusions: "In these cases [Cases 8 & 9] the most manifest advantage was derived from the Epsom salts and the effervescing draught....In the second [case 9], the calomel and tepid drinks were persevered in longer, but, while free bilious evacuations were induced, the patient was not relieved....I should say, that these cases were cured by the saline purgatives and refrigerating drinks. Calomel, so far as could be judged by the medical attendants, was nugatory....How far a similar change in the treatment of the little boy [case 6] might have affected the issue of his case, cannot now be determined; but it is impossible to repress a feeling of regret that the experiment was not made." Regrettable indeed, for *the little boy (case 6) was his son Willie; case 8, his wife Susan; and case 9, a young female friend of the family.*[233]

The City Hospital and the Work House

A description of the City Hospital appears in the 1838 and 1839 publications of the *Directory of Lexington and County of Fayette:*[234]

> *"The City Hospital and Work House"* is a plain Block Building of 2 stories. It was erected in 1836. The object of the Institution is to provide an asylum for the poor and sick; and also for the confinement of persons, sentenced to hard labor, for drunkenness, rioting, vagrancy, et. cetera. The number confined in the Hospital since its creation, is 64, of whom 63 were white, and 1 black. The room appropriated to

> the Hospital is spacious and well aired, measuring 100 by 18 feet, and having 17 windows. It is a wing detached from the main building, and Work House. In the latter Institution, pauper children are furnished with board, raiment and education, and when properly qualified, are apprenticed to trades. The discipline reflects much credit on Mr. Jas. Peel. The building was erected and supported by the City.

Although hospitals in the Americas can be traced to those constructed by the Spanish Conquistadors during the sixteenth century, the famed Pennsylvania Hospital in Philadelphia (1751), conceived by Dr. Thomas Bond and aided principally by Benjamin Franklin, was the first general hospital to open its door in the British colonies. The New York Hospital first opened in 1773, then burned and reopened in 1791; however, similar institutions were slow to develop in the new nation, primarily because there were "few cities and large towns."[235] The fact that Lexingtonians saw fit to erect a city hospital and workhouse in 1836 testifies to their belief in themselves and in their city, the Metropolis of the West, as a medical center *par excellence.* American hospitals during the early nineteenth century were altogether different institutions than are our hospitals today. The early hospitals were for *care* of the sick poor, the aged, the handicapped, and the victims of contagious disease, and they sometimes housed sick strangers. Patients were there to be housed and fed, at times isolated, and to some degree comforted. Self-reliant patients were customarily treated in their homes, and so it remained until the latter part of the nineteenth century. With the discovery of anesthesia by Crawford Long (1842) and William Morton (1846), the development of modern nursing by Florence Nightingale (1854-56), the discoveries of Louis Pasteur (1860-85) and Robert Koch (1880-90) leading to the development of the science of bacteriology, the advent of antiseptic surgery by Joseph Lister (1867), and the introduction of aseptic surgery by Ernst Von Bergman (1891), the emphasis shifted from care to therapy and to cure: the hospitals were no longer solely the domain of the poor and deranged.[236]

Eastern State Hospital

Another group of patients, the mentally ill, were in dire need of being saved from the public, and the public, from the deranged. Being the responsibility of the family, such unfortunate individuals, in ancient times, were customarily kept at home. During the Medieval period, Christian concern for the sick and poor did not embrace the mentally ill, for the latter, it was believed, were "possessed by devils," and insanity was a sin. The Moslems had a much more lenient, even enlightened view of the mentally ill, treating them compassionately and as the responsibility of society some several hundred years before the West did so. Likewise, the first institutions built solely for the care of the mentally ill were built in Moslem lands. Conversely, in Europe, the mentally deranged were expelled from the cities, or "shipped to sea, locked up in jails or madhouses, and treated with contempt or worse.[237] By the sixteenth and seventeenth centuries, Europeans transferred the obligation of caring for the poor and the "deranged" to society, with the directors of facilities holding absolute power, the key to the lock. This break in tradition was not for the benefit of the insane but to permit a more orderly society to divorce itself from the afflicted. Not until the action of the French psychiatrist Philippe Pinel (1755 1826) at the Paris hospital for the insane, Bicetre, in 1792, when he set inmates free of their chains and free of their tormentors, did society begin to seriously consider the plight of the insane and their humanity.[238] In the early to mid-nineteenth century, Americans likewise shifted their method of care for the mentally ill to a more humane and scientific endeavor; they too placed the burden on society and placed the mentally ill in institutions.

For the citizens of Lexington, from the birth of the city and through the first two decades of the 19th century, the only institution available for suitable care of the insane was the Lunatic Asylum at Williamsburg, Virginia, founded in 1773. The risk and burden of transporting an insane person from Lexington, day after day, through the wilderness and keeping him safe from Indians, therefore, meant that the asylum in Williamsburg was rarely used by Kentuckians.

On May 8, 1818, an advertisement for a *Lottery for the Benefit of the Fayette Hospital* appeared in the *Kentucky Gazette.* Following the particulars of tickets and prizes, the managers appealed to the sensibilities of the public: "Every benevolent heart, whose sensibilities are alive to the sufferings of the poor, the sick and the infirm, and to the most efficient means of affording them permanent comfort and relief, will cordially unite with the managers in the promotion of the speedy success of this lottery." Evidently, the managers had considerable faith in their fellow citizens, for the building of the hospital was in progress at the time of the lottery announcement. The "Panic of 1819," however, made it impossible to complete the hospital, and the state eventually took over the building and converted it into a lunatic asylum.

The origin of the Lunatic Asylum in Lexington is described (October 1869) by its second medical director, W. S. Chipley, M.D.[239]

> This Institution owes its origin to private benevolent enterprises. The center building of the present development for males was commenced on 1817, under the name of "The Fayette Hospital." The building committee consisted of Stephen Chipley, Thomas January, Andrew McCalla and Sterling Allen.
>
> About the same time this building was roofed in, there burst upon the country one of

> those terrible financial storms which prostrate the most substantial, uproot all confidence, and utterly defeat the best natural plans of the most discreet and prudent. The building committee, unfortunately for themselves, had assumed heavy liabilities in anticipation of means which, it was confidently believed, would be promptly contributed by their associates. The members of the committee were, at that time, men of property; but this could avail little in the payment of a large cash debt, when the city lost, in a brief space of time, nearly half of its population, and the value of real estate became merely nominal. I know of houses that will now rent for from $500 to $700 a year that were then unoccupied, the windows and doors broken down; the building failing at that time, to yield a sufficient amount to keep them in repair.
>
> The liabilities alluded to continued to press upon the committee until 1822, when they tendered the property to the State, to be converted into a Lunatic Asylum, expecting no more than an extinguishment of outstanding debts. In 1823 the General Assembly appointed commissioners, and made an appropriation to provide a hospital for the insane.

The asylum was built within a mile of Transylvania University, a distance close enough to permit members of the medical faculty to treat physical ailments of the inmates in a timely fashion. For the most part, only the dangerous and the raving "mad" were admitted to the institution during its first twenty years. The Lunatic Asylum in Lexington was the second such state mental institution in America. The Lunatic Asylum came of age with the appointment of Dr. John Rowan Allen in 1844, for it was principally through his efforts that a more compassionate and humane regimen was begun, "moral treatment."

The asylum housed the eldest son of Lexington's leading statesman, Henry Clay. As related by Collins: Thomas Wythe [Clay], born in 1802, lost his reason in his young manhood, from an accidental blow on the head with an ax in the hands of a negro boy, and died, in 1869, in the Insane Asylum at Lexington of which he had been an inmate for forty years.[240]

Surgery

Various factors stymied the progress of surgery during the first half of the nineteenth century, namely, pain and the lack of anesthesia, the almost inevitable infection, and inadequate anatomical knowledge; yet, had all these obstacles been met, there still would have been but minor gain because of the lack of a rational surgical pathology. The humoral system of the Ancient Greeks was still in vogue in Lexington as elsewhere in the early years of the nineteenth century, and this system held that diseases were of a general nature, that disease as an entity, with rare exceptions, did not exist. How could one surgically correct an imbalance of the humors? How could one operate upon the blood?[241] One could not and did not. Such was the intellectual climate of physicians at this time. How did change come about?

Giovanni Battista Morgagni (1682-1771) of Padua, Italy, reasoned that at some point the machinery of the organism misfires and that this precise spot marks the seat and the cause of a disease. He insisted on obtaining good clinical histories, first ascertaining the sex, next the age and locality, and then particulars such as marital status and occupation. In his classic work, *The Seats and Causes of Diseases Investigated by Anatomy*, published in 1761, the clinical symptoms and their corollary, the anatomical lesion, run like a thread throughout the book. Diseased organs, he noted, "differ in their structure from normal organs and since their structure is different their function is different," and it is this abnormal function that we recognize as symptoms. Disease started locally, he believed, and the seat of an illness was an organ or organs. The anatomical lesion in that organ represents the effects, not the basic cause, of the disease.[242]

Although the idea of disease specificity was enunciated in the seventeenth century, acceptance did not come for almost two centuries.[243] The process of disease localization was hastened by the discovery of percussion by Leopold Auenbrugger (1761) and by the invention of the stethoscope by Rene Theophile Laennec (1819), for now symptoms and physical signs in living patients could be matched with the post-mortem findings, thus confirming the diagnosis.[244] The next important step in disease localization was made by the Frenchman Marie-Francois Bichat (1771-1802), who believed that the living body was not merely made up of organs but could be studied on the basis of an intricate network of tissues. Subsequently, Theodore Schwann (1810-82) and Matthias Jacob Schleiden (1804-81) developed the cell theory. It was Rudolph Virchow (1821-1902) in Germany, creator of the "master science of pathology," who later pointed out the fundamental role of the cell and, in turn, did away with the last vestige of the humoral theory. Surgeons could now make a diagnosis before the operation, could identify and remove the "footprints"[245] of disease, and could do so precisely.

Benjamin W. Dudley, Surgeon

When we speak of surgery as it was practiced in Lexington, Kentucky and in the West during the first half of the nineteenth century, we speak of Dr. Benjamin W. Dudley (1785-1870).[246] Surgery in the latter part of the eighteenth and the first half of the nineteenth century was all too often identified with pain, infection,

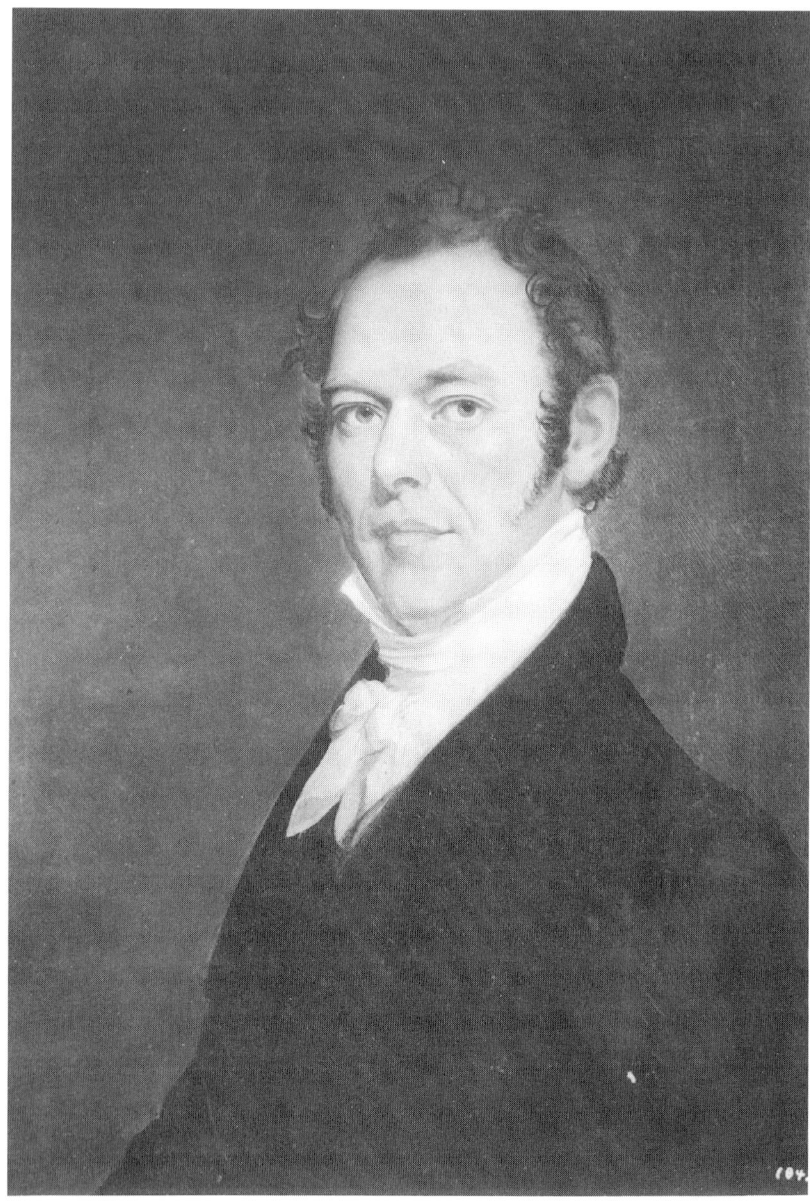

Benjamin Winslow Dudley, M.D. (1785-1870)
Courtesy of Transylvania University Library

speed, and death, and in the course of his lifetime, Dr. Dudley became intimate with each. As we have previously noted, all American physicians at this time were surgeons, physicians, preparers of medications, et cetera; however, there were a few who by their training and expertise dealt principally with surgery. One such was Dr. Dudley. As a young boy, Dudley became an apprentice under the tutelage of Dr. Frederick Ridgely of Lexington. He later received his medical degree at the University of Pennsylvania (1806) and then returned to Lexington in association with Dr. Joseph Fishback for a period of four years. The need to reach beyond the customary practice of medicine and to excel in the field of surgery convinced Dudley that he must remove to Europe, specifically to Paris and London, for training with surgeons. Dudley spent three years in Paris (1810-13) under the tutelage of Dr. Jean Dominique Larrey (1776-1842) and about one year (1813-14) in London with the celebrated Sir Astley Cooper (1768-1841) and Dr. John Abernethy (1764-1831). On his return from Europe in 1814, he resumed his medical and surgical practice in Lexington and, with the contemplated re-establishment of the Transylvania Medical Department, was appointed to the Chair of Surgery and Anatomy. The double appointment did not necessarily please his colleagues because it also secured for him double pay. Even so, the combined chair of surgery and anatomy had its origin in Europe several hundred years before, at which time surgery was but an "appendix" of anatomy.

The abdominal, chest, and cranial cavities were banned to surgery.[247] Trephining of the skull and plastic surgery had been applied from ancient times; amputations were essential, especially in wartime; superficial growths could be removed and abscesses drained; "crossed-eyes" and clubfeet could be repaired; and particularly in the Bluegrass there were bladder stones. It was through the removal of the latter that Dr. Dudley first gained regional and then national fame. Two of his cases, in 1817 and 1818, were of such interest to the public that they were reported in the *Kentucky Gazette:*

THE TRANSYLVANIA

JOURNAL OF MEDICINE,

AND THE ASSOCIATE SCIENCES

VOL. I. FEBRUARY, 1828. NO. I.

ORIGINAL COMMUNICATIONS.

ART. I.—*Observations on Injuries of the Head.* By BENJAMIN WINSLOW DUDLEY, M. D. Professor of Anatomy and Surgery in Transylvania University, Member of the Royal College of Surgeons, London.

THE great authorities of Europe and of our own country have laid down certain principles by which practitioners are generally governed in the treatment of injuries done to the scalp, cranium and brain. Since the publication of Mr. Abernethey's invaluable paper on injuries of the head, it might seem that little remains to be done in that department of surgery, while it is more than probable that under the present organization and management of the crowded hospitals of the large cities in Europe, no interesting and salutary innovations will be suggested: whereas in the United States, and especially in the valley of the Mississippi, where there is comparatively no human misery, no remarkable excesses in luxury, no crowded manufactories, and no large cities; where every individual partakes of nourishment equally healthy and invigorating, the fairest prospect is offered of giving new and increasing interest to this subject.

B

The Transylvania Journal of Medicine and the Associate Sciences
Vol. I., No. I. – February, 1828
The first article of Journal (It was by Benjamin Winslow Dudley, M.D.)
Courtesy of Transylvania University Library

> The operation of *lithotomy* was performed by Dr. Dudley on Mr. S. Owens, of this place, on Wednesday last, and a stone was taken from him one and three fourths of an inch in length, and one and a half inch in thickness, weighing nearly two ounces. The patient is doing well. This is the first operation for stone that has been performed in Lexington. The skilful and eminent operator on the present occasion, extracted a stone from a little boy in the town of Paris some time ago....Our Medical College, Kentucky, the western country at large may well be proud of a professional man of the skill and talent of Dr. Dudley.[248]

The following year a second operation for stone was reported:

> Dr. Dudley last week, again performed the operation of *lithotomy* with success on a boy about 10 years of age, from whose bladder two stones of magnitude were extracted, and who is already walking about.[249]

To a great extent, Dudley's fame has been tied to the large number of lithotomies that he performed with but three deaths, an amazing feat. His reputation was further enhanced by (1) trephination in the treatment of traumatic epilepsy, an operation that he pioneered; (2) ligation of the subclavian artery for the cure of an axillary aneurysm, the first of its kind in the west (1825); and (3) ligation of the carotid artery for an intracranial aneurysm with pulsating exopthalamus, the first of its kind in this country. A. Scott Earle, in his rendition of *Surgery in America,* refers to Dudley's efforts as follows: "These cases represent an early series of patients for whom craniotomy was performed for the relief of epileptiform seizures. As such they are a pioneer (and often overlooked) contribution to neurosurgery." [250] The first cases were reported in the first issue of the *Transylvania Journal of Medicine* in 1823.

In March 1849, Dr. Dudley's nephew, Professor E. L. Dudley, gave the valedictory address to the graduates at the Commencement of the Medical Department of Transylvania University in which he spoke of his uncle. Graduates reported and published the following passages from his lecture:[251]

> You may recollect an allusion to a young man, 21 years of age, who had been blind from the moment of his birth, and came to this place in order to have the film removed from before his sight, that he might look out upon the world around him, of which he had heard so much, and which he had often endeavored to picture to his imagination by the assistance of the senses of touch and hearing. Life had been one long, dreary night to him, the loneliness of which had only been relieved by the kind offices of his friends. He was operated upon by Professor Dudley, in the presence of the medical class, and after the expiration of a few days was brought before those again to have the bandages removed and the blessed light of heaven let in upon his brain for the first time. With the eagerness and simplicity of a child and with that touching expression of hopelessness and dependency which is the associate of blindness, he awaited the anxious moment, while the struggling emotions of hope and fear were plainly visible upon his features. Here was a sight to touch the soul of the coldest cynic that ever steeled his sensibilities against the appeals of sympathy. The patient had never looked upon the face of a friend, was a stranger to all the delightful

> impressions depending upon the sight and had only learned to detect the loved presence of parents and friends by the quick induction's of the dark. The bandages were finally removed, and he desired that the first image impressed upon his vision might be that of the surgeon to whom he owed the precious boon which it had pleased nature to withhold. At first he seemed paralyzed by the rush of unaccustomed impressions that crowded upon his brain, and stood trembling with excitement, turning his eyes from face to face of the crowd who gathered around him with feelings almost as excited as his own; but finally with a cry of delight which thrilled through the heart of every one present like an electric spark, he exclaimed that he could see. Objects were presented before him, and with the old instinct still upon him, he hesitated to express an opinion until he had felt them, and thus secured the aid of that sense which had until then been as eyes to him...of all the strange and beautiful objects he saw, none produced so rapturous an impression as "the ladies."

A Half Century Ahead

It is essential now to take a further look at Dudley's accomplishments, to equate his talents with those of the first order of surgeons, with the father of American Surgery, Philip Syng Physick (1768-1837) of Philadelphia and the celebrated Valentine Mott (1785-1865) of New York.[252] In 1892, Dr. Bedford Brown, of Alexandria, Virginia, reported "Personal Recollections of the Late Dr. Benjamin W. Dudley, of Lexington, Ky., and of His Surgical Methods and Work."[253] Brown remarks that Dudley "was a half-century ahead of the profession." He justifies his opinion with the disclosure that Dudley used "sterilized water as a dressing for wounds ... and used it to the exclusion of all other dressings. Not a drop of non-sterilized water was permitted to touch a wound. [Dudley] believed that unboiled well- or spring-water contained poisonous materials...that the purest form of water, next to the boiled or distilled, was cistern, which was used exclusively for drinking purposes in his family and office. [This remark suggests why not one of Dudley's family had cholera in the outbreak of 1833.] His use of boiled water in all wounds, except those healing by first intention, was profuse and abundant...Preliminary to and after operation he practised a system of asepsis and antisepsis consisting of absolute regard for cleanliness in every detail." Dudley's principles of wound care were practiced many years before the advent of bacteriology and the introduction of antisepsis.

Why did Dudley take such care of his patients with sterile preparations together with cleansing of the wounds with boiled water? He, himself, gives no answer; it was just his practice and "never departed from." Dudley has been described as a man with strict habits of neatness and cleanliness, yet these qualities were shared by many of his contemporaries who, unlike Dudley, prided themselves on wearing their blood-stained aprons. Were his precautions learned from abroad or through trial and error at home? Possibly they were fortuitous, similar to the chance observation of Ambrose Paré (1545), the great French Renaissance surgeon, that unattended gunshot wounds heal more readily than those treated with burning oil. Strangely, Dudley never wrote on this subject; our only knowledge comes through his juniors. To speculate further on his reasoning would be unrewarding. For the most likely scenario, we return to the reflections of his apprentice, Bedford Brown: "...he knew that all dirt and filth contained the seeds of disease, and to place his patient beyond the pale of disease was to preserve him in an absolute state of cleanliness."[254]

Though skeptics may question the authenticity of Dudley's innovative use of boiled water in the preparation of the patient and the surgical instruments, he was, even so, not the first to proclaim such a practice. Indeed, the concept of cleanliness meandered through many surgical theatres from the fourth millennium BC to the nineteenth century AD. Physicians of Babylon and Egypt were, in turn, followed by the Persians of the tenth century and thirteenth century Europe in precautions to prevent infection. We quote the famous surgeon Henri de Mondeville (c. 1260-1320).[255]

> Needles are to be clean, or they will infect the wound. When your dressings have been carefully made, do not interfere with them for some days; keep the air out, for a wound left in contact with the air will suppurate.

The French surgeon Claude Poteau (1725-75) preceded Dudley's regimen by almost one-hundred years "stressing cleanliness" with impressive results (120 lithotomies with the loss of but three patients).[256] Such gigantic intellectual leaps are not uncommon in medicine, but unlike Dudley's and Poteau's contributions, they often are so far ahead of the times that their use or proof cannot be entertained or validated by the existing science. For example, Girolamo Fracastoro's (1484-1553) treatise *De Contagione* (1546) "was a precursor of the modern theory of infection by invisible microorganisms."[257] Further scientific insight was demonstrated by the Lexington Medical Society member and president, Daniel Drake, who in the year 1832, writing about cholera asserted, "the mode in which that disease spreads, was more fully explained by the animalcule hypothesis than any other." Even so, Drake could not demonstrate the organisms.[258] Not until the germ theory was indelibly imprinted in the medical mind in the latter part of the nineteenth century did these various century-spanning concepts of disease and its prevention find certain proof. Within a span of three decades medicine moved from the concept of cleanliness to the proof of microorganisms to the advent of antisepsis and thence to asepsis.

Indeed in America and in Europe some three or more decades before the Civil War (1861-65) sanitarians led in America by Benjamin W. Crealy in 1837 and John W. Griscon in 1842 steadfastly sought to correct the harbingers of disease and death, namely: filthy streets; overcrowded housing; inadequate sewerage; poor lighting; insufficient ventilation; and unsanitary food.[259] Cleanliness called for water. Water was essential to drink; to clean the body; to cleanse wounds especially with the use of boiled water applied to local inflammation; to clean the streets. Even a new therapy namely hydrotherapy (use of water both internally and externally) was often preferred by citizens sickened by the heavy-handed heroic medicine advocated by the regular physicians.

Great as these exploits were, another custom of Dudley's practice may have been even more important than those just described: his concern for the patient's "constitution," yesterday's term for preoperative and postoperative care: "Thus the condition and action of every organ was carefully scrutinized, and if not up to the desired standard, they were to be placed in that condition by a well-regulated system of diet and medicine....the patient was deprived of all stimulants, as coffee, tea, tobacco, or alcohol....Under his system of diet and medication patients who came to him broken down by disease, with loss of appetite and digestion, would improve with astonishing rapidity." Having attended to his patient's "internal" affairs, Dr. Dudley did not neglect the necessity of his patients being cheerful and hopeful. The external body likewise came in for its share of attention, "his [the patient's] entire body was carried through a thorough cleansing and renovating process by means of soap and water, in a warm bath." When placed on the "operating" table, the patient was covered with warm blankets. Postoperatively, the wounds were managed once again by the same strict regimen of compresses dipped in boiling hot water and thorough cleansing of the wound with boiled water, Dudley's purpose to realize healing by first intention (healing without the formation of pus). Nutrition and nursing care were emphasized.

It is of particular interest that Bedford Brown does not give the reader the precise duration of the lithotomy operation.

Because of the agony (anesthesia was not available until the late 1840s) and shock experienced by the patient, together with blood loss, time was of the essence.[260] Most surgical procedures of the day were, of necessity, completed in less than fifteen minutes. Beyond that time, shock was almost always irreversible. From the description of the procedure as given by Brown, we can believe that Dudley required a few minutes, at most. Before the incision was made, an assistant introduced a grooved staff into the bladder. "Then the [left] lateral incision was made by the scalpel down to the groove in the staff, the beak of the gorget[261] inserted and rapidly plunged through the prostate into the bladder, giving vent to a sudden rush of urine; the finger of the left hand was then introduced into the bladder, and making a quick exploration, he introduced his forceps with the right, grasped the stone, and in an instant he had it in his left hand....After the operation the patient was placed on his left side for complete drainage, and only hot-water applications used on the wound."[262]

Dudley chose Sunday as the day on which to perform his most important operations.[263] Beginning the process from his office, he counseled his staff, "Young gentlemen, be ready to move to a certain house by the ringing of the last church bells." Some boarding house or hotel served as his surgical amphitheater. Sunday had its own religious relevance, both for the patient and for the surgeon; it was also quiet. Dudley's mastery of surgery closely matches the innate qualities of the great composers; *to know intuitively the unknown.*

Prevailing Diseases in Lexington

A source of prevailing disease topics in Lexington comes from the Transylvania University Medical Library, housing the dissertations of many Transylvania Medical Students graduating during the years 1820-59, a total of 1758 dissertations.[264] By far the largest number (240) of dissertations were under the heading "fever." Various fevers were described, namely, continuous, remittent, unremitted congestive, typhoid, typhus, and bilious (Yellow Fever is not included in this list). Other frequently listed topics include cholera (45); dysentery (55); scarlatina (27); and blood-letting (17). Additional diseases included pneumonia, hepatitis, amenorrhea, dyspepsia, syphilis, milk sickness, and curved spine.

Additional data on the prevalent diseases were published by physicians writing in the *Journal of Transylvania and Associated Sciences.* Dr. Lloyd Warfield comments on the diseases prevalent in Lexington in November 1836, and we learn of the presence of *Cynanche Maligna,* or putrid sore throat, which he said prevailed in Paris, Kentucky, and surroundings for several years after 1821 in epidemic form.[265] The disease was controlled by the use of general and local remedies; however, those cases treated with antiphlogistics (non-inflammatory) and calomel proved fatal. Other cases consisted of patients having *Phrenetic State of Fever,* "chilling pains in the head, fever and other derangement's.... Remedies-General blood-letting from the arm; one pint taken in the morning:-blood-letting repeated in the evening, now from the temporal artery on each side, and again from the arm; in all about a pint. The bleeding in the morning had little effect; that from the head diminished the force of the pulse very much."

An 1837 report in the *Transylvania Journal of Medicine* gives us an insight into the particular diseases affecting the citizens of Lexington during the month of September 1837. The reporter, Dr. David Bell, relates:[266] "As far as my observation extended, I was induced to believe that the last month, [September] was pregnant with more diseases, that were malignant in their nature and fatal in their tendency, than any preceding month since the organization of this college." He lists the following: typhus fever, bilious fever, diarrhea, and *Cynanche Maligna.* Referring to the *Cynanche Maligna,* he recounts that he had one such patient and had heard of several others, and that the disease "baffled all skill, resisted all remedial agents, and proved fatal within a few days."[267] Dr. Bell gives us a glimpse of the malady and the measures he used for remedy:

> I was called upon to treat several cases of *Cynanche Maligna*, in the family of Mr. Petit, a worthy farmer. The first person attacked was his elder son, aged six years, who had been the subject of phthsic from his infancy, and was supposed to be labouring under that disease at the time I was sent for, which was on the third day of his illness. I had scarcely taken my seat before I perceived their fatal mistake.
>
> His breathing was hurried and very laborious; every inspiration could be heard fifty yards from the house; his cough was incessant; tongue coated far back, with yellow fur, red at tip and edges; tonsils very much swollen, inflamed, and ulcerated; covered here and there with ash-coloured scabs. The caliber through which he breathed, was not larger than that of a quill; pulse too weak and rapid to be counted; lungs deeply affected. I applied blister plasters to the nape of the neck and over the sternum; gave an emetic of tartar, which was followed with calomel and rhubarb; had his lower extremities bathed in hot salt water; used a gargle of red pepper and alum;-but all to no purpose, death having put an end to his sufferings in a few hours.

Dr. Bell comments that he attended a younger brother of the Petit family, having the same problem but treated in a similar fashion and earlier in the disease process with recovery. The continuous bilious fever was treated by blood-letting, emetic, and nauseating potions of tartar, calomel, aloetic, saline, and oleaginous purgatives, and in each instance "the fever yielded."

Although smallpox, cholera and other epidemic diseases

often terrorized the populace, they were not the most prevalent diseases and certainly not among those causing the greatest number of deaths in nineteenth century America. Lexingtonians, for example, were frequently subject to respiratory diseases namely bronchitis, pneumonia, and tuberculosis (consumption/phthisis). Other common diseases included the various fevers—intermittent, remittent, and continued (probably malaria)—pneumonia, scarlet fever, croup, whooping couch, chicken pox, dysentery, enteritis, and measles. A high infantile mortality is affirmed by noting the average age of death of Kentuckians in 1859; white males—20.95; white females 21.48; and blacks 17.08 and 19.47 respectively.[268]

Although accounts of diseases were chronicled by physicians and students alike, there were, nevertheless, few statistical tabulations of the frequency of particular diseases and the causes of death until a pioneering report issued in 1852 for the state of Kentucky.[269] The leading causes of death as listed in 1852 were: Dysentery—18.39 percent; various fevers—15.47 percent; consumption—9.20 percent; cholera—6.94 percent; pneumonia—5.74 percent; croup—4.43 percent; whooping cough—3.19 percent; and measles—3.18 percent. By 1857 the cholera had dropped to 0.21 percent and dysentery to 4.67 percent, while consumption had risen to 11.93 percent from 9.20 percent.[270]

Tuberculosis (consumption), known as the "White Plague" was the supreme killer of the nineteenth century.[271] Measles, too, often proved fatal. Daniel Drake, in his classic *A Systematic Treatise, Historical, Etiological, and Practical on the Principal Diseases of the Interior Valley of North America* (1854), commented that measles "prevails from the [Great] Lakes to the shores of the Gulf affecting the inhabitants of both town and country." And, he added, "This disease dates from the first settlement of the interior."[272] Scarlet fever, he reported, was extremely fatal in Kentucky where it was called "putrid sore throat."[273] He observed that scarlet fever had become endemic and at "no time been absent from the Valley of the Mississippi and the Lakes."[274] In 1851 Dr. W. S. Chipley, Lexington physician, concluded: "The prevailing diseases of Fayette County, of a serious character, are typhoid fever and pneumonia." Other leading causes of death included: consumption, dysentery, accidents and "unknown."[275]

The whole number of deaths in the state of Kentucky for the year, ending June 1, 1852, was 15,211—being 1 in 64.46 persons, or 1.65 percent, "...a very favorable state of the public health."[276] Nevertheless, the mortality varied greatly in the different counties. Four classes of counties were identified by mortality rates:

Classes	**Number of Counties**	**Average Population Density**	**Mortality Rate**	**Percent**
First Class (Mortality: over 2.0 percent)	18	55 persons to square mile	1 in 41.90	2.38
Second Class (Mortality: 1.5 to 2.0 percent)	20	30 persons to square mile	1 in 58.92	1.69
Third Class (Mortality: 1.0 to 1.5 percent)	30	29 persons to square mile	1 in 79.16	1.23
Fourth Class (Mortality: below 1.0 percent)	32	21 persons to square mile	1 in 122.35	.81

Lexington, the "garden spot of Kentucky," took its place in the first class, a dubious distinction. Statistical returns were available for Lexington for twenty-one consecutive years, from 1831 to 1851:

Year	**Mortality Rate**	**Percent**
1817	1 in 90.88	1.10
1820	1 in 64.71	1.54
1831-51	1 in 79.16	2.73

The births for the same period 1831-51 were 4,331, scarcely more than the number of deaths. Only one year of these twenty-one gave as many as two births to one death. During one of the twenty-one years, 1833, when cholera prevailed, the mortality was 1 in 9.70, or 10.30 percent. The lowest mortality for any one year was 1837, 1 in 110.79 or .90 percent. The mortality in the last year of the study, 1851, was 1 in 31.84 persons or 3.14 percent. Two years earlier the author of the report, Dr. W. S. Chipley of Lexington, expressed the opinion that the mortality of Lexington did not exceed 2 percent; however, he had not seen the figures for the twenty-one consecutive years when he gave that opinion.[277] The Standing Committee on Vital Statistics of the Kentucky State Medical Society concluded that there had been, in Lexington, for some years past, an increasing mortality, the causes of which demanded a thorough and prompt investigation. Sanitary reform was suggested as the most likely remedy.

Because of the distance, the difficulty of travel and other restraints, it was not always possible for the doctor to see a patient but once or twice during the course of an illness. A diagnosis first given, therefore, often "stuck" even though its accuracy may or may not have been later confirmed had the entire course of the illness been observed. Even in the 1852 Annual Kentucky Report on Disease and Cause of Death it is likely that the accuracy of diagnosis (cause of death) could be called into question.[278] Referring to the report, Rawlings asserts, "It does not meet modern practice but it served a highly useful purpose. Inaccuracies crept in."[279] Even so, this remarkable report on vital statistics for the state of Kentucky was the first of its kind for the Western States and of such note that a review was occasioned in the *Boston Medical and Surgical Journal of April*, 1853.[280]

144 James Thacher, *American Medical Biography or Memoirs of Eminent Physicians Who Have Flourished in America* (Boston, 1828; reprint ed., New York: Milford House, Inc., 1967), 14-15.

145 Felix Marti-Ibanez, *Centaur: Essays on the History of Medical Ideas* (New York: MD Publications, 1960), 632; Richard Harrison Shyrock, *Medicine and Society in America, 1660-1860* (New York: New York University Press, 1960), 55. Mather held that disease "was ultimately caused by sin and was to be cured by prayer and forgiveness."

146 John B. Beck, *Medicine in the American Colonies,* 2d ed. (Albany, N.Y.: Horn and Wallace Publishers, 1850; reissue Albuquerque, N. M., 1966), 18-22; and Joseph M. Toner, *Contributions to the Annals of Medical Progress and Medical Education in the United States Before and During the War of Independence* (Washington, D.C.: Government Printing Office, 1874), 35-37.

147 James Wilkinson (1757-1825) served on the staffs of Benedict Arnold and Nathaniel Greene during the Revolutionary War. His participation in the Conway Cabal, a movement to remove General Washington, led him to resign his commission. He moved to Lexington, Kentucky in 1784 and soon became embroiled in the "Western discontent over proposed American concessions to the Spanish." His later involvement with the treacherous Aaron Burr caused his removal as territorial governor of Louisiana by President Jefferson. John A. Garraty, ed., *Encyclopedia of American Biography* (New York: Harper & Row, Publisher, 1974), 1203-04.

148 Genevieve Miller, "Medical Schools in the Colonies," *Ciba Symposia 8,* no. 10 (Jan 1947) : 523-532. John Morgan, in his *A Discourse Upon the Institute of Medical Schools in America* (1764), proposed the British system of separation of physician, surgeon and apothecary for Americans; however, such policy went against the grain of American Medicine.

149 Richard H. Shyrock, "European Backgrounds of American Medical Education (1600-1900)," *J.A.M.A.* 194, no. 7 (1965) : 119-124.

150 Levi Todd was the grandfather of Mary Todd Lincoln.

151 For example, *Kentucky Gazette,* 20 June 1789. "On Sunday evening last 2 Indians came to Mr. Jacob Stucker's on North Elk Horn, near Lebanon, and stole 3 horses; on Monday a party of about 12 Indians killed a lad about 2 or 3 miles from Colonel Johnson's, near Captain Herndon's; Capt. Herndon, who heard the guns, having a horse saddled, immediately rode to the place, and seeing the lad killed, alarmed the neighborhood, and in a very short time raised about 15 men and pursued the Indians; a number of others who collected after Capt. Herndon started, followed after; Capt. Herndon and his party, after following some distance, they discovered the trail of those who had stole Stucker's horses to cross those they were in pursuit of, and much easier to follow. Capt. Herndon tho't proper to leave the former and pursue the latter; in short time they came upon them, killed 2 and wounded the other (there being only three) and recovered all the horses."

152 Robert Peter, *A Brief Sketch of the History of Lexington, Kentucky and of Transylvania University* (Lexington, Ky.: D. C. Wickliffe, Printer, 1854), 5.

153 The first practicing physician in Kentucky was Dr. George Hartt, who settled at Harrods's Station (Harrodsburg) in May 1775. He later moved to Louisville and subsequently settled at Bardstown. John H. Ellis, *Medicine in Kentucky* (Lexington, Ky.: The University of Kentucky Press, 1977), 6-7.

154 Charles R. Staples, *The History of Pioneer Lexington 1779-1806* (originally published in 1939) (Lexington, Ky.: The University of Kentucky Press, 1996), 318-321. Staples cites his source in each instance, most being from the *Kentucky Gazette.* I have not found such a collective listing of these early "Medicine Men" in any other periodical.

155 Lewis Collins, *History of Kentucky*, vol. I, rev. by his son Richard H. Collins (Frankfort, Ky.: Kentucky Historical Society, 1966), 5.

156 *Kentucky Gazette*, 8 August 1798.

157 William Shippen (1736-1808) A contemporary of John Morgan (1735-1789), Father of American Medical Education, and with Morgan, a professor in the first medical school in America, 1765, The College of Philadelphia.

158 *Kentucky Gazette,* 11 September 1806.

159 "Report on the Committee on Surgery," *Transactions of the Kentucky State Medical Society* (Louisville, Ky.: Webb & Levering, 1853), 102.

160 Dumas Malone, ed., *Dictionary of American Biography,* Vol. VIII, Platt-Seward (New York: Charles Scribners Sons, 1935), 229.

161 Richard Harrison Shyrock, *Medicine and Society in America,* 1660-1860 (Ithaca, N.Y.: Cornell University Press, 1960), 74.

162 John S. Haller, Jr., *American Medicine in Transition* (Urbana: University of Illinois Press, 1981), 43-52.

163 Lunsford P. Yandell, "Notices of the Diseases of the Summer and Fall of 1832," *Transylvania Journal of Medicine and the Associate Sciences,* Vol. V (1832) : 500-506.

164 L. P. Yandell, "A Memoir of the Life and Writings of Dr. Benjamin Dudley," in J. N. McCormack, ed., *Some of the Medical Pioneers of Kentucky* (Bowling Green, Ky.: Kentucky State Medical Association), 60-61.

165 Haller, *American Medicine in Transition,* 80.

166 James C. Cross, "An Essay on Scarlatina," *Transylvania Journal of Medicine and the Associate Sciences,* Vol. II (1838) : 29-98; Elisha Bartlett, *Essay of the Philosophy of Medical Science* (Philadelphia: Lea and Blanchard, 1844), 237-241; Emmet Field Horine, *Daniel Drake* (1785-1852) *Pioneer Physician of the Midwest* (Philadelphia: University of Pennsylvania Press, 1961), 330-332.

167 The practice of smallpox inoculation was introduced into America by the Reverend Cotton Mather (1663-1728) and the physician Zabdiel Boylston (1680-1766) in 1721 in the city of Boston. Mather had become aware of the practice of inoculation through English publications and also from the tales of slaves brought from Africa. George Rosen, *A History of Public Health,* with a foreward by Felix Marti-Ibañez (New York: MD Publications, Inc., 1958), 186-187.

"During the sixth epidemic of smallpox in Boston, Massachusetts, Zabdiel Boylston courageously inoculated his son, and two Negro slaves on June 26, 1721, and had inoculated 244 persons before its close, exciting great opposition and even threats of hanging." Fielding H. Garrison, *An Introduction to the History of Medicine* (Philadelphia: W. B. Saunders & Co., 1922), 387.

168 Rosen, *A History of Public Health*, 99.

169 Although the American Indians were sacrificed to the European infectious diseases, they, in turn, introduced the Europeans in the latter part of the fifteenth century to syphilis. The French called it the Neapolitan disease; the Spanish named it the French disease, et cetera.

Frederick D. Cartwright, *Disease and History* (N.Y.: Thomas Y. Crowell Co., 1972), 58-59.

170 The idea (inoculation) was introduced into England by Timoni's and Pilarini's communications to the Royal Society in 1713-16, and was afterward taken up by Sir Hans Sloane (1717). On March 18, 1718, Lady Mary Wortley Montagu had her three-year-old son inoculated in Turkey, and her five-year-old daughter was inoculated in England in April 1721.

Garrison, *An Introduction to the History of Medicine,* 387.

171 "The skepticism that appeared, even among the most enlightened of medical men when my sentiments on the important subject of cow-pox were first promulgated, was highly laudable. To have admitted the truth of a doctrine, at once so novel and so unlike any thing that had ever happened in the annals of medicine, without the test of the most rigid scrutiny, would have bordered upon temerity; but now, when that scrutiny has taken place, not only among ourselves, but in the first professional circles of Europe, and when it has been uniformly found in such abundant instances that the human frame, when once it has felt the influence of the genuine cow-pox in the way that has been described, is never afterwards at any period of its existence assailable by the small-pox, may I not with perfect confidence congratulate my country and society at large on their beholding, in the mild form of the cow-pox, an antidote that is capable of extirpating from the earth a disease which is every hour devouring its victims; a disease that has ever been considered as the severest scourge of the human race." Edward Jenner.

Daniel F. Roses, "Vaccinations Bicentennial: A Surgical landmark," *Bulletin of the American College of Surgeons* 8, no. 5 (May 1996) : 30-33.

172 William G. Rothstein, *American Physicians in the Nineteenth Century* (Baltimore: The Johns Hopkins University Press, 1985), 30-31; and H.J. Parish, *A History of Immunization* (Edinburgh: Livingstone, 1965), 25-26.

173 "It had long been a countryside tradition in Gloucestershire [England] that dairy-maids who had contracted cow-pox through milking did not take smallpox. On learning of this fact from a milkmaid, Jenner early conceived the idea of applying it on a grand scale in the prevention of the disease. ...on May 14, 1796, [he] performed his first vaccination upon a country boy, James Phipps, using matter from the arm of the milkmaid....The experiment was then put to the test, by inoculating Phipps with smallpox virus on July 1st, and the immunization proved successful."

Garrison, *An Introduction to the History of Medicine,* 387.

174 Frank L. Dewey, *Thomas Jefferson Lawyer* (Charlottesville, Va.: University of Virginia Press, 1986), 46-47.

175 In 1777, Virginia enacted a law allowing inoculation if a majority of the neighbors consented and if a quarantine was maintained. Jefferson was a member of the legislative committee and under this law had his children inoculated. Many of the earlier settlers in Kentucky were Virginians and, therefore, familiar with the laws of that state regarding inoculation. The first paragraph of Section three of the Kentucky Statute regarding inoculation is similar to the Virginia law in its purpose with but a change in the consent to read from two miles (Va.) to three miles (Ky.). In 1792, when Kentucky separated from Virginia, the Kentucky Legislature had no hesitancy in adopting *Acts of Parliament and of Virginia of a General Nature,* i.e., they simply left certain acts to which they had been subject to as Virginians in force in the state of Kentucky. Sentiments were little changed by the turn of the century.

176 John Gunn, *Gunn's Domestic Medicine,* with an introduction by Charles E. Rosenburg (Knoxville: The University of Tennessee Press, 1830, facsimile ed.; new ed., 1986), 259.

"SMALL POX is known by the following symptoms:—A few days before its appearance, you feel restless and uneasy, and a great dislike to motion of any kind. Cold chills steal over you, followed by flushing of heat, and accompanied by a slight fever all of which end as the disease gradually increases. You have a pain in the head, a dull heavy pain in the small of the back, great thirst, increase of stupor—until about the third day, when the eruptions or spots on the skin, something like flea-bites, make their appearance on the face, neck, breasts and arms, and gradually extend over the whole body. These spots gradually increase in size, until about the fifth or sixth day, when they begin to turn white at the tops, and feel painful. Your voice then becomes hoarse as if you had a severe cold; your face becomes much swelled; and your features appear much changed.—Your eyelids particularly swell to a considerable extent and a spitting takes place as if you were salivated. On the eleventh day, these pustules or pimples have increased to about the size of a common pea, and instead of white contain a yellow matter, on the tops of which pustules or pimples, you will discover a small black spot, whilst all the rest is filled with this yellow matter. About the twelfth day they burst, and discharge their contents, with a horrible stench which is almost insupportable; nor dare you attempt to wash this matter—the slightest touch giving the most excruciating pain. If the matter dries quickly, it leaves no marks; but if, from any unhealthy constitutional defect, it lingers for some time on the body it generally leaves those marks behind it, which disfigure the countenance for life."

177 William Littell, *The Statute Law of Kentucky; with notes, praelections, and observations on the public acts,* vol. II (Frankfort, Ky.: Johnston & Pleasants, 1810), 46-50.

178 Smallpox had a devastating impact among the American Indians, indicating their susceptibility to this newly acquired infection; whole tribes were wiped out. "A favor of providence, so thought the Puritans." Shyrock states that not only villages but tribes themselves were decimated, an early and successful form of "biologic warfare." He adds that such acts were usually unintentioned; however, other investigations show a very different and less salutary interpretation.

Shyrock, *Medicine and Society in America 1660-1860,* 83-84.

"It is also during the eighteenth century that we find written reports of American Indians being intentionally exposed to smallpox by Europeans. In 1763 in Pennsylvania, Sir Jeffrey Amherst, commander of the British forces...wrote in the postscript of a letter....suggesting that smallpox be sent among the disaffected tribes."

Russell Thornton, *American Indian Holocaust and Survival: A Population History Since 1492* (Norman, Okla.: University of Oklahoma Press, 1987), 78-79.

179 William G. Rothstein, *American Physicians in the Nineteenth Century* (Baltimore: The Johns Hopkins University Press, 1985), 30-31; and John B. Blake, *Public Health in the town of Boston 1630-1822* (Cambridge, MA.: Harvard University Press, 1959), 239-244; and Solon S. Bernstein, "Smallpox and Vaccination: Their Historical Significance in the American Colonies," *Journal of the Mt. Sinai Hospital* (1951) : 237.

180 Staples, *The History of Pioneer Kentucky 1779-1806,* 323.

181 Robert McAfee, Journal, *Kentucky State Historical Society Register* 25 (1927) : 127.

"My father seemed to be set upon my Education, and to make Provision for my future welfare, and Mr. John Breckinridge having heard that I was a boy of some promise, and being also a warm friend of my fathers he had proposed to take me into his office and complete my Education, and on my part I was to copy any papers he might need, by this I understood that I was to be a Lawyer, which pleased me very much, as my father had often taken me to Harrodsburgh where I was seated in the Bar for hours to hear the Lawyers plead, I was delighted with the idea as it was an honorable profession and I felt ambitious to rise to distinction and give proof that my Father and his friend would not be disappointed, my whole heart was in the matter and I then resolved to devote myself to the subject I was however not aware of the long road I had to Travel and how much I yet lacked in my Education before I could get a fair start—

(1794). In the month of February of this year I was taken from Mr. Dunlavys school and after having the best clothes my father and mother could procure made up I was sent to Lexington with my Uncle James McAfee who was going there to get some Linseed and other necessaries to paint his house he had several packhorses with flour to sell, I rode one of them, but rode into town behind him and went to Mr. Breckinridges house, he lived in one which Thomas Hart afterward lived in (Mr. Clays father in law) I will never forget his fine carpets which were new furniture to me, I hestitated to walk on it until my uncle seeing my embarrassment ordered me to walk on. Mr. Breckenridge was not in at the time but came in soon after & after inspecting me very closely he told my uncle that Small Pox had made its appearance in town & that he thought he ought not to have me as his own family had not had it and he thought it would be dangerous, The small pox originated in the army then stationed at Cincinnati and was then spreading all over the county[.] I was glad to hear this, as notwithstanding my high anticipations, I was truly glad to get back home, as I had left with a heavy heart, so much so that I had slept none the night before but lay and tossed all night, and when the cocks began to crow for day I had taken a hearty cry, I thought I was doomed to a hard lot & all my ambition had evaporated my mental sufferings were extreme, but when I heard that I could return home I was supremely happy as the thoughts of my kind & indulgent parents rose before—

We staid that night at a Mr. Keisers on the hill on high street, and next morning the ground was coverd [sic] with snow, but I was happy, My uncle had to go about two miles East of the Town to the oil mill owned by a Mr. _____ and we had to pass through the Transylvania Seminary lot which was then uninclosed & we had to pass near the old Brick Seminary, I was mounted on a packsaddle and in this style rode over the lott, (something like Franklin when he first entered Philadelphia) the school boys were out snowballing each other & as I approached I *good* several at me which I thought very unmannerly of them, I took a good view of the house as I knew I was destined to go to school there as it was agreed that I should return as soon as the small pox ceased, It came to Lexington sure enough and the town suffered severely as all who could not get away were innoculated, The Kine Pox was not then known, Mr. Breckenridge was near dying with it and I made a fortunate escape as it ravages were princi*ply* confined to the North side of the Kentucky river, As soon as I returned home I went back to my school dressed in my fine clothes as I was anxious to show off to the best advantage to my pretty Miss Curry—which added to my enjoyments—" Ibid., 127-128.

182 F. A. Michaux, *Travels to the West of the Allegheny Mountains in the States of Ohio, Kentucky and Tennessee* (London: B. Crosby and Co., 1805), 205.

183 John B. Blake, *Benjamin Waterhouse and the Introduction of Vaccination,* a Reappraisal (Philadelphia: University of Pennsylvania Press, 1957), 14. "In the United States, the Harvard professor of medicine, Benjamin Waterhouse (1754-1846) made the first vaccinations upon his four children in July, 1800, procuring his virus from Dr. Haygarth of Bath, England. He was speedily followed by Crawford and Smith in Baltimore, James Jackson in Boston, David Hosack in New York, and John Redmond Coxe in Philadelphia....Waterhouse said that, before the introduction of

vaccination, the fear of the smallpox compelled the New Englanders, 'the most democratic people on the face of the earth,' to endure 'restrictions of liberty such as no absolute monarch could have enforced.'" Garrison, *An Introduction to the History of Medicine,* 389.

184 "During my stay at Lexington I frequently saw Dr. Samuel Brown, from Virginia, a physician of the college of Edinburgh, and member of the Philosophical Society, to whom several members of that society had given me letters of recommendation. A merited reputation undeniably places Dr. S. Brown in the first rank of physicians settled in that part of the country. Reviewing regularly the scientific journals from London, he is always in the channel of new discoveries, and turns them to the advantage of his fellow-citizens. It is to him they are indebted for the introduction of the cow-pox. He had at that time inoculated upward of five hundred persons in Kentucky, when they were making their first attempts in New York and Philadelphia."

Michaux, *Travels to the West of the Allegheny Mountains,* 205.

185 *Kentucky Gazette* (Lexington), 25 May 1801.

186 Ibid., 8 June 1801.

187 In 1800, the population of Lexington was 2400.

188 *Kentucky Gazette,* 1 June 1801. Dr. Basil Duke (1766-1828) settled in Lexington, Kentucky, in 1791 and developed a large practice. Born in Calvert, Maryland; studied medicine in Baltimore. Removed in 1798 to Mason County, Ky. [The correspondent, Basil Duke, is believed, by the author, to be the same person as Dr. Basil Duke of Lexington. The identical name and the fact that he also plans to inoculate with the smallpox matter plus the nearness of Washington to his birthplace in Calvert, Md. support this contention.—author]

189 The following newspaper clipping from a Fredericksburg Paper was printed in the *Kentucky Gazette,* 27 July 1801:

The President [Thomas Jefferson] of the United States lately received some new vaccine or cowpox matter from Dr. Waterhouse of Boston, which he has put into the hands of Dr. Gantt of Georgetown, in order to have its effects tried there. Experiments which have resulted unfavorably, have been made in several parts of the United States—but the want of success, it is highly probable, has arisen from the quality of the matter, for this mode of inoculation has been practiced to great advantage in different parts of Europe. The vaccine is said to be a much milder disease than the smallpox, not infectious, and to prevent a subsequent infection of either species of disorder.

Jefferson acknowledged the value of Dr. Jenner's discovery in a letter to him:

Monticello, May 14, 1806

"SIR,—I have received a copy of the evidence at large respecting the discovery of the vaccine inoculation which you have been pleased to send me, and for which I return you my thanks. Having been among the early converts, in this part of the globe, to its efficiency, I took an early part in recommending it to my countrymen. I avail myself of this occasion of rendering you a portion of the tribute of gratitude due to you from the whole human family. Medicine has never before produced any single improvement of such utility. Harvey's discovery of the circulation of the blood was a beautiful addition to our knowledge of the animal economy, but on a review of the practice of medicine before and since that epoch, I do not see any great amelioration which has been derived from that discovery. You have erased from the calendar of human afflictions one of its greatest. Yours is the comfortable reflection that mankind can never forget that you have lived. Future nations will know by history only that the loathsome small-pox has existed and by you has been extirpated.

Accept my fervent wishes for your health and happiness and assurances of the greatest respect and consideration. "

Thomas Jefferson, *Thomas Jefferson Writings* (New York: Library Classics of the United States, Inc., 1984), 1162-63.

190 A. H. Barkley, "Dr. Samuel Brown, The First Professor of Medicine West of the Alleghenies," *Annals of Medical History*, III, no. 4 (July 1931) : 366.

191 Caleb W. Cloud, "An Account of the Small-Pox, as it appeared in the city of Lexington and county of Fayette, Ky., during May and June, 1837 *Transylvania Journal of Medicine* 10 (1837) : 442.

192 Ibid.

193 J. M. Bruce, "Smallpox in Lexington," *Transylvania Medical Journal* I, no. 4 (Feb. 1850) : 337-343.

194 Ibid.

195 William H. McNeill, *Plagues and Peoples* (Garden City, N.Y.: Anchor Press/Doubleday, 1976), 230-231. "This disease (cholera) had long been endemic in Bengal, and spread thence in epidemic fashion to other parts of India and adjacent regions from time to time. It was caused by a bacillus that could live as an independent organism in water for lengthy periods of time. Once swallowed, if the cholera bacillus survives the stomach juices, it is capable of swift multiplication in the human alimentary tract, and produces violent and dramatic symptoms—diarrhea, vomiting, fever, and death, often within a few hours of the first sign of the illness. The speed with which cholera killed was profoundly alarming."

196 Rev. Robert Davidson, *History of the Presbyterian Church in the State of Kentucky* (Lexington, Ky., and New York: Charles Marshall, 1847), 333-334.

197 "The limestone formation of Lexington is catacombed by underground streams and caverns which are readily tapped by the wells. The vicinity abounds in sink holes through which surface water readily reaches, undisturbed, the underground streams. Drainage from the privies and latrines could easily reach, through the sink holes and without the filtering action of the soil, these underground streams; tapped by wells these streams supplied the drinking water of the city. No more suitable conditions for the contamination of the water supply could have been found." John S. Chambers, *The Conquest of Cholera* (New York: The Macmillan Co., 1938), 176.

198 *The Lexington Observer and Kentucky Reporter,* 15 November 1832.

199 Calomel is mercurous chloride, a white tasteless, crystalline powder, used in medicine as a cathartic.

Clarence L. Barnhart, ed., *The World Book Dictionary* (Chicago: Doubleday & Co., Inc., 1967), 271.

200 C.W. Short, "A Brief Historical Sketch of the Origin and Progress of Cholera Asphyxia," *Transylvania Journal of Medicine* 11, no. 1 (August 1837), 11-21.

201 Davidson, *History of the Presbyterian Church in the State of Kentucky*, 334.

202 Ibid., 334-335

203 C. W. Short, "A Brief Historical Sketch," 20.

204 *Frankfort Commonwealth,* 18 June 1833. Orlando Brown was the nephew of Dr. Samuel Brown.

205 *Niles Weekly Register,* 22 June 1833.

206 During the Yellow Fever epidemic in Philadelphia in 1793, many of the local physicians abandoned their patients and fled the city. The most notable among this group was Dr. William Shippen.

207 Chares E. Rosenberg, *The Cholera Years* (Chicago: The University of Chicago Press, 1962), 72.

208 Drs. Dudley and Bush with members of their immediate families remained free of cholera, presumably because of their use of cistern water for drinking, the only two cisterns in the city.

Bedford Brown, "Personal Recollections of the Late Dr. Benjamin W. Dudley, of Lexington, KY., and of His Surgical Methods and Work," *Transactions of the Southern Surgical and Gynecological Association* (1892) : 11, 26.

209 Specialization, to the extreme of limiting one's practice to surgery or otherwise, was not accepted by patients or regular American physicians during the first fifty plus years of the 19th century. Indeed, specialization would have made the physician an outcast. In 1876, the celebrated American surgeon Samuel Gross said that it was "safe to affirm that there is not a medical man on the continent who devotes himself exclusively to the practice of surgery."

Rothstein, *American Physicians in the Nineteenth Century,* 252. The author's impression as given above and that of Dr. Gross are at odds with that of Earle, who states: "His [Dudley's] practice was restricted to his own specialty, a decided rarity in that day." A. Scott Earle, ed., *Surgery in America; From the Colonial Era to the Twentieth Century* (New York: Praeger Publishers, 1983), 156.

210 Benjamin W. Dudley, "Letter (22 June 1833) of Professor Dudley, of Lexington, on the Cholera," *National Gazette and Literary Register* (Philadelphia), 4 July 1833.

211 *Niles Weekly Register,* 22 June 1833.

212 *Transylvania Journal of Medicine* (1833) : 305.

213 Thomas H. Appleton, Jr., "William Solomon," in John E. Kleber, ed., *The Kentucky Encyclopedia* (Lexington, Ky.: The University of Kentucky Press, 1992), 832; Burton Milward, *William (King) Solomon,* 1775-1854 (Lexington, Ky.: The King Library Press, 1974).

214 Short, "A Brief Historical Sketch," 20.

215 *The Commonwealth,* Frankfort, 18 June 1833.

216 Chambers, *The Conquest of Cholera,* 226.

217 Ibid., 176.

218 Julius P. Bolivar MacCabe, *Directory of the City of Lexington and County of Fayette for 1838 & '39* (Lexington: J. C. Noble, 1838), 22.

219 *Lexington Observer and Reporter*, 29 October 1847.

220 Ibid., 20 December 1848.

221 Ibid., 13 June 1849 and 7 July 1849.

222 Ibid., 2 June 1849.

223 Chambers, *The Conquest of Cholera*, 228.

224 Charles-Edward Amory Winslow, *The Conquest of Epidemic Disease; A Chapter in the History of Ideas* (Madison, Wisc.: The University of Wisconsin Press, 1980), 66.

Great wood fires were first used in Ancient Greece to control epidemics; however, in cities such as Philadelphia in 1793, their use had to be abandoned because of hazards to the entire city. The great wood fires were the first means of an attempt to control the epidemics in ancient Greece, and they were also used in Philadelphia before turning to guns and cannon; however, the fires proved too dangerous.

225 On January 12, 1824, a circular appeared on page two of the *Kentucky Gazette* requesting the public to respond to an inquiry specific to the different accounts of the autumnal fever. The report, requested by order of the (Lexington Medical) Society, was to be submitted to the Physicians of the Western and Southern states. Communications were to be addressed to Dr. Daniel Drake, President of the Society.

226 Ibid., 244-248; and Roderick E. McGrew, *Encyclopedia of Medical History* (New York: McGraw-Hill Book Co., 1985), 286-287.

This theory of the origin of the disease, i.e., that filth and squalor ripened into poisonous vapors, was held well into the mid-nineteenth century and, ironically, led to the public health movement in mid-nineteenth century America, especially to clean water, clean streets, and expeditious disposal of sewage.

227 Chambers, *The Conquest of Cholera,* 229.

228 *Lexington Observer & Reporter,* 18 August 1849.

229 Frederick F. Cartwright, *Disease and History,* 154-157.

230 Kenneth Dewhurst, "Sydenham on 'A Dysentery,'" *Bulletin of the History of Medicine* XXIX (Sep-Oct, 1955) : 393-400.

231 Lunsford P. Yandell, "Cases of Dysentery, with Remarks," *Transylvania Journal of Medicine and the Associate Sciences* 9, no. 1 (1836) : 240-250, quotations from 245-250.

232 Ibid., 245-250.

233 Steven M. Stowe, "Seeing Themselves at Work; Physicians and the Case Narrative in the Mid-Nineteenth-Century American South," *The American Historical Review* 101, no. 1 (February 1996) : 41-79.

234 Julius P. Bolivar Mac Cabe, *Directory of the City of Lexington and County of Fayette for 1838 &'39* (Lexington, Ky.: Hunts Row, 1838), 21.

235 George Rosen, *A History of Public Health* (New York: MD Publications, Inc., 1958), 148-150.

236 John R. Green, *Medical History for Students* (Springfield, Ill.: Charles C Thomas, Publisher, 1968), 137-54.

237 "Some towns [in Europe] turned their mental cases over to sailors or even hired a ship to carry them away. Thus the ship of fools *(Narrenschiff)* became a persistent image in literature and art, a symbol of humanity's follies and restlessness."

McGrew, *Encyclopedia of Medical History*, 193.

238 Ibid., 195.

239 W. S. Chipley, "Summary of the Beginning of Eastern State Hospital in 1824 through 1869," a typed copy of the original, Archives, Eastern State Hospital, Lexington, Ky, 1-14.

240 Lewis Collins, *History of Kentucky*, rev. Richard H. Collins (Louisville, Ky.: published by Richard H. Collins, 1877), 217.

241 Shyrock, *Medicine and Society in America:* 1660-1860, 59.

242 Giovanni Battista Morgagni, *The Seats and Causes of Disease,* trans. Benjamin Alexander (New York: Hofner, 1960), xxx.

243 McGrew, *Encyclopedia of Medical History*, 69-70.

244 Referring to pneumonia in the lower lobe of the right lung, Drake commented: "Percussion is of little value, except when the inflammation ascends beyond the region rendered obtuse by the position of the liver….Auscultation is here of great value." Drake, *Interior Valley of North America,* 860. Not surprisingly, Drake was one of the few American physicians using such techniques before the 1870s.

Although the stethoscope was invented in 1819 and palpation of the chest was introduced in 1761 and resurrected in 1808, few American physicians made use of such diagnostic tools, and such instruments as the otoscope and ophthalmoscope were still distant as were the chemical and bacteriological exploits of Pasteur and the discovery of antisepsis by Lister. Green, *Medical History for Students,* 114-15, 141-42.

245 Stanley Joel Reiser, *Medicine and the Reign of Technology* (Cambridge: Cambridge Press, 1978), 17.

246 Dr. George G. Greene, "The Life & Times of Dr. Benjamin Winslow Dudley," May 1985,

Archives of Transylvania University.

247 Philip Rhodes, *An Outline History of Medicine* (London: Butterworths, 1985), 107; and McGrew, *Encyclopedia of Medical History*, 112. Ephraim McDowell (1771-1830) of Danville, Kentucky is known as the father of abdominal surgery. Surgical penetration of the peritoneal cavity of the abdomen, before his series of ovariotomies (1809-18) was so feared and so deadly that surgeon and patient alike shunned any such action. By the latter part of the nineteenth century, with the benefit of anesthesia and asepsis, surgical opening into the abdominal cavity was well established.

248 *The Kentucky Gazette*, 29 November 1817.

249 Ibid., 22 May 1818.

250 "Trephination was one of the first operations performed, and skulls bearing the marks of healed trephine wounds have been found dating back to the Neolithic age. The operation apparently has been used continuously since; deterioration after head injury has always been an indication for trephination. Excellent results frequently followed the removal or elevation of depressed bone fragments or the evacuation of clot or fluid. Trephination, in the days before antisepsis, was but one of the most important procedures in the surgeon's armamentarium." Earle, *Surgery in America; From the Colonial Era to the Twentieth Century*, 154-156.

251 *The Lexington Observer and Reporter*, 7 March 1849.

252 John H. Talbott, *A Biographical History of Medicine* (New York: Grune and Stratton, 1970), 370-371. Phylip Syng Physick (1768-1837) is the Father of American Surgery. A native of Philadelphia, Physick, at the age of 20, became an apprentice of the renowned John Hunter in London. He later transferred from London to Edinburgh. Returning to Philadelphia in 1794 he became a member of the staff of Pennsylvania Hospital. By 1805 Physick became professor of surgery at the University of Pennsylvania where his surgical skills, the application of Hunter's physiological principles and teaching process, designated him as the premier American surgeon.

253 Brown, "Personal Recollections of the Late Dr. Benjamin W. Dudley of Lexington, Ky., and of His Surgical Work," *Transactions of the Southern Surgical and Gynecological Association* (1892), 11-28.

254 Ibid., 16.

255 Brian Inglis, *A History of Medicine* (Cleveland and New York: The World Publishing Company, 1965), 150.

256 McGrew, "Surgery," *Encyclopedia of Medical History*, 323.

257 Ira M. Rutkow, *Surgery An Illustrated History* (St. Louis: Mosby Year Book Inc., 1993), 123.

258 Daniel Drake, *An Account of the Epidemic Cholera, as it Appeared in Cincinnati* (Cincinnati: O. E. Deming, 1832).

259 Rosen, *A History of Public Health*, 237-238.

260 "Robert Liston (London) was the fastest knife in the West End. He could amputate a leg in 2 1/2 minutes....Time me, gentlemen, time me," he called to students holding pocket watches. In one of his most famous cases, he amputated a leg in 2 1/2 minutes; however, in his haste he also amputated the testicles. In another instance he amputated a leg under 2 1/2 minutes. His knife also severed the fingers of his young assistant who died of gangrene. "He also slashed through the coat-tails of a distinguished surgical spectator, who was so terrified that the knife had cut his vitals he dropped dead from fright....When anesthesia was unknown—you had the choice of fuddling with opium or rum, or biting on a cloth-wrapped peg—surgery was a matter of more haste, less pain."

Richard Gordon, *Great Medical Disasters* (New York: Stein and Day, 1983), 19-21.

261 The gorget was "a curious instrument" of fine steel, composed of a handle and blade all of steel without any extraneous material, and when dipped in hot water, which was always done, was really an antiseptic instrument. The blade has a beak, a cutting edge, and back, the beak fitting in the groove of the staff. The steel handle is turned slightly to the right, which adapts to the lateral operation.

Brown, "Personal Recollections of the Late Dr. Benjamin W. Dudley," 11-28.

262 Ibid., 19-20.

263 Dr. Ephraim McDowell (Danville, Kentucky) chose Sunday to operate upon Jane Todd Crawford in 1809 because "he wished for the prayers of the church to be with him as he performed the operation (ovariotomy)." No mention was made by McDowell as to anesthesia of any type for Mrs. Crawford; however, for his second case, he provided his patient with cherry bounce (bourbon whiskey in which ripe cherries are soaked) to prevent shock."

Laman S. Gray, *The Life & Times of Ephraim McDowell* (Louisville, Ky.: V. G. Reed and Sons, 1987), 59-60.

264 *Catalogue of the Transylvania University Medical Library* (Cincinnati: C. J. Krehbiel Co., 1987).

265 Lloyd Warfield, "Diseases Prevalent in Lexington and its vicinity in the month of November, 1836; with cases," reported to the College of Physicians and Surgeons, Lexington, Ky. *Transylvania Journal of Medicine* 10 (1837) : 636-645.

266 David Bell, "Report on the Prevailing Diseases in Lexington, Kentucky, during the month of September, 1837," read to the College of Physicians and Surgeons, *Transylvania Journal of Medicine* 10 (1837) : 213-216.

267 Ibid., 213.

268 Kenneth W. Rawlings, *Medicine and Its Development in Kentucky* (Louisville, Ky.: The Standard Printing Co., 1940), 308.

269 *First Annual Report to the General Assembly of Kentucky Relating to the Registry and Returns of Births, Marriages and Deaths, from January 1, 1852, to December 31, 1852,* (Frankfort, Ky.: A. G. Hodges, State Printer, 1853).

270 *Medicine and Its Development in Kentucky,* Appendix IV, "Classified Causes of Death for the Years 1852-1859."

271 René and Jean Dubos, *The White Plague* (New Brunswick, N.J.: Rutgers University Press, 1952).

272 Drake, *Diseases of the Interior Valley of North America,* 586.

273 Ibid., 594.

274 Ibid.; William Pawling, *The Transylvania Journal of Medicine and Associate Sciences,* X (1837) : 455-56.

275 "The Sanitary Conditions and Vital Statistics of Fayette County, Kentucky," *The Western Journal of Medicine and Surgery* (December 1851) : 363-96.

276 "Report of the Standing Committee on Vital Statistics," *Transactions of the Kentucky State Medical Society* (1851), 461-97.

277 "The Sanitary Condition and Vital Statistics of Fayette County, Kentucky," *The Western Journal of Medicine and Surgery* (1851) : 461-97.

278 Rawlings, *Medicine and Its Development in Kentucky,* Appendix IV.

279 Ibid., 308.

280 "Vital Statistics in Kentucky," *Boston Medical and Surgical Journal,* XLVII, 10 (1853) : 188.

Chapter IV

MEDICAL EDUCATION IN ANTEBELLUM LEXINGTON

Address to Medical Students (1806)

Perhaps I am now addressing the gentleman who shall, from the chair I now occupy, or from the press, expose the errors of my system of medicine. Did I know who was to be that person, I would take him by the hand and cordially wish him success in his noble undertaking. Perish my name and the memory of my labors from the records of time, provided that the science I have loved and cherished be advanced and perfected in the world.[281]

Benjamin Rush

A Public Responsibility

With the ending of the Revolutionary War, the new nation had to rely on its people to preserve its republican character. Only an educated people could govern. Thus, "the Revolutionaries insisted that education must become a public responsibility."[282] "Wisdom and knowledge, as well as virtue, diffused generally among the body of the people, being necessary for the preservation of their rights and liberties...[it is the] duty of legislatures and magistrates [to extend the] opportunities and advantages of education in the various parts of the country," declared the Massachusetts Constitution of 1780.[283]

The advancement of education and the province of medicine went hand in hand throughout the first four decades of nineteenth-century Lexington. For years education continued to be the primary concern of medicine throughout the nation, as documented by the words of Dr. Nathan Smith Davis, founder of the American Medical Association,[284] who identified the deterioration of medical standards as the leading concern of those who originated and carried into effect the Convention of May, 1846. The 1846 Convention led to the establishment of the American Medical Association in Philadelphia in May 1847.

Education in Pioneer Lexington

In all likelihood, the beginning of education in Lexington took place within the confines of the fort. The first evidence of formal schooling occurred in 1782, when the settlers built a small log house outside the fort, "sited in the middle of the public square, on the east side of Cheapside Street, west of the present courthouse."[285] "That the initial building consciously implanted on the layout of Lexington fostered education indicated the high regard for knowledge that the community maintained."[286] By 1788, other schools were offering to the public the education of their children. One schoolmaster was John Filson,[287] companion of Daniel Boone and noted pioneer historian, who proposed a seminary in Lexington. His advertisement appeared in the *Kentucky Gazette* on January 19, 1788:[288]

> Tuition five pounds per annum, one-half cash, one-half produce. Boarding and lodging within one mile of town at 9 pounds per annum. Those who wish to secure lodging will apply to Mr. Barr and Mr. Coburn in Lexington. Begin sometime in April, and French language with all sciences and arts will be taught. In the beginning of April all students will apply for entrance, as I shall be constantly in Lexington from that time.
>
> John Filson

Beyond grammar school, the new republic had little to offer. Along the Eastern seaboard there were colleges: Harvard (1636); William and Mary (1691); Yale (1700); Princeton (1746); Philadelphia (1754); and King's, now Columbia, (1754),[289] but only a small number of students had the opportunity to study at them.

The Apprenticeship

During the seventeenth, eighteenth, and nineteenth centuries, American youths who sought a medical career were indentured to an active practitioner. There were no medical schools in America until 1765; thus, before that date, the apprenticeship was the only means of securing a medical education. The age of the apprentices varied, with some entering into a contract at the age of fifteen or younger. Their services had a wide latitude, not always confined to medical training, e.g., grooming horses, running the master's errands, sweeping the office, building fires, and caring for the children. On the other hand the apprentices' experience in the "office" customarily included mixing medicines, spreading plasters, and, later, pulling of teeth, bleeding patients, nursing patients, and finally joining in the doctor's daily routine. For many of the earlier practitioners, this was their only training.

The apprenticeship system survived because it was the only means of becoming a physician in America until the mid-eighteenth century, and it continued to be the only means, except for a select few, into the nineteenth century. It also boosted the income of the physicians and freed them from menial chores.[290] Duties and rights were carefully negotiated by each party, apprentice and preceptor. Although there were modifications to the contract, the apprentice usually spent three to five years with his tutor, with a fee to the preceptor of about $100 per year. For this amount the apprentice received his room and board, books and equipment, and, upon completion, a certificate.[291] The apprentice method, and possibly a few lectures, was the sole means by which the first ten or so physicians in Lexington, with the exception of Samuel Brown, took their training.

Daniel Drake (1785-1852), one of the foremost medical educators of the nineteenth century, began his own medical education under a reputable preceptor, Dr. William Goforth of Cincinnati. Drake was but 15 years old when he began his apprenticeship in Cincinnati, a town of 1,000 people in 1800. Once settled in his preceptor's home, "his first assigned duties were to read John Quincey's *Dispensary*, and grind quicksilver into unguentum mercuriable; the latter of which, from previous practice on a Kentucky hand-mill, I found much the easier of the two."[292] At the end of the allotted time, Drake was given a certificate from his preceptor:[293]

> I do hereby certify, that Mr. Daniel Drake has pursued under my direction, for four years, the study of Physic, Surgery and Midwifery. From his good Abilities and marked Attention to the

> Prosecution of his studies, I am fully convinced that he is qualified to practice in the above branches of his profession.
>
> William Goforth, Surgeon General
> 1st Division Ohio Militia
> Cincinnati, State of Ohio, August 1, 1805

After his apprenticeship, Drake traveled by horse to Philadelphia,[294] arriving on November 9, 1805. Following six months of study in Philadelphia, Drake returned to Kentucky. On the departure of Dr. Goforth from Cincinnati to New Orleans (1807), Drake took over his practice and continued to serve the people of Cincinnati until 1815 at which time he returned to Philadelphia and received his medical degree from the University of Pennsylvania in May 1816.[295] Within a year, he accepted the chair of Materia Medica at Transylvania University, Lexington, Kentucky. "I am now going to astonish you," [Drake] wrote to a friend, "so cling hold of every support within your reach. *I am a professor!* Yes, incredible as it may appear to you and my other intimate friends, I am really and bona fide appointed a professor, and I repeat it on this side of the sheet to save you the trouble of turning back to see whether your eyes did not deceive you. I am, let me repeat, unquestionably a professor." Then he had a sobering thought. "But you must not suppose by this that I am a great man. For a professorship to confer greatness it must be a professorship in a great institution. But this [Transylvania] does not happen to be the case in this instance."[296] In 1830, Drake was offered the Chair of the Theory and Practice of Medicine, Jefferson Medical College, Philadelphia, a position he accepted to become the first Western physician to be invited to a professorship in an Eastern medical school.[297]

In 1844, Drake complained about "The almost total absence of discipline in the period of private pupilage; the preceptor seldom laying down any rules, and the student, for the most

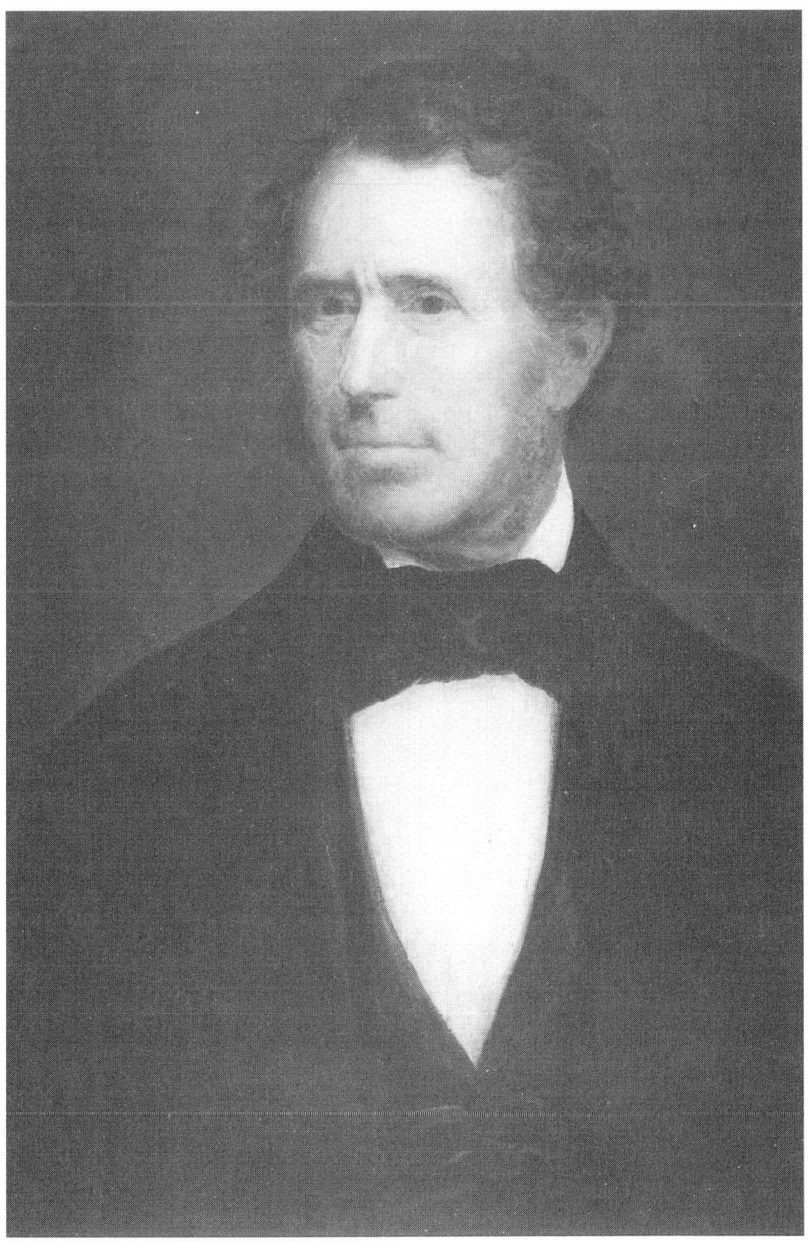

Daniel Drake, M.D. (1785-1852)
Courtesy of Fayette County Medical Society

part, coming and going at his pleasure, not even making his intended absence known to the preceptor. Reading on one topic today, and leaving it unfinished, taking up another tomorrow."[298] He added:

> The situation and circumstance in which a pupil should prosecute his studies deserve to be considered. In the country and all the smaller towns of the United States, the fashion is for the student to reside and study in the shop or office of his preceptor, and often to become a member of his family. The latter has its advantages, as contributing to preserve him from dissipation; but his time is often wasted in labors foreign to his studies, and he is apt to be introduced more frequently into company, than is compatible with his interests as a student.[299]

Choice of Preceptor

Records indicate that students who chose to study medicine under the direction of Lexington preceptors such as Frederick Ridgely had much to gain. Two of Dr. Ridgely's students, Drs. Walter Brashear and Benjamin Dudley, became internationally known. But because any physician could serve as a preceptor if he could attract apprentices, there was no standard of training. If the preceptor had been poorly trained, it was altogether likely that his apprentice would share the same deficiencies. Thus, there were those "physicians" who took on young men primarily to provide cheap labor, and, too, there were those young men who were equally incompetent and yet stayed on with the preceptor and "secured" their certificate. That the preceptorial method, generally speaking, was severely lacking is evident in the writings of Daniel Drake in 1832: "the physicians of the United States, are culpably inattentive to the studies of their pupils; and...this is one of the causes which retard the improvement, and arrest the elevation of the profession. Exceptions...are frequently met with, especially in the great cities; but still they are only exceptions."[300]

Drake recommended that the following tenets be considered when parents determined the choice of preceptor:[301]

> 1. It is not *necessary* that the preceptor should be a man of genius; but it is indispensable that he should possess a sound and discriminating judgment, or he will be a blind guide....
>
> 2. A preceptor should be learned, at least in his profession. If a father wishes to make his son a skillful mechanic, he places him with a good workman-not a botch....
>
> 3. It is not sufficient that a private preceptor has talents and learning. He must be devoted to his profession, jealous of its character, and ambitious of its honours....
>
> 4. The preceptor should be conscientious in the performance of his duties; that is, he should feel the responsibilities of his office, and studiously endeavor to discharge them....
>
> 5. The private preceptor should, if possible, be a man of business:-Punctual to his pecuniary engagements, accurate in his accounts, and systematic in all his affairs....
>
> 6. Finally, sound morals and chastened habits are not among the least of those qualifications, which an anxious father would require in the man, whose deportment and precepts are to exert so great an influence on the character of his son....

Drake did not limit his criticism of the preceptorship to that of the method or that of the preceptor. He cited deficiencies in the age of entry, stating that a pupil entering the study of medicine at age fifteen "generally sets up for himself" at the age of nineteen or twenty, "a time of life when he lacks *judgment*." Seventeen or eighteen was for Drake "the most proper age to commence study."[302] He recommended that students spend four years, not two or three, in their pupilage. At the age of twenty-one and after such experience, they would then be sufficiently mature, he believed, to begin practice.[303] He had no sympathy for parents who showed minimal discrimination "when about to put their sons to the study of medicine..." And because so many parents were themselves illiterate, they were unaware of the "importance of early intellectual discipline."[304] Drake stated, "The current opinion, that men of slender abilities are competent to the practice of physic, is, obviously, a great cause why so many feeble minded boys are dedicated to its study."[305] It is said that Drake wrote with both clarity and ease, garnished by a robust, incisive, and vigorous style. In reading his impression of his colleagues, we would agree:[306]

> Another cause of the evil which we deprecate, is the liberal proportion of inferior men, who unfortunately belong to the profession [medicine], and so often succeed in acquiring business and popularity. An observation of this fact, not a little mortifying to the more talented members of the profession, encourages parents to set apart for the study of medicine, those sons who are least remarkable for strength of mind; reserving, the better class, for pursuits which in their opinion require more vigour of intellect, or promise greater distinction.

The preceptorship system was practically the only opportunity for medical training, however inadequate, for well over two hundred years. To condemn the preceptorship would be equivalent to condemning the log cabin and the stage-coach. Each played a core role in the nation's growth, and, although each had its faults, what would we have done without them? In his foreword to Norwood's *Medical Education in the United States Before the Civil War*, Henry Sigerist, Johns Hopkins Medical Historian, quoted with approval a statement by Richard Shyrock that had just appeared in the *Isis*: "The value of studies in the history of American Science is not to be found primarily in contributions to the history of science as such, but rather to the history of the United States...."[307] This assertion, Sigerist thought, could be extended: "Shyrock's statement fully applies to the history of medicine....Medical education as it was practiced in the United States before the Civil War had certainly nothing to give the world and yet it was undoubtedly an important factor in the life of the nation."

Study Abroad

The opportunity for study abroad was limited to very few students. Indeed, not until 1718 did anyone from the colonies dare to take passage to Europe to study medicine.[308] But to study abroad was not without risk. Travel on the seas was subject to the mercy of the elements. And several young American students fell ill and died, victims of smallpox and other epidemic diseases rampant in England. A few of the early Lexington and Kentucky doctors attended the University of Edinburgh. The exodus of medical students to Europe continued into the nineteenth and early twentieth centuries; students went principally to Edinburgh or London in the eighteenth century, and then to Paris in the first half of the nineteenth century. During the last half of the nineteenth century and the first decade of the twentieth century, the medical institutions of Austria and Germany were the most popular choices of Americans for completing their training abroad. Abraham Flexner has this compliment for those who dared to go overseas:[309]

> Beginning early in the eighteenth century, having served their time at home, they resorted in rapidly increasing numbers to the hospitals and lecture-halls of Leyden, Paris, London and Edinburgh. The difficulty of the undertaking proved admirably selective; for the students who crossed the Atlantic gave a good account of themselves. Returning to their native land they sought opportunities to share with their less fortunate or less adventurous fellows the rich experience gained as they "walked the hospitals" of the old world....

First American Medical Schools

Although there were faculties of medicine in the Italian Universities of Padua and Bologna in the twelfth century, the medical school as a formal entity developed in Holland and extended through the disciples of Herman Boerhaave (1668-1738) into London, Edinburgh and Vienna. The London medical schools remained a part of the hospital system unassociated with the universities.

The founding of medical schools was under way in the colonies (Philadelphia) by 1765, under the leadership of a young Philadelphian, Dr. John Morgan (1735-1789), a medical graduate of Edinburgh (1763). At the age of thirty, Morgan expounded the basic principles for the integration of the medical discipline into the university system:[310]

1. A medical school ought to be an integral part of a college or university.

2. Hospital instruction should form

an integral part of instruction in a medical school.

3. Young men should come to the instruction of medicine with a liberal education.

4. The curriculum should follow a graded order from anatomy to clinical instruction and experience.

5. Teachers should have time to experiment and search for the secrets of nature.

We have noted the birth of the medical school in Philadelphia principally through the efforts of John Morgan. The importance of this event, however, is not simply the existence of a medical school itself but the fact that it was associated with a university.[311] It was this happy combination that made the sum of the two far greater than anything each could have possibly attained individually.

The University of Pennsylvania's medical school had its origin in Edinburgh as a consequence of Morgan's experience. Kings College (Columbia University) at New York followed suit in 1768 with its association with a medical school, once again founded by graduates of Edinburgh. Five university-affiliated medical schools were established in America by the end of the eighteenth century, namely, the College of Philadelphia (1765), (later united with the University of Pennsylvania), Kings College (1764), (later to become the Medical Faculty of Columbia College), Harvard University (1783), the Medical School of Dartmouth College (1798) and Transylvania (1799).[312] This highly productive relationship, the union of the medical schools and the universities, set the precedent for medical training in America, which today remains solidified and prosperous, the medical benefits flowing not only to its citizens but also to the world.

What John Morgan had envisioned in his historic address in 1765, namely that a medical school should be part of a college or university, seemed to be secure by 1800. Yet beginning in the 1820s and extending to the end of the nineteenth century, the university-affiliated medical schools were substantially outnumbered by the non-affiliated proprietary schools.[313] The latter schools arose principally on the conviction "that in a free country every one should have the right to follow any occupation he likes, and employ for any purpose any one whom he selects, and that each party must take the consequences."[314] The conflict, however, was not limited to these two broad categories, for the medical faculties of one university fought with those of another for students. Fees were lowered and the term shortened, all to attract those students who desired a degree more than an education.

The period from 1820 to 1910 was one of chaos and change in the field of medical education. In 1900, Henry Bowditch of Harvard Medical School, summed up nineteenth century medical education, namely, the transition from dependence on the apprenticeship to that of the medical school:[315]

> In those early days it was in the office of his preceptor and at the bedside, as his actual assistant, that the embryo physician was initiated into the mysteries of his calling. Then followed a period when it was clearly perceived that the trained mind is necessary to interpret the data of observation, and that mental training is essential to correct observation. Hence schools were established to provide this training by means of systematic didactic lectures covering all the departments of medicine and usually extending over not more than four months. These schools were intended at first

> merely to supplement the work of the preceptors, but in the process of time the relative importance of these two educational agencies was reversed and the work of the preceptors became supplementary to that of the schools. The function of the preceptors finally became so subordinate that their names no longer appeared in the catalogues, though this did not always indicate that they had ceased to afford students opportunities for practical clinical work.

In referring to the period of the American Medical Association's founding, Dr. Nathan Davis, founder of the A.M.A., states: "[A]t the end of the period we have under consideration, between 1840 and 1850, among all the forty or more colleges then existing, not one of them required of the student any standard of preliminary education, and the longest lecture terms were embraced in sixteen weeks of the year, while in several of them it was reduced to thirteen weeks, in which the student was to go over the whole field of medical science.…Some of the most vivid pictures of the evil effects that had been produced, are to be found in the writings of that eminent man of the Mississippi Valley, Dr. Daniel Drake."[316]

In 1820, Drake set forth his views on medical schools in his *Inaugural Discourses on Medical Education.*[317] Among several recommendations, he advocated a full complement of professors ("every medical school should have eight professors"),[318] a more thorough and liberal preparatory education, bedside teaching and hospital training, and the removal of the "existing evil of so many lectures each day" by lengthening the school term from four to five months. It has been said that there would have been no necessity for the Carnegie Report on Medical Education in the United States had Drake's principles of education been implemented by later medical educators.[319]

When Charles Eliot, the newly elected President of Harvard University in 1869, tried to initiate written examinations for medical degrees, he was resisted by the director of the medical school, who complained that most of the students could hardly write.[320] In 1891, David Starr Jordan, President of the University of Indiana, addressing the relation of medicine to the work of the college, stated:[321] "...for the number of college-bred men in medicine is lower than in almost any other profession. Statistics...show that in the United States at present, about one clergyman in four, one lawyer in five, and one physician in twelve, has had a college education.....Taking the country over, of all classes of students, those in medicine are as a rule (and such a rule admits of many individual exceptions) the most reckless in their mode of life and the most careless of the laws of hygiene and of decencies in general of any class of students whatsoever."

Transylvania Medical Department

Transylvania University was the first to found a medical department West of the Alleghenies. The founding of the medical school (1799) and the founding of the Lexington Medical Society (1799) had much in common, namely, their almost identical dates of origin, originators, and membership. This does not imply that the Society was an extension of Transylvania University, for this was not so. Membership in the Society included physicians practicing in Lexington who were unattached to the University, together with members of the University Faculty and their apprentices (also Transylvania medical students beginning in 1817). Transylvania, therefore, offered the Society not only refuge for meetings but also the stimulus of its renowned professors and the excitement of student members. That this cordial relationship of town physicians, medical faculty, and students continued through the mid-1830s is documented. The lack of substantive records pertaining to the Society after that time negates further speculation.

For medical students throughout the South and West, the presence of Transylvania University Medical School was a dream come true. Throughout this region, the opportunity to study medicine was limited both by the lack of schools and by the number of reputable physicians practicing in the rural areas who could act as preceptors.[322] In 1799, two distinguished physicians, both citizens of Lexington, made up the faculty. Dr. Samuel Brown was named professor of Chemistry, Anatomy, and Surgery; and Dr. Frederick Ridgely, Professor of Materia Medica, Midwifery, and the Practice of Physick. Dr. Ridgely was the first professor West of the Alleghenies to deliver lectures to medical students. In addition to Drs. Brown and Ridgely, the Board, on Thursday, October 7, 1802, unanimously elected Dr. Walter Warfield as professor of Medicine.[323] Although lectures were given to a small group of medical students by Professors Brown and Ridgely, who were also members of the Lexington Medical Society,[324] the school remained essentially one in name only for the next several years. Medical students at the time were apprentices to the town physicians; there were no Transylvania University medical students until 1817.

At the meeting of the Transylvania Board on Thursday, December 11, 1799, the Board authorized Dr. Brown to import medical books and other means of instruction for an amount not to exceed five-hundred dollars. Appointed as Professor of the Theory and Practice of Physic in 1805, Dr. James Fishback became the fourth member of the Transylvania Medical Department.[325] An announcement in the *Kentucky Gazette* of November 3, 1806, states: "A COURSE of Lectures on the Theory and Practice of MEDICINE, in the Transylvania University, will commence on the third Monday of the present month, (signed) JAS. FISHBACK, P.M., October 3, 1806." During the medical school's developmental phase, the medical apprentices evidently matched the faculty, being few in number. Presumably, the newness of the medical department, the small size of the Transylvania medical faculty (no more than three to four professors consistently from 1799 to 1809), inadequate facilities for lectures, and lack of chemistry equipment and anatomy specimens, hindered the growth of the Medical Department. By 1807, the founding fathers of the medical department, Brown and Ridgely, had left Lexington, Ridgely moving to Richmond, Kentucky in 1806, and Brown joining his brother James in New Orleans in 1807.

Although there was a brief flurry of activity relating to the Faculty of Medicine at Transylvania in 1809, little came of it other than the announcement. Dr. Benjamin Dudley, a Lexingtonian and a recent graduate of the University of Pennsylvania Medical School (1806), returned to the practice of medicine in Lexington and, together with Dr. James Fishback and the newly appointed Drs. James Overton and Elisha Warfield, attempted to restore some semblance of organization. Dr. Dudley, at the age of twenty-four, was appointed to the chair of Anatomy and Physiology; Dr. Warfield to Surgery and Obstetrics; and Dr. Overton to Materia Medica and Botany. There is no record at this time of the number of students, the delivery of lectures, the number of graduates, if any, or the other specifics of instruction. Dr. Warfield resigned his faculty appointment in 1809. The final blow came in 1810 with the departure of Dr. Dudley to Europe to study surgery in both Paris and London.

Reorganization of the Medical School

We know little of the medical activities taking place in Lexington between the years 1810 and 1815. Dr. C. C. Graham, a medical student at that time, relates the following:[326] "What few private students there were in Lexington went from shop to shop (at that day so called) and got three only, Dudley, Richardson, and eccentric Overton to give us a talk." We likewise have no account of the Lexington Medical Society during this period and extending until 1817. If the Society did meet, such meetings probably came about through the efforts of these three private physicians and the small cluster of students. Dr. Dudley recounts teaching anatomy and surgery to a group of twenty to twenty-five students in 1815 in "Trotters Warehouse" situated at the corner of Main and Mill

Streets, and the following year having fifty or sixty students attend.[327] This period of transition actually set the stage for the rejuvenation of the Transylvania Medical School that took place in 1817.

The first step toward reorganization of the medical school began with the resignation of the University president, James Blythe, to accept the Professorship of Chemistry in 1817. Other appointments followed:

> Dr. Benjamin Dudley, Professor of Anatomy and Surgery
> Dr. Daniel Drake, Professor of Materia Medica and Medical Botany
> Dr. William H. Richardson, Professor of Obstetrics
> Dr. James Overton, Professor of Theory and Practice

Twenty pupils attended the course of lectures in 1817, and in the spring of 1818 the degree of M.D. was conferred for the first time in the West. "John Lawson McCullough, of Lexington, was the first graduate of medicine in the valley of the Mississippi."[328] In March 1817 a group of Transylvania University medical students offered this public announcement:[329]

> *To James Overton, M. D., professor of the institutions and practice of physic; Dr. [Benjamin] W. Dudley, M.D., professor of anatomy and surgery, and the Rev. J. Blythe, D. D., professor of chemistry, in the Transylvania University.*
>
> Gentlemen- The undersigned having been appointed a committee by the Medical students of this place, to express their approbation of the courses of Lectures which they have lately had the honor to attend, beg leave, as organs of your

respective classes, to return their most grately acknowledgments, for the attention you have bestowed to the various duties which you voluntarily engaged to perform, and which has greatly contributed to increase their information.

With the most indefatigable perseverance you have succeeded in establishing your courses, against obstacles heretofore considered insuperable—and have been instrumental in giving character to an institution, which seems to ensure success, commensurate with the most sanguine expectations of all lovers of MEDICAL SCIENCE, in this important section of the union—an institution which in its progress to extensive popularity and usefulness, nothing short of the most casual and unforeseen events can oppose.

For your zeal in the diffusion of medical knowledge; for your kind attention to your respective classes, and the able assistance rendered to their exertions, permit us, gentlemen, to tender to you, our warmest gratitude, and to assure you that we shall ever remember you with the respect which your exertions have so richly merited.

Committee
David J. Ayres
Thos. J. Garden
Charles H. Warfield

The following tribute to members of the Transylvania Faculty was published on November 15, 1817, in the *Kentucky Gazette:*

TRIBUTE OF GRATITUDE
INTRODUCTORY LECTURES.

We have heard this week, with peculiar pleasure, the introductory lectures delivered by the professors of the MEDICAL COLLEGE; and, so far as we are competent to judge, we think that great professional talent was displayed. Certain we are, that the composition of the lectures, and the general information which they comprised, would do credit to any institution, however long established.

Dr. OVERTON'S lecture was distinguished by that beauty of style, those fine effusions of fancy, and that sound discriminating sense, which belong to superior genius and cultivated intellect.

Dr. DUDLEY'S lecture exhibited that learning, those solid professional acquirements, and that ardent devotion to medical science, which have rendered him decidedly the first anatomist and surgeon in the western country, and one of the best in the United States.

Of Dr. DRAKE'S lecture, we may truly pronounce, that it was one of the most finished performances we have ever witnessed, and showed him to be a master of his branches of the profession, and a man of general science.

Dr. RICHARDSON'S lecture, particularly the conclusion of it, was very good.

Dr. BLYTHE is universally acknowledged

> to be fully adequate to the duties of *chemical professor.* His introduction was learned and eloquent; and if at any time heretofore *"the foul hand of party spirit"* has profaned *"the temple of science, let us forget and forgive the past."*
>
> Upon the whole, our MEDICAL COLLEGE bids fair to become, and that soon, one of the best in the union; and we imagine that even now it is superfluous for western students to travel over the mountains to finish their professional education. The favorable opinion here entertained of the abilities of the faculty, can only incite them to redoubled exertions, in order to elevate and render permanent and general their good fame.

Transylvania—Lexington Bond

The respect that the Lexington community held for Transylvania University and for the professors of the Medical College is evident in this newspaper report March 10, 1821:[330] "$17,000 are to be expended in Europe this year for the [Transylvania] Medical Department. Doctor [Charles] Caldwell [the agent] is already on his way. $5,000 only is the gift of the Legislature, while $6,000 rest upon the responsibility of Lexington alone and $6,000 upon that of *six individuals* in the town who have generously stepped forward in this manner to anticipate the too cautious bounty of the Legislature." (Indeed, on several occasions the citizens of Lexington came to the rescue of Transylvania University and especially to that of the Medical Department.) The growth of the Medical Department of Transylvania University was a communal effort. The citizens of Lexington took considerable pride in the University and were ready to play their part in tangible contributions to aid its every success.

Medical Faculty Duels

Although duels were outlawed in Kentucky (1799) there were certain confrontations for which any alternative resolution by the participants would have been perceived as demeaning. Physicians were often in attendance in a professional capacity. In 1809, Drs. Warfield and Overton acted as surgeons in a duel fought by David Trimble and Henry Daniel, both attorneys, of Winchester, Kentucky. Mr. Trimble escaped unhurt; Mr. Daniels was dangerously wounded.[331] One of the more memorable events to occur after the reorganization of the medical school took place in 1817 and involved three members of the Lexington Medical Society and Transylvania Faculty, Benjamin Dudley, Daniel Drake, and William Richardson. The incident was a duel fought between Dudley and Richardson; however, the duelists were not necessarily the principal adversaries. As one would expect of such a heated controversy, there was more than one version. The following version is that of Dr. Robert Peter:[332]

> A difficulty having originated between himself [Dudley] and Doctor Drake, in relation to the resignation of the latter and some matters connected with a postmortem examination of an Irishman who had been killed in a quarrel, sharp pamphlets passed between them and a challenge to mortal combat from Dudley to Drake, which the latter declined, but which was vicariously accepted by his next friend, Doctor William H. Richardson. A duel resulted in which, at the first fire, Richardson was seriously wounded in the groin by the ball of Dudley, severing the inguinal artery. Richardson would have speedily bled to death—as it could not be controlled by the tourniquet—but for the ready skill and magnanimity of Dudley. He immediately asked permission of his adversary to

> arrest the hemorrhage, and by the pressure with his thumb over the ilium gave time for application of ligature by the surgeon of Richardson—thus converting his deadly antagonist into a lifelong friend.

In his biographical sketch of Dr. Drake in *Pioneer Life in Kentucky*, Emmet Field Horine offers a contrasting view:[333]

> Dissension arose in the medical Faculty—Dr. Benjamin Dudley and William H. Richardson quarreled throughout the session and Drake resigned at its close. Dudley then accused Drake of a breach of faith in addition to many charges of lesser importance. Drake issued a defense in pamphlet form addressed to the *Intelligent and Respectable People of Lexington* (1818) in which, with unanswerable logic, he refuted all charges. Some biographers of Drake have erroneously asserted that he refused to accept a challenge to a duel. Contemporary sources disclose that Drake was not challenged but boldly announced his positive intention of accepting any challenge proffered. Probably Dudley had had enough of dueling, having shortly before Drake's retort, fought with pistols in response to the challenge of William H. Richardson.

Dudley and Drake continued with an exchange of "pleasantries" and it was Drake who had the last and public word with his character assassination of Dudley: "In my first interview, I perceived the ensigns of Paris foppery to have nearly obscured the slender stock of intellect on which they were engrafted,-while a closer inspection soon convinced me, that egotism, ignorance, and sycophancy had formed within him an unholy alliance, and alternately guided the helm of his destinies."[334] After this barrage, the two men never brought their animosity to the public in this manner again, and when Drake returned to Transylvania in the mid-twenties their differences remained but were held within bounds of civility.

The duel fought between Drs. Dudley and Richardson arose from dissension between the two with respect to the latter's appointment as a professor in the Transylvania Medical Department (1817). Dr. Richardson did not have a medical degree. Dr. Drake became involved through his urging of Dr. Richardson's appointment. As Drake puts it: "I did not insist that Dr. Richardson, in particular, should be recognized as a Professor, though I strongly advised it." This incident was the root cause of a number of subsequent conflicts between the participants. One of the disagreements involved the Lexington Medical Society, however, before relating the specifics it is necessary to comprehend the general. For this purpose the *Note* by Dr. Drake at the close of his second pamphlet to the "Intelligent and Respectable People of Lexington" will suffice:[335]

> In the summer or autumn of 1815….Dr. Brown was elected Professor of the Institutes and Practice of Physic; Dr. Dudley of Surgery and Anatomy; Dr. Richardson of Obstetrics; Dr. Short of Materia Medica & Botany and Dr. Rogers adjunct Professor of Anatomy. Drs. Brown, Short and Rogers refused; but Drs. Dudley & Richardson accepted their appointments; and Dr. D. in the ensuing winter, delivered a course of lectures on anatomy and surgery. Dr. Overton, who was a candidate for the chair refused by Dr. Brown, proceeded at the same time to deliver a course on the institutes and practice of physic; and Dr. Blythe another on chemistry. In the following autumn a second election was held, which resulted in the choice of

> myself as Professor of Materia Medica and Botany; but the two other vacant chairs were not filled. In the ensuing winter, that of 1816-17, Doctors Dudley, Overton and Blythe resumed their courses; and, before the expiration of the season, the two latter were, by a union of their friends, elected, and signified their acceptance.

The unveiling of the incidents as given thus far by Drake are consistent with reports by others relating to the same events. It gives us the sequence of events occurring with the return of Dr. Dudley from Europe (1814) and the measures taken to revive the Medical Department. In this effort, Dudley played the leading role. The many medical apprentices in Lexington constituted sufficient audience to attract Drs. Dudley, Overton and Blythe to lecture on many occasions between 1815 and 1817. Indeed, the lectures were of such interest as to attract medial apprentices from Ohio. It did not take long, however, for disharmony to infect this incipient group.

We return to Drake's *Note:*

> The friends of Dr. Rogers, meanwhile, insisted that Dr. Dudley should relinquish to him one of his professorships; but this he refused [Dr. Dudley received a salary for each of the two professorships]. Dr. Richardson was among the number who urged this separation, and to this is to be attributed, in a great degree, the unfortunate differences between him and Dr. Dudley. About that period Doctors Overton and Dudley became united in their views; and although Dr. Richardson had been eminently instrumental in the election of the latter [sic], he joined Dr. Dudley in the technical objection to Dr. Richardson, that he had not grad-

> uated. Doctor Richardson believed, that, as Dr. Dudley was elected at the same time with himself, and made no objections to him; and as Dr. Overton had manifested a strong desire for admission into the College, not withstanding this circumstance, their objections were the result of hatred, inspired by his efforts in favor of Dr. Rogers, and refused, therefore to resign. A violent animosity was the consequence, and in that state they continued till the following October, when Doctors Dudley and Overton agreed to associate with Dr. Richardson, provided he would sign no diplomas until he graduated. Soon after this [1817], I arrived at Lexington, and the professors elect held a meeting. Dr. Richardson was recognized as a colleague, under the above condition, and leave of absence was granted him, in the winter of 1818-19, for the purpose of graduating in one of the eastern schools.

When Drake arrived in Lexington he was invited by Dr. Richardson to lodge at his home until his family arrived. Drake refused this kind invitation because to do so would have suggested his siding with Richardson in the latter's ongoing conflict with Dudley. Drake rightfully perceived that the truce between Dudley and Richardson was but temporary. And he did not want to "come to Lexington as a partisan." The matriculation for the school year 1817-18 now was at hand, and the faculty realized that any further delay, whatever its merit, would not be in the interest of Transylvania University. A meeting was called. Drake continues:

> This was the first meeting of the Faculty, and before that time, although Lectures had been delivered for two years, there was no Medical College organized; and our resolutions expressly

> declared that the students, who attended those courses, should not thereby be rendered eligible for degrees. I state this fact explicitly, because Doctor Dudley has blamed the recognition of Doctor Richardson (which he ascribes to my influence, although it had been agreed to before my arrival) for the loss of a brilliant student from the state of Ohio, who was a personal enemy of Dr. Richardson, and would not, therefore, we are given to understand, return to Lexington. We thus lost, says Dr. Dudley, the opportunity of conferring a diploma on "a young man who might have given as much eclat to our school as a graduate, as you have done in the capacity of professor." Now, by the resolutions of the Faculty just referred to, although this young man had attended some Lectures in Lexington the preceding winter; he could not have graduated until he went through two other full courses; but that he would not have done this under any circumstances, is evident from the fact, that he has since engaged in the practice of physic without visiting any Medical School.

With the admission of twenty medical students to the fall session of 1817, Transylvania Medical School was, at last, underway with a full faculty and its glory days dawning. Even with the smoldering antipathy between members of the faculty, the first year was a huge success, with one student, John Lawson McCullough of Lexington, the first graduate of the College of Medicine (1818). The calm was shattered, however, when in the spring of 1818 Drake announced his resignation. The confrontation that arose with Drake's resignation was but one of many clashes beginning to surface between Drake and Dudley. In a pamphlet by Drake, namely, *An Appeal to the Justice of the Intelligent and Respectable People of Lexington*, Drake denounced some fourteen charges brought by Dudley against him.[336] "That not a single charge, however trifling, may remain unrefuted."[337] He then proceeds with a point by point denunciation of each charge. Drake introduces the affairs of the Lexington Medical Society by quoting from extracts received in the way of an "affectionate and approbatory address" from his students:[338]

> We fear, however, from information derived from other sources, that you intend to resign. We intreat you to look around you, upon us and the Institution. We expected much from you, and our expectations have been surpassed...the lustre and fame you must shed upon our rising Institution by your superior talents—these call forth our deepest interest, as well as highest admiration.
>
> Be assured that we cannot find words to express our gratitude for your attentions to us, the smallest of which will never be forgotten.

Drake's devotion to his students and to the Lexington Medical Society are clearly set forth in the following passage:[339]

> To this I shall only add, that I attended the meetings of the Medical Society regularly, and was the only Professor of the College that attempted to meet and encourage the young men in that mode of prosecuting their studies. This can be testified by the whole society.

Drake held that formal lectures, even experience in medical practice itself, must be supplemented by the give and take of differing opinions and the exchange of ideas. Such beliefs were put into practice by debates between Drake and Caldwell, two of the leading medical educators of the day. In his *Appeal,* Drake relates:[340] "The Medical Society was in a very irregular state. I suggested to Dr. Dudley the importance of having it reorganized, and made an auxiliary institution to the College—a theatre for the Professors to appear upon in discussion before the students. He assented to the whole. The Constitution was revised, and at my suggestion, Dr. Dudley was elected President, and then utterly neglected to attend the meetings."

Among many broadsides delivered by Drake were the following:[341] "True it is, that while I have the disadvantage of being unknown to many of you, Dr. Dudley labours under the greater disadvantage of being well known…." And in closing he leaves the reader with no doubt whatever of his opinion of Dr. Dudley. "How far the preceding facts are adequate to this end, is not for me to decide. But I may be permitted to remark, that in proportion as they establish *my* innocence, they inevitably demonstrate Dr. Dudley to be a base and unprincipled villain, who has wantonly and wickedly attempted to destroy my reputation."[342] And to be certain that the reader did not miss his intent, Drake concludes: "Although I cannot like the Grecian Hercules, boast of having vanquished a monster, I may at least claim some praise for having ferreted out one of the vermin which infest our modern Attica."[343]

In contrast to the twenty-three page pamphlet by Dr. Drake, Dr. Dudley confines his reply to a mere eighteen pages.[344] The biting passages of Drake are met with an equal ferocity if not an equal pen. He chides Drake for the latter's pamphlet[345] "…unprecedented for its low vulgarity, unequaled for its abuse of individual character." He also strikes a blow at Drake's on again, off again relationship with the people of Cincinnati:[346] "I sincerely believe that, although 'comparatively a stranger,' your domestic virtues, your feelings of sympathy, affection, and humanity for those with whom you stand in close relationship, are more highly estimated even in Lexington, than in Cincinnati." Midway through the pamphlet, Dudley addresses the statement made by Drake referable to the Medical Society.[347] "I call on you," he says "to read the following certificates, handed me by the members of the society."

> WE, the undersigned, members of the Lexington Medical Society, do certify, that doctor Dudley did, during last winter, attend the meeting of said society as often as appeared consistent with his professional engagements; and further, that we have, on different occasions, heard doctor Dudley and doctor Drake discuss the same subjects in the society together.
>
> (Signed) CHRISTO. GRAHAM,
> JONA. STOUT,
> S. P. RUSSELL,
> J. H. ROYLE

> WE, the undersigned members of the Medical Debating Society, being called upon to certify concerning the attendance of doctor Dudley and Drake at the said society during last winter—state, that we recollect to have seen doctor Dudley at four, and doctor Drake at eight meetings. We further certify, that we recollect once to have heard doctors Dudley and Drake discuss the same subject.
>
> SAM. P. RUSSELL
> JOHN T. PARKER
> GEORGE W. VENABLE
>
> *Lexington, July 25th, 1818*

Several pages later, Dudley returns to the affairs of the Medical Society.[348] "Your assertion in regard to your being the only professor who attended the meetings of the Medical Society, is controverted by the positive testimony of the members of that body." He then refers to the process of the nomination of himself to the presidency of the Medical Society.[349] "That you have perverted the truth in relation to the presidency of the Medical Society, is clear from the certificate of Mr. Graham. That you have perverted the truth in regard to my attendance on the society, we have ample testimony, in the certificates of different members of the society."

In reply to Dr. Dudley, Drake issued a thirty-one page *Second Appeal.*[350] In this second pamphlet Drake reiterates his recommendation that the Lexington Medical Society be reorganized and made an auxiliary institution to the Transylvania University. Drake then proceeds to attack the "good for nothing" certificates:[351] "But if I had not already seen how little sagacity Dr. Dudley possesses relative to certificates, I should be very much surprised to find that of Mr. Graham introduced. I never made a *nomination* in that Society, nor did I know who nominated the officers. All that I said was, that Dr. Dudley was elected at my *suggestion.*" To prove his point Drake introduces a letter from Mr. Venable, one of the signers of the certificates:[352]

> I recollect very well (says he) that you requested me to use my influence in procuring the election of Dr. Dudley, as President, and Dr. Richardson as Vice President, for the purpose of *conciliating the differences* between those two gentlemen. Mr. Royle is very certain that you spoke publicly in favor of the election, of Drs. Dudley and Richardson, the evening on which it took place: Mr. Russell is perhaps equally certain.

Drake takes credit for the election of Dudley as President of the Lexington Medical Society because the election of Dudley took place "not long after my *suggestion*, it was quite natural to attribute to it the influence which I did. This will be sufficient for all who comprehend the difference between the words *suggestion* and *nomination*; to those who, like Dr. Dudley, are too ignorant for such distinctions, I have nothing to say."[353] He then proceeds to breakdown the substance of the first certificate by casting doubt as to the veracity of the signers' elusive account of Dudley's attendance at the Society's meetings namely that he attended " as frequently as *in their opinion*, was consistent with his professional engagements." Drake concedes that this "might have been once or twice." He adds that two of the signers, Royle and Russell, acknowledge that they had testified to more than was correct and that they "made an earnest application to have their names taken off; and were surprised and mortified to find that it was not done."[354] Drake then asserts that the other subscribers, Messrs. Graham and Stout were Dr. Dudley's favorite students.[355] Dr. Drake does not take issue with the second certificate, acknowledging that Dr. Dudley may well have been present at society meetings on four occasions "But considering that he [Dudley] was the President, that he had placed himself at the head of the Medical College, and that the meetings of the Society were held at his own *shop*, his attendance was absolutely a minimum; that, in short, in comparison with the claims of the Institution upon him, it was utter neglect." He continues to solidify his position by recalling: "I never saw him [Dudley] in the Society but twice, and was really surprised that he could so contrive to be from home when it assembled." Drake obviously believed that clarifying the record of attendance of the President, Dudley, was of prime importance. "I have deemed it necessary to dwell for some time on this subject (altho' no part of the original dispute) that it might be correctly understood, before a final decision on my veracity is awarded by those to whom I am personally unknown…."[356]

Daniel Drake left Lexington for Cincinnati in 1818, where he founded the Medical College of Ohio. Following a bitter controversy in Ohio, Drake resumed his professorship in Lexington from 1823 to 1827.[357] The author has observed that to a considerable degree the decision to favor Dudley or Drake in this famous dispute rests on the distance the particular writer resided from

Lexington or Cincinnati. And as in most disputes the truth is apt to rest about midway.

Speaking on the merits of Daniel Drake, Dr. David W. Yandell,[358] twenty-fourth President of the American Medical Association, said, "As a lecturer Doctor Drake had few equals. He was never dull. His was an alert and masculine mind. His words are full of vitality. His manner was earnest and impressive. His eloquence was fervid." Drake was such a gifted physician, writer, teacher, and consummate member of the medical communities of Lexington, Louisville,[359] and Cincinnati[360] that each city can revere and share in the time that he spent in each of their medical schools. The great William Osler said of Drake, "In many ways Daniel Drake is the most unique figure in the history of American medicine."[361] His accomplishments and person loom ever larger in the epic of medicine.

New President and Medical Faculty

A series of events in 1819 ushered in the period that was soon to put Transylvania University among the elite of American medical schools. First, there was the appointment of the Reverend Horace Holley to the Presidency of the University. The highly acclaimed Dr. Charles Caldwell (1772-1853) of Philadelphia was called to the Chair of the Institutes of Medicine and Materia Medica, and Dr. Samuel Brown, at the very last moment, was lured away from the invitation to join Dr. Drake in Cincinnati to take the chair of the Theory and Practice of Medicine. Also the noted naturalist, C. S. Rafinesque,[362] was persuaded to lecture on Botany and Natural History. Added to this distinguished group were the on-site professors, Benjamin Dudley, James Blythe, and William H. Richardson. A rapid increase in the number of students took place at this time, beginning with twenty students and one graduate in 1817 and then escalating to two hundred students and fifty-six graduates in 1823-24.[363]

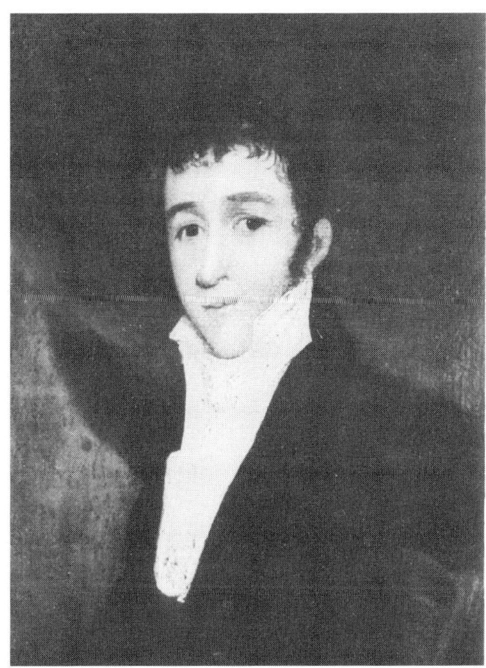

James Overton, M.D.
(1785-1865)
Courtesy of Transylvania University Library

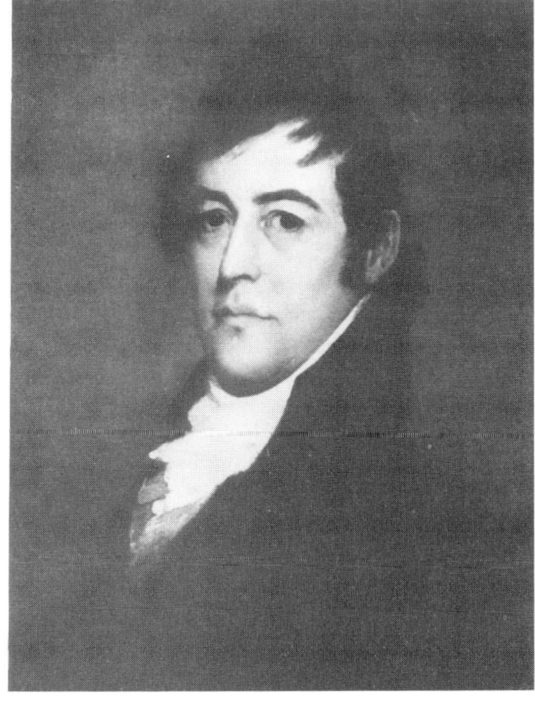

William Hall Richardson, M.D.
(1785-1845)
Courtesy of Transylvania University Library

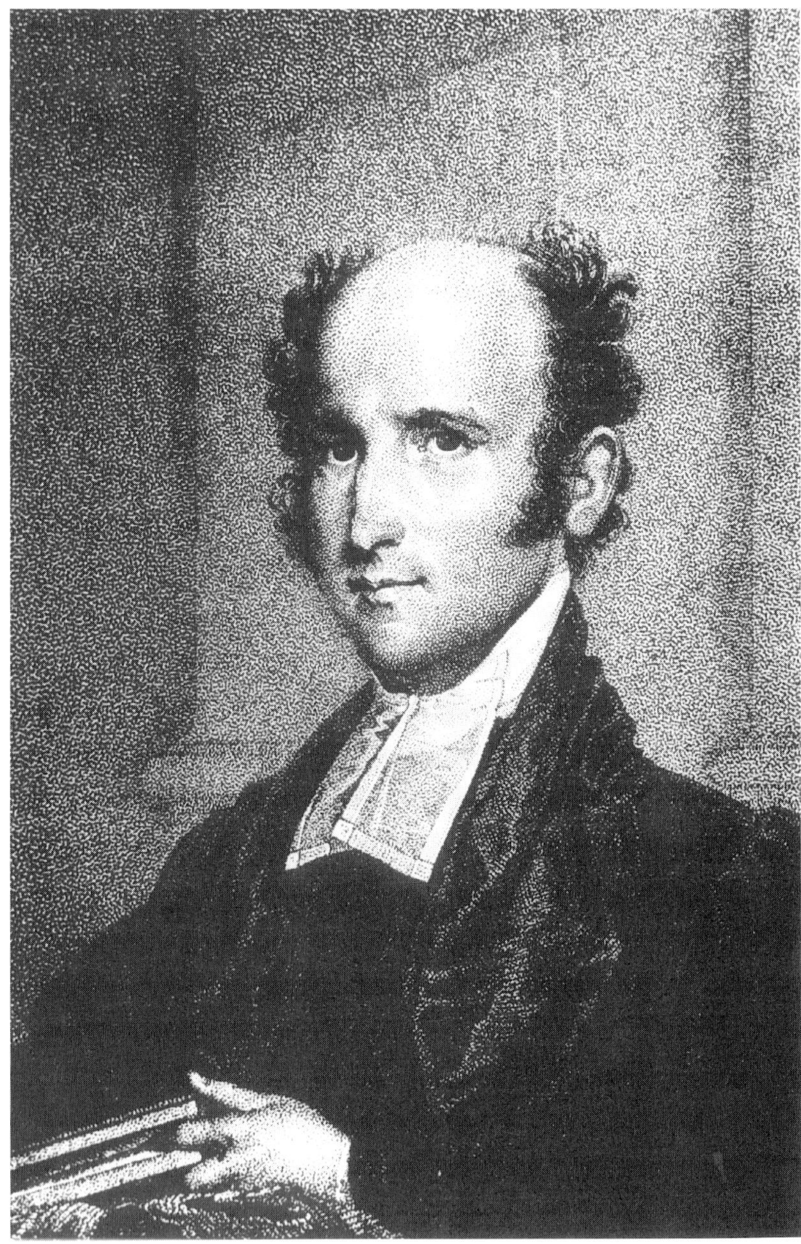

Horace Holley, A.M., A.A.S.,
President, Transylvania University 1819-1827
Courtesy of Transylvania University Library

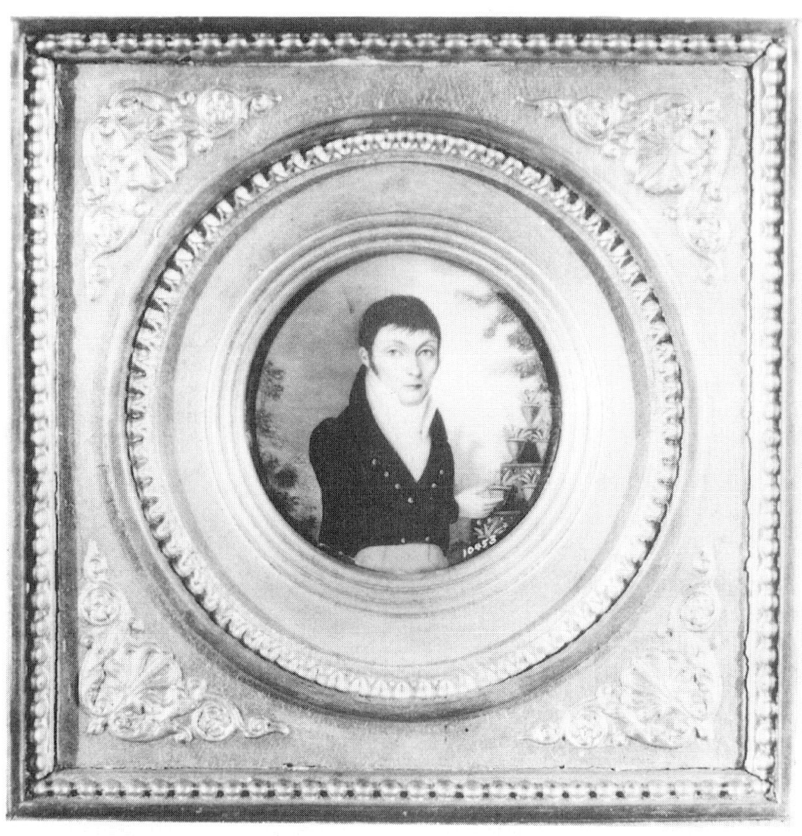

Constantine S. Rafinesque (1784-1840)
Professor of Natural History and Botany of Transylvania University
Courtesy of Transylvania University Library

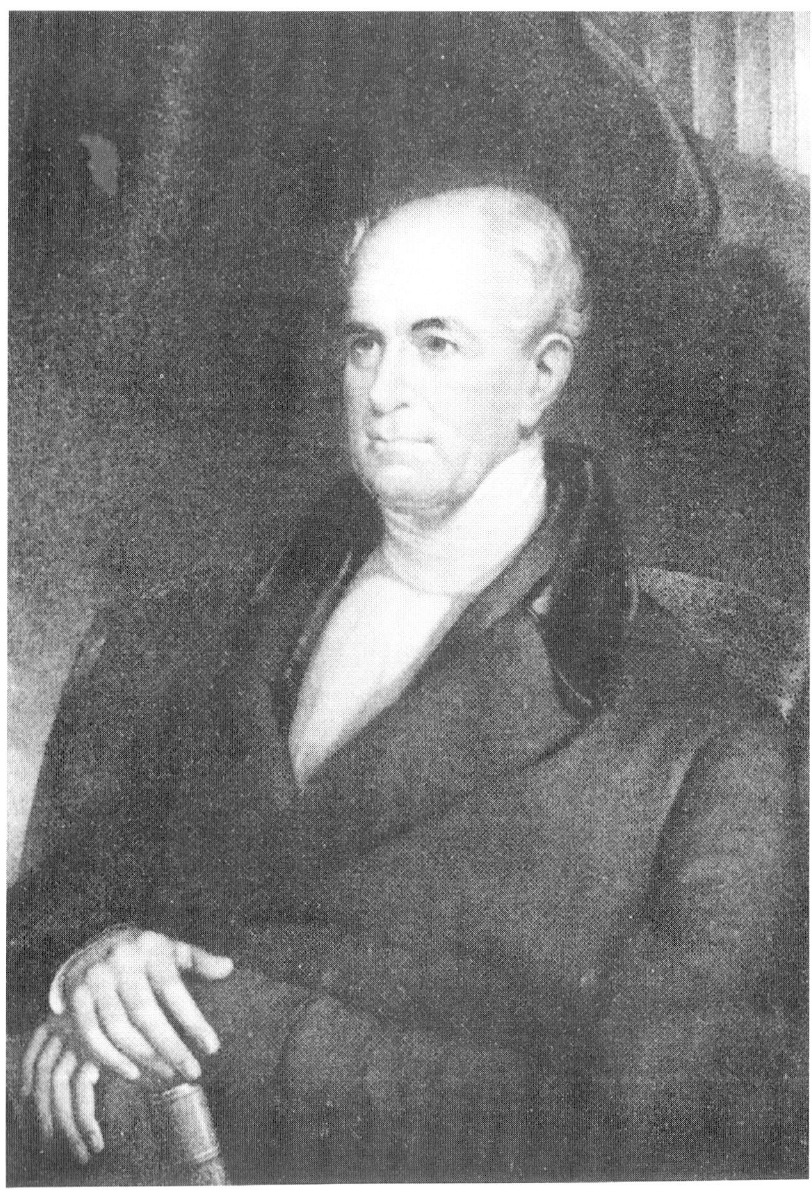

Charles Caldwell, M.D. (1772-1853)
Courtesy of Transylvania University Library

Before leaving Philadelphia in 1819 for the Chair of Medicine at Transylvania University, Dr. Charles Caldwell had been a rival of Dr. Nathaniel Chapman(first president of the AMA) for the Chair of the Institutes of Medicine ("the chair of Benjamin Rush") at the University of Pennsylvania, Philadelphia.[364] Known as Transylvania's "superlative egotist," Caldwell fed on controversy.[365] His personal appearance was that of a monarch "with scepter waving in his hand, he moved majestically along."[366] Caldwell's major contribution unquestionably is the many rare and valuable works [bought in Europe] which made the Transylvania Medical Library superior to any other at that time in this country."[367]

Dr. Caldwell was the first honorary member of the Tennessee State Medical Association. He was in Nashville for a scheduled address on phrenology and was characterized, at the time, by a local newspaper as "an enthusiastic as well as an ingenious and eloquent defender."[368] A humorous tale of Caldwell's boundless ego is told by Dr. Samuel Gross: In lecturing to an audience in Lexington, Dr. Caldwell announced "There are only three great heads in the United States, one is that of Daniel Webster, another that of Henry Clay, and the last," pointing to his own, "modesty prevents me from mentioning."[369]

On December 8, 1821, in one of his several letters to his friend, Thomas Jefferson, Dr. Samuel Brown gave the following account of Transylvania University and the Medical Department:[370]

> The number of Students in this university, including the Preparatory school which is immediately attached to it, as will appear in the Report of the President 366— The Medical Department, of which I know more, consists of 135 regular Medical Students who will practice Medicine as a profession—Previous to the establishment of this Medical Institution Kentucky never sent to the Atlantic Schools more than 10 or 12 Medical students annually-By examining our Matriculation

> list it appears that this state alone furnishes our classes with 90-the rest are collected from ten different states-I mention this fact to show how important it is to increase the number of our Medical institutions & to bring Education more into the reach of the lower & middling classes of society, whose habits of industry & labour so often advance them to the highest ranks of professional usefulness & reputation-From what I have seen of the Med. Students here & in Philadelphia, & N York, I have no hesitation in affirming, that with *equal means of instruction* double the amount of information would be acquired here in an equal time-We have no amusements to attract, few dissipations to tempt our young men from regular study & we have no *fame* as a school which can be substituted for individual merit. When Medical Schools become very large the Professors & not the Pupils are the gainers-Two hundred is as great number as can profit in one class, from the Anatomical Demonstration of the Clinical case—Why do not Virginia establish a Medical School at Richmond or Norfolk?

Jefferson founded the University of Virginia's medical school in 1825. "In contrast to the medical school at Transylvania, that at Virginia first taught medicine as a cultural rather than as a professional study."[371]

The Medical Department of Transylvania and other medical schools of the time customarily received students after their completion of an apprenticeship. The Transylvania Faculty did not consider the two-term curriculum as a replacement for the preceptorship but rather as a supplement. There was no test of accomplishment, i.e., "...no examination for promotion from the office of the preceptor to the benches of the lecture room."[372] Obviously, there were minor to major differences in the abilities of the entering students, yet the first-year students might sit alongside the more senior students, the latter having had the advantage of one or more years of apprenticeship and a full term of courses. At Transylvania, as in all medical schools in the United States during Drake's lifetime, "the lectures of each preceding year, (were), as to topics, the same with the last."[373] Many students alternated, i.e., would enter the school without having fulfilled the requirements of the apprenticeship, take a course of lectures, and then return to the apprenticeship for another period of time before returning to the school for further lectures. Graduated courses, those moving from a lower level of study to succeeding higher levels, did not come into play until the latter third of the nineteenth century.[374] To attend a lecture, students had to buy tickets from the professors, and attended as many courses during the first term as they felt profitable.[375] The remaining courses were taken on return to the medical school. Drake considered the idea of classifying the students as juniors and seniors; otherwise, he suggested that a student "direct his attention, chiefly, during the first course, upon Descriptive Anatomy, the Institutes of Medicine and of Surgery, Chemistry, Pharmacy, and the Natural History of Medicine." The second year, he suggested, should be reserved for "General and Surgical Anatomy, Operative Surgery, Therapeutic Materia Medica, Obstetrics, and the Diseases of Women and Children." [376]

There also were problems, namely the lack of roads and the lack of funds. Trails, not roads, led to Lexington from any direction. Many students attended but one term, and others would drop out for a period of time to better their finances and then return for the second term. We can glimpse the travails of travel in the experiences of Professor Charles Caldwell, on his visit to Europe to purchase books and apparatus for the Medical Department of Transylvania University in 1820.[377] The trip from Lexington to Maysville was an adventure. Caldwell had one servant and three horses, one a pack-horse for luggage. "The animals were all powerful and active," but "so deep and adhesive was the mud that they did not reach Maysville-only sixty miles distant-until an early hour on the fourth day." We now can only partially appreciate the danger, the toil, and the sweat shared by medical students and others who traveled for hundreds of miles to attend Transylvania. Yet, Transylvania was so much more appealing than Philadelphia because of the cost and added difficulties of travel that the number of westerners attending Transylvania was several-fold those attending the medical schools of Philadelphia. By the school year 1825-26, the student enrollment at Transylvania Medical School (235)[378] was second only to that of the University of Pennsylvania (480). In a letter of February 1826 to Horace Holley, the departing president of Transylvania, Henry Clay wrote: "The catalogue with which you have favored me exhibits a highly prosperous condition of the Medical School, which, in some measure, compensates for the less flattering situation of the College."[379]

Transylvania Medical School

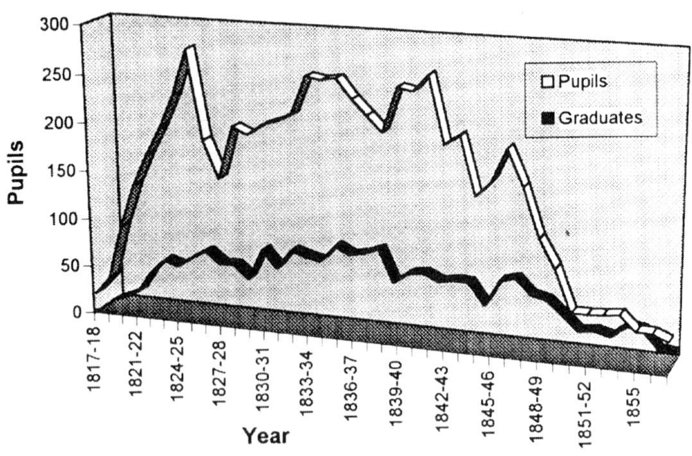

Chart depicting the pupils and graduates of Transylvania University Medical Department
Information taken from:
The History of The Medical Department of Transylvania University
by Doctor Robert Peter

Grave Robbers

Anatomical instruction and dissection were integral parts of medical education in 1817, as they are today. However, the source and ready availability of anatomical specimens were invariably in doubt. Dr. C. C. Graham gave an account of his first-hand student experience in Lexington:[380]

> Dead bodies at that day were not articles of commerce, so we, the students, had to disinter them; and we once had a battle, so published in the newspapers, at the old Baptist graveyard-The Battle of the Graveyard, so-called-when taking up the Irishman that caused the duel (between Dudley and Richardson). We were taken prisoners by an armed guard and hauled up to the court-house for trial, but there was no law to make the dead private property, so the declaration of Scripture that from dust we came and unto dust we must return let us off by paying one cent damages for taking that much clay or soil. At another time, near Nicholasville, we were pursued when making our way to our horses hitched outside an orchard fence, and one ball of several fired lodged in the subject, on my back.

For those who could afford private lessons and lived where such were available there was the chance of limited individual training in anatomy. Indeed, one of the best things a preceptor could do for his students was to instruct them in practical anatomy; however, if the preceptor's familiarity with anatomy came primarily from the textbook, then its usefulness was curtailed. However essential anatomy was to the study of medicine, autopsies were seldom requested or sanctioned. Occasional hangings afforded a legal dissection, but generally bodies were "imported" or sometimes stolen.[381]

Lexington Medical Society

What happened to the Lexington Medical Society during the latter decades of the first half of the eighteenth century? The last extant record of the Society was the previously reported address by Dr. Caldwell to the Lexington Society in 1834. As previously intimated, the fortunes of the city of Lexington, Transylvania University, and the Lexington Medical Society were closely bound. With the departure of Drs. Caldwell, Yandell, Cooke, and Short to Louisville in 1837-38, perhaps the interest and the time that the remaining faculty members of Transylvania had to devote to the Society was decreased. From 1834 to 1869, the activities of the Society were either non-existent or its records were lost, probably the latter.

The Demise of the Medical School

The Medical School lost two of its leading professors in the mid-1820s. In a letter of 20 February 1825, Daniel Drake reported to Henry Clay: "We have had the misfortune to lose Profr [sic] Brown. He delivered a final valedictory to the class on Friday and will send in his resignation perhaps tomorrow. I did all in my power to prevent such a consummation; and greatly fear that we shall suffer from it, by a diminution in our future classes."[382] Drake, himself, left Lexington in 1827 and returned to Cincinnati.

Many factors were responsible for the downfall of the Transylvania University Medical School. The Medical Faculty debacle of 1837-38, with the transfer of four outstanding members, played its part; however, there were events long before, many of which were unrelated to the machinations within the University and which were even more irreparable. Some of the events were local, whereas others were regional and national. The City of

Lexington, which had been so magnanimous in its support of Transylvania University, was no longer the "Metropolis of the West." Without question the most damage to Lexington was the lack of river transportation. Before the steamboat, the advantage of the river highways was not sufficient to overcome the attraction of the interior cities such as Lexington, but with the emergence of the two-way river traffic by steamboat navigation, Lexington's destiny was foretold. Cincinnati and Louisville, both of which were villages when Lexington was a vibrant and growing city, now had surpassed Lexington. One problem fed another; population in Lexington declined from about 8,000 in 1814 to a discouraging 4,000 in 1820. Businesses left the city for the more profitable river towns; the city attracted fewer people, and property values plummeted. The population of Cincinnati, which was but 2,000 in 1810, had risen to 24,000 in 1830, compared to Lexington's 5,000.

Relief seemed to be at hand in 1831 when a railroad, "The Lexington & Ohio," was begun. The opening ceremony was a celebrated event, with the illustrious Dr. Caldwell prophesying to the audience the great benefits to be derived. Unfortunately, the railroad was slow to progress, having reached only as far as Frankfort by 1835. The railway itself "was composed of stone sills laid side by side, with a dressed surface on the portion upon which the wheels were to run. The cars resembled an old pattern of streetcar and were drawn by horses."[383] Unfortunately, relief by the railroads lay decades ahead. By the twenties and thirties, Louisville and Cincinnati were no longer content to stand aside; they, too, had visions of medical grandeur. And so, the medical schools of neighboring cities, more advantageously situated on the navigable rivers, drew students who heretofore would have matriculated at Transylvania. The population decline of Lexington, beginning in 1810 and continuing into the twenties, had an unforeseen and detrimental effect: the withering away of anatomical specimens. What had already been a very difficult problem was now exacerbated.

The action of the Transylvania president, Dr. Holley, in bringing about the emergence of a medical faculty second to none in the United States, an improved medical library, additional instruments for teaching, and the attraction of students from ten states other than Kentucky, ran counter to the tide of events in Lexington, undercutting the institution even as it reached new heights in education. The flair and the genius of the Transylvania Medical Faculty (Dudley, Drake, Caldwell, Brown and others) could not, in the end, slow or reverse the inexorable decline of the city and its university.

Although the reasons as given above are sufficient to bring nearly any undertaking to its knees, there were two additional causes that led to the demise of the city itself, the undoing of Transylvania University, and the declining fortunes of the medical community and its affiliate, the Lexington Medical Society. The two factors were the Cholera epidemic of 1833 and the failure of the Kentucky Legislature to adequately fund Transylvania University, which was at the time the state university.

The Cholera Epidemic

The Cholera epidemic of 1833 brought about the deaths of hundreds of people in and near Lexington. Life and property were decimated, but the destruction did not end there, for the disease also put an end to the myth of Lexington as a paradise of health, a sanctuary somehow divorced from the fevers and dysenteries of the East. No longer was Lexington a haven for the invalid; its vaunted medical professors were as inept at diverting or stopping the ravages of this ghastly plague as were quacks and Indian doctors.

The Legislature

In a speech to the Kentucky Legislature in 1836, Dr .

Caldwell made a plea for an endowment to the Transylvania Medical School.[384] He outlined to the Legislature the gifts by other states to their universities of $100,000 to $150,000. "In New Jersey, a State far behind Kentucky in population and wealth, an arrangement is made to raise one hundred thousand dollars, for the improvement of education in the college at Princeton....Even Indiana and Illinois, which in their capacity of States, are but the creations of yesterday, are fast taking the lead of us in the career of education." This was an outstanding speech, and Dr. Caldwell evoked every emotion to sway the Legislature. "If you demand work from your colleges, you must fit them for that work. You must give them strength and the means that are required." And to their pride he prodded "We all pride ourselves on the Independence of the Union, and boast of it as loudly and earnestly as the people of any other State. But where, let me ask you, *in a literary and scientific point of view*—where is the proud and manly spirit of KENTUCKY INDEPENDENCE?...the spirit of Kentucky independence is no where to be found...." Dr. Caldwell was well known for saying what he wanted to say as he wanted to say it. He continues:

> ...there appears to be, among the people of Kentucky, a disposition to begin Education, if they begin it at all, at the *wrong end.* The loudest if not the only call is for *Common School* education. How, I ask, can that be obtained, and diffused through the Commonwealth, without *competent teachers*, in number to supply the demand? And where can they be formed, but in the *higher* seats of learning. I say, *"competent teachers;"* for if they be *incompetent*, they are an *evil* rather than a good, and should be treated accordingly. Kentucky must either *form able teachers* herself, or *procure ordinary* ones from other States. Accomplished instructors will be retained elsewhere, where they are more esteemed, and better paid."

Louisville Bound

Dr. Caldwell's appeal went unanswered. A year later his name no longer appeared on the list of Transylvania University faculty; he had moved to Louisville to join the faculty of the new medical college, the Louisville Medical Institute. Dr. Caldwell's departure was not without acrimony. Dr. Dudley also had considered making the move to Louisville, and when he withdrew, Dr. Caldwell became incensed, setting off a public tongue-lashing culminating in the dismissal of Professor Caldwell from Transylvania University.[385] The loss of Drs. Caldwell, Yandell, Short, and Cooke to Louisville in 1837-1838 severely impaired the prestige of Transylvania. The impact of the loss of these eminently qualified professors, namely their ability to draw students, was not immediate, for the Transylvania medical class size remained above 200 during the next five years, decreasing to 120 in 1848-49, and then sinking to 32 at its last term 1856-57.[386] Although the Faculty was reorganized in 1838 with the addition of Drs. John Eberle, Thomas D. Mitchell, and James C. Cross, the Medical Department never regained its previous eminence.[387]

281 John A. Schutz and Douglass Adair, eds., T*he Spur of Fame: Dialogues of John Adams and Benjamin Rush,* 1805-1813 (San Marino, CA: The Huntington Library, 1980), 50.

282 Jack P. Greene and J. R. Pole, eds., *The Blackwell Encyclopedia of the American Revolution* (Cambridge, Mass.: Basil Blackwell, 1991), 412-13.

283 Ibid.

284 N. S. Davis, "Address on the Present Status and Future Tendencies of the Medical Profession in the United States," *JAMA*, vol. 1, no. 2 (July 1883).

285 Clay Lancaster, *Vestiges of the Venerable City; A Chronicle of Lexington, Kentucky,* (Lexington, Ky.: Lexington-Fayette County Historic Commission, 1978), 11.

286 Ibid. "It has been said that the first school in Lexington was started to keep the younger boys occupied so that they would not be roaming through the forests where they might be picked up by prowling Indians." Workers of the Federal Writers' Project of the WPA, *Lexington and the Bluegrass Country* (Lexington, Ky.: E. M. Glass, Publisher, 1938), 14.

287 Ibid. John Filson, surveyor, adventurer, and first historian of Kentucky.

288 Charles R. Staples, *The History of Pioneer Lexington,* 1779-1806, with a foreward by Thomas D. Clark (Lexington, Ky.: The University Press of Kentucky, 1939), 298.

289 James Thacher, *American Medical Biography or Memoirs of Eminent Physicians Who Have Flourished in America* (Boston: 1828; reprint, New York: Milford House, Inc., 1967), 16.

290 "Some practitioners had a veritable band of students. Dr. Thomas Hubbard of Pomfret, Conn., rode fast and furiously over the country followed by a pack of apprentices, known by his disapproving colleagues as 'his hounds.'"

Rosemary Stevens, *American Medicine and the Public Interest* (New Haven: Yale University Press, 1971), 13, note 6.

291 William G. Rothstein, *American Physicians in the Nineteenth Century* (Baltimore and London: The Johns Hopkins University Press, 1985), 85.

292 Rothstein, *American Physicians in the Nineteenth Century,* 85-86.

293 Daniel Drake, *Practical Essays on Medical Education and the Medical Profession in the United States,* with an introduction by David A. Tucker (Baltimore: The Johns Hopkins Press, 1952) ix.

294 One writer [Charles D. Aring, ed., *Daniel Drake, M.D., Frontiersmen of the Mind* (Cincinnati: Crossroads Books, 1985), xviii.] states that the trip by horseback took eighteen days from Cincinnati to Philadelphia.

295 Ibid., xviii-xx.

296 James Thomas Flexner, *Doctors on Horseback* (New York: The Viking Press, 1937), 193.

297 Daniel Drake, "Biographical Sketch of Daniel Drake, MD (1785-1852)," *Pioneer Life in Kentucky* 1785-1800, Emmet Field Horine, ed. (New York: Henry Schuman, 1948), xxii-xxiii.

298 Henry D. Shapiro and Zane L. Miller, eds., *Daniel Drake, Physician to the West* (Lexington, Ky.: University Press of Kentucky, 1970), 297.

299 Drake, *Practical Essays on Medical Education,* 25.

300 Ibid., 41.

301 Ibid., 21-22.

302 Drake, *Practical Essays on Medical Education,* 24.

303 Ibid., 24-25.

304 Ibid., 17.

305 Ibid., 8.

306 Ibid., 9.

307 Ronald L. Numbers, *The Education of American Physicians: Historical Essays* (Berkley: University of California Press, 1980), 2.

308 Elizabeth H. Thomson, "Thomas Bond, 1713-84, First Professor of Clinical Medicine in the American Colonies," *Journal of Medical Education* 33, no. 9 (1958) : 614-624.

309 Abraham Flexner, *Medical Education in the United States and Canada: A Report to the Carnegie Foundation for the Advancement of Teaching,* Bulletin no. 4, with introduction by Henry S. Pritchett (New York City: The Carnegie Foundation for the Advancement of Teaching, 1910; reprint, 1960), 5. Flexner played a definitive role in medical education with the publication of the Carnegie Report.

310 Morgan's basic principles as stated here are formulated by William F. Norwood in "Critical Incidents in the Shaping of Medical Education in the US," JAMA, 15 November 1965, vol. 194, no. 7 : 715. John Morgan expounded his principles in *A Discourse Upon the Institution of Medical Schools in America* (Philadelphia: William Bradford, 1765; Reprint, New York: Arno Press, 1975).

311 David R. Goddard, "Medicine and the Universities," *JAMA* 194, no. 7 (1965) : 133-136.

312 The number of medical schools existing before the end of the eighteenth century is variously listed depending upon the writer, the definition of what constitutes a medical school and the number of faculty and graduates. In other instances, Transylvania is not recognized as established until 1817, because there was not a "full faculty" (a full faculty at the time was made up of six professors) and no medical graduates. On occasion, Transylvania Medical School has been erroneously described as "second in the whole United States." Robert S. Peter, *History of the Medical Department of Transylvania University* (Louisville, Ky.: John P. Morton & Co., 1905), Introduction, x.

313 "Between 1810 and 1840, twenty-six new medical schools sprang up; between 1840 and 1876,

forty-seven more; and the number actually surviving in 1876 has been since then much more than doubled. First and last, the United States and Canada have in little more than a century produced four hundred and fifty-seven medical schools, many, of course, short-lived, and perhaps fifty still-born. ...The city of Cincinnati brought forth about twenty, the city of Louisville eleven. These enterprises—-for the most part they can be called schools or institutions only by courtesy—-were frequently set up regardless of opportunity or need: in small towns as well as in large, and at times almost in the heart of the wilderness."

Flexner, *Medical Education in the United States and Canada*, 6.

314 Frank Bradway Rogers, ed., *Selected Papers of John Shaw Billings* (Baltimore: Waverly Press, 1965) Medical Library Assoc. Publication No. 2, "Ideals of Medical Education" delivered at Yale University, 1891, 1965 : 208.

315 H. P. Bowditch, "The Medical School of the Future," *Boston Medical and Surgical Journal* CXLII, no. 18 (May 3, 1900) : 445, 449.

316 Davis, "Address on the Present Status and Future Tendencies of the Medical Profession in the United States," JAMA vol. 1, no. 2 (1883) : 33, 36.

317 Daniel Drake: *An Inaugural Discourse on Medical Education;* delivered at the opening of the Medical College of Ohio (Cincinnati, Ohio: Locker, Palmer and Reynolds, 1820), 31.

318 Drake, *Practical Essays on Medical Education and the Medical Profession in the United States,* 46; and George W. Corner, "Beginnings of Medical Education in Philadelphia, 1765-1776" (Philadelphia: American Philosophical Society) *JAMA* 194, no. 7 (Nov 15, 1965) : 131. [read before the 61st annual Congress on Medical Education, Chicago, Feb. 7, 1965.]

319 David A. Tucker, Jr. "Daniel Drake and the Origin of Medicine in the Ohio Valley," *The Ohio State Archaeological and Historical Quarterly* XLII, no. 4 (October 1933) : 451-68.

320 James G. Burrow, AMA: *Voice of American Medicine* (Baltimore: The Johns Hopkins Press, 1963), 9.

321 David Starr Jordan, "The General Education of the Physician," *Bulletin of the History of Medicine* 50 (1891) (Baltimore: The Johns Hopkins University Press, 1976), 14-22.

322 Peter, *The History of the Medical Department of Transylvania University*, 55. From a delivery to the Lexington Medical Society in 1834, "On the Impolicy of Multiplying Schools of Medicine," Dr. Charles Caldwell described the success of the medical school: "It is believed from this view of it that for its vigorous prosperity and the rapid increase of its classes, the Medical Department of Transylvania is without a parallel. Certainly in the United States there is nothing comparable to it...In *thirty-three* years, then, that school [University of Pennsylvania] has added about 200 to its classes, while *in less than half that time* the school of Transylvania has *formed* a class of 262. This is the highest eulogy the institution can receive."

323 Dr. Peter in his *The History of the Transylvania Medical Department,* 11, states that Dr. Warfield was made Professor of Midwifery.

324 In the *Kentucky Gazette* of 14 February 1804, there was notice of a lottery, "600 Dollars for 5!!!" "to build a house for the *Kentucky Medical Society* in the town of Lexington." 277 prizes were

offered, a total value of $4000 dollars. First prize was $600. The *Kentucky Medical Society* should have read *Lexington Medical Society* (author).

325 A notice appearing in the *Kentucky Gazette* on September 10, 1802, announced that Dr. Ridgely and Dr. Fishback had united in the practice of Physic. The *Lexington City Directory* of 1806 includes the following physicians: Richard W. Downing, Michael Schaag, Samuel Brown, William Patrick, James Fishback, and Elisha Warfield.

326 Peter, *History of the Medical Department*, 27, note 1.

327 Ibid., 29.

328 Lewis Rogers, *Facts and Reminiscences of the Medical History of Kentucky*, an address before the Kentucky State Medical Society (Louisville: John P. Morton & Co., Publishers, 1873), 6.

329 *The Kentucky Gazette,* 10 March 1817.

330 *Lexington Observer-Reporter*, 10 March 1821. In 1839 the City of Lexington donated $70,000 to build a new medical college and enlarge the library. In 1839 an additional $3000 was given by Lexingtonians to purchase a lot for the site of the medical college
Peter, *The History of the Medical Department of Transylvania University*, Appendix, 168.

331 *The Kentucky Gazette*, 5 September 1809.

332 Peter, *The History of the Medical Department of Transylvania University*, 24-25.

333 Horine, ed., *Drake's Pioneer Life in Kentucky, 1785-1800*, xvi-xvii.

334 Horine, *Daniel Drake (1785-1852)*, 131.

335 Daniel Drake, *A Second Appeal to the Justice of the Intelligent and Respectable People of Lexington* (Cincinnati: Looker, Reynolds & Co., 1818), 33-34.

336 Daniel Drake, *An Appeal to the Justice of the Intelligent and Respectable People of Lexington* (Cincinnati: Looker, Reynolds & Co., 1818).

337 Ibid., 11.

338 Ibid., 15-16.

339 Ibid., 16.

340 Ibid., 21.

341 Ibid., 12.

342 Ibid., 23.

343 Ibid.

344 Benjamin W. Dudley, *To Dr. Drake* (Cincinnati: Looker, Reynolds & Co., 1818), 18 p.

345 Ibid., 1.

346 Ibid., 4.

347 Ibid., 8-9.

348 Ibid., 16.

349 Ibid., 16.

350 Daniel Drake, *A Second Appeal to the Justice of the Intelligent and Respectable People of Lexington* (Cincinnati: Looker, Reynolds & Co., 1818), 34 p.

351 Ibid., 11.

352 Ibid.

353 Ibid., 12.

354 Ibid., 12-13.

355 Ibid., 13.

356 Ibid., 14.

357 Peter, *The History of the Medical Department of Transylvania University,* 41.

358 Ibid., 42. Dr. Yandell was a graduate of the University of Louisville Medical School from which he graduated in 1846. Dr. Drake was professor of the Louisville Medical Institute and later the University of Louisville.

359 It was during his time as a medical professor in Louisville that Drake wrote his invaluable work, *A Systematic Treatise, Historical, Etiological and Practical on the Principal Diseases of the Interior Valley of North America, as they appear in the Caucasian, African, Indian and Esquimaux Varieties of its Population.* The masterpiece was hailed as "...a durable monument to his own name, and to the medical reputation, not only of the Great Valley, but to the Greater Union."
Alfred Stillé: [Chairman]—Committee on Medical Literature [for 1849-50], *Transactions of the American Medical Assn,* (Philadelphia, 1850), vol. III, 166. Time has only confired this appraisal.

360 Donovon F. Ward, "Presentation Remarks," *JAMA* 194, no. 7 (1965) : 132. "Dan Drake founded the first hospital in this country (Cincinnati) devoted primarily to teaching while at the same time offering medical care to the needy." [read at the 61st annual Congress]

361 Sir William Osler, *Aequanimitas With other Addresses,* 3d ed. (Philadelphia: The Blakiston Company, 1944), 307.

362 Billy Reed, "A Collection of Bicentennial Columns from *The Courier-Journal*," in *Famous Kentuckians*, Nancye J. Kirk, ed., with a foreward by A. B. Chandler (Louisville: Data Courier, Inc., 1977), 28-29.

363 Peter, *The History of the Medical Department of Transylvania University*, 46.

364 Burton A. Konkle, *Standard History of the Medical Profession of Philadelphia*, 2d ed. (New York: AMS Press, 1977), 155. Dr. Chapman later became the first President of the A.M.A. Ibid., 184.

365 Waller O. Bullock, "Dr. Benjamin Winslow Dudley," *Annals of Medical History*, vol. 7, no. 3 : 201-213

366 Lewis Rogers, "Address of the President," Kentucky State Medical Society (1873), 24-53.

367 George W. Ranck, *History of Lexington* (Cincinnati: Robert Clarke & Co., 1872), 293-294.

368 Philip M. Haner, ed., *The Centennial History of the Tennessee State Medical Association, 1830-1930* (Nashville: Tennessee State Medical Association, 1930), 30.

369 *Medicine and Its Development in Kentucky*, 40; citing Samuel D. Gross, *Autobiography*, vol. 2 (Philadelphia: 1887), 282-287.

370 James A. Pagett, ed., "The Letters of Doctor Samuel Brown to President Jefferson and James Brown," *Register of the Kentucky State Historical Society*, vol. 35, no. 111 (April 1937) : 120. The University of Virginia Medical School was established by Jefferson in Charlottesville in 1825. He chose a Scotsman, Dr. Robley Dunglison, to head the faculty.

371 Charles S. Sydnor, *The Development of Southern Sectionalism*, 1819-1848, Volume 5 of *A History of the South* (Baton Rouge: Louisiana State University Press, 1948), 73.

372 Charles McIntyre, "Medical Education in the United States: From Chaos Towards Cosmos," *Bulletin of the American Academy of Medicine* (1893) : 462.

373 Drake, *Practical Essays on Medical Education and the Medical Profession in the United States*, 47.

374 "By 1870 only two colleges had a graduated course of lectures occupying three winter sessions, Chicago Medical College (formerly Lind Univ, and later Northwestern Univ) and the Woman's Medical College of the New York Infirmary."

C. D. O'Malley, ed., *The History of Medical Education* (Los Angeles: University of California Press, 1970), 487-488.

375 "Miscellaneous Notices," *Transylvania Medical Journal* 12, no. 1 (1838-39) : 243. "The charge for a full course of lectures, is *one hundred and five dollars*. The matriculation fee is five dollars, and gives the right to use the library. This ticket must be taken first, and be exhibited to each professor, in order to procure his ticket. The dissecting ticket is ten dollars, and may be taken or omitted at pleasure.…In order to become a candidate for graduation, the pupil must be 21 years of age, must have been the student of a regular physician for at least two years, and must have attended two full courses of lectures in a chartered medical school, the last of which to be in this institution."

376 Drake, *Practical Essays on Medical Education and the Medical Profession in the United States,* 47.

377 Peter, *The History of the Medical Department of Transylvania University,* 31. The quotations are from Dr. Caldwell's *Autobiography* as quoted by Dr. Peter. Robert Wickliffe described the Transylvania Medical School library in 1837: "The Medical Library of the Institution, now contains more than *four thousand volumes,* embracing all the standard works in medicine, and many of those in the collateral branches of Science. There is among them, a full portion of all the *text books* to the various courses." The Transylvania University Medical Library was the envy of medical educators throughout the land. Robert Wickliffe, Chairman of the Board of Trustees of Transylvania University, "To the Public," *Transylvania Journal of Medicine* 10 (1837) : 596-600.

378 James Thacher, *American Medical Biography* (Boston, 1828; reprint ed., New York: Milford House, 1967), 78.

379 Henry Clay to Horace Holley, 21 February 1826, in James F. Hopkins and Mary W. M. Hargreaves, eds., *The Papers of Henry Clay,* (Secretary of State) (Lexington, Ky: University of Kentucky Press, 1973), Vol. V, 124.

380 Peters, *The History of the Medical Department,* 33, note 1, quoting a letter from Dr. Graham.

381 "Beginnings of Medical Education In and Near Chicago," *Bulletin of The Society of Medical History of Chicago* iii (1925) : 339-383.

382 Daniel Drake to Henry Clay, 20 February 1825, in James F. Hopkins, ed., *The Papers of Henry Clay,* (Secretary of State) (Lexington, Ky.: The University of Kentucky Press, 1972), Vol. IV, 79.

383 Peter, *The History of the Medical Department of Transylvania University,* 58-60.

384 Charles Caldwell, "A Report made to the Legislature of Kentucky, on the Medical Department of Transylvania University, February 15th, 1836," *The Transylvania Journal of Medicine* Vol. 9 (1836), 25-28.

385 Robert Wickliffe, "To the Public," *The Transylvania Journal of Medicine* 10 (1837) : 596-600. Wickliffe, Chairman of the Board of Trustees offered this explanation to the public: "For the space of eighteen years, the Medical Department of Transylvania University advanced in reputation and extended its usefulness, with unprecedented rapidity. Its wide spread fame had already made it not only an object of affectionate regard to the citizens of Lexington, but of pride to the State, and of interest to the West. That any circumstances should occur, calculated to threaten its existence, or even to circumscribe its usefulness, may be readily supposed well calculated to excite the liveliest interest among its friends, and to cause such measures to be adopted by its guardians as would counteract such influences. Without pausing here to enquire into the particulars of these circumstances, it is sufficient to say, that they were of such a nature as to render a dissolution of the Faculty by the Board of Trustees imperative...After a protracted and thorough investigation of the circumstances above alluded to, which threatened a destruction of our Institution, it was found necessary to dismiss one of the Professors (Caldwell),and to dissolve the remainder of the Faculty."

386 Peter, *The History of the Medical Department of Transylvania University,* 167.

387 Ibid., 57-60.

Chapter V

1850 to 1900

Contemplating [Kentucky's] condition, we find its agricultural interests in most part deplorably neglected, its soil washing away or being worn into utter unproductiveness; its education system, though much improved, still in a most deplorable state of backwardness. Our state abounding in the richest minerals, we spend the gleanings of our tired soil for imports of the very class that should be to us a source of munificent income. Arts and manufactures are shamefully languishing, while in the higher walks of statesmanship and learning the sons of Kentucky are retreating from the high position of leadership once cheerfully accorded them to a position painfully subordinate.[388]

D. T. Smith (1873)

The mourning for the decline and fall of the Medical Department of Transylvania University did not end with its closure in 1857. The bells continued to toll throughout the remainder of the nineteenth century and into the twentieth. Even before its closure, the declining relevance of the medical school and of Lexington were conspicuous. We find evidence of the medical decline as early as the meeting of the Kentucky State Medical Society in 1852. Dr. W. L. Sutton, the president of the Kentucky State Medical Society in 1852 commented, "that the profession as a body, and physicians as individuals, are less respected now than they were thirty years ago," and he adds, "Now the whole country is crowded with physicians, armed with diplomas."[389] In his "Report of the Committee on Improvements in Surgery," (1852) the chairman, Dr. Samuel Gross, laments: "The committee is expected to report on 'Improvements in Surgery.' On what Improvements?....Were the Committee to confine itself to the duty prescribed by the Society its labors would, indeed, be light and unimportant; for no one will pretend to assert that Kentucky has effected much 'improvement in surgery,' however rich and creditable may be her exploits in this branch of the health art."[390] Although the closure of the Medical Department lay some five years ahead, the author acknowledged its fallen state, referring to it as "the oldest, and, for a number of years, the most celebrated and successful school of Medicine in the valley of the Mississippi." He then proceeds to devote several pages to the surgical preeminence of Benjamin W. Dudley, concluding that there was nothing to show in the surgical literature of the West before his rather limited but impressive writings (Dudley's initial article appeared in 1828, in the first volume of the *Transylvania Journal of Medicine and the Associate Sciences*). Dr. Gross then cites other writings by Dr. Dudley and his surgical disciples. He also relates the history of the illustrious Ephraim McDowell and his celebrated ovariotomy but adds that McDowell "never contributed anything to any Western periodical."

We have sought to show the close ties between the well-being of the state and the well-being of medicine. Medicine flourishes in the prosperity of the government, of manufacturers, of agriculture and mining, of progressive educational systems, of culture, of up-to-date transportation and communication. Although medicine does not take the lead in this enterprise, it does follow close on and accentuates the grandeur of each component. On the other hand, it is apt to be one of the last to fall by the wayside.

The End of an Era

In 1857 the "Athens of the West" lost its last vestige of fame with the closing of the Medical Department of Transylvania University.[391] The once proud city would no longer harbor its prestigious medical faculty, nor be favored by the armada of eager medical students who had converged on Lexington from the vast reaches of the South and West. The Wednesday evening meetings of the Medical Society no longer took place; there was no medical society. Physicians would continue to come to Lexington, to live, to practice, and to die, but not one of them would approach the professional stature of their forbears.

The 1850s were years of great upheaval, of economic and social unrest, and of growing divisions between the North and the South. It was the eve of the Civil War, and the people of Lexington, centered within the border state of Kentucky, had to fight, as did other Kentuckians, their battles not only on the field but also in their homes; neighbors were divided, friendships shattered, and families torn apart. The dissolution of the medical school and the diminished state of medicine in general in Lexington became somewhat irrelevant in the larger picture of a nation at war with itself. For the Civil War shaped the postwar destiny of Kentucky and of other southern states for well over a half-century, making a mockery of the intellectual, commercial, scientific, and artistic ambitions of its people. The historian C. Van Woodward interprets the words of the renowned Kentuckian geologist, Nathaniel Southgate Shaler.[392]

> Distressed at the poverty of Southern Achievement in the arts and sciences during this period, Nathaniel Southgate Shaler speculated on the reasons for "the failure of the Kentucky People to make good on their promise." He ascribed it to a "peculiar combination of circumstances, of which the Civil War was the most potent," especially the resulting sacrifice of life. "This sacrifice," he wrote, "was in peculiarly large measure from the intellectual, the state-shaping class," and it was made in the South "in far larger proportion than the Northern states." Before the war he had seen evidence that the "men and women were seeking, through history, literature, the fine arts, and in some measure through science, for a share in the higher life. Four years of civil war... made an end of this and set the people on a moral and intellectual plane lower than they occupied when they were warring with the wilderness and the savages."

The Medical Hall

The Medical Hall of Transylvania, built in 1839 by the philanthropic action of the citizens of Lexington at a cost of about $35,000, reverted to the city in 1860. Located at the corner of Broadway and Second Street, the building was commandeered by the federal government during the Civil War as a hospital for Union soldiers and burned on May 22, 1863, while occupied, another casualty of war.

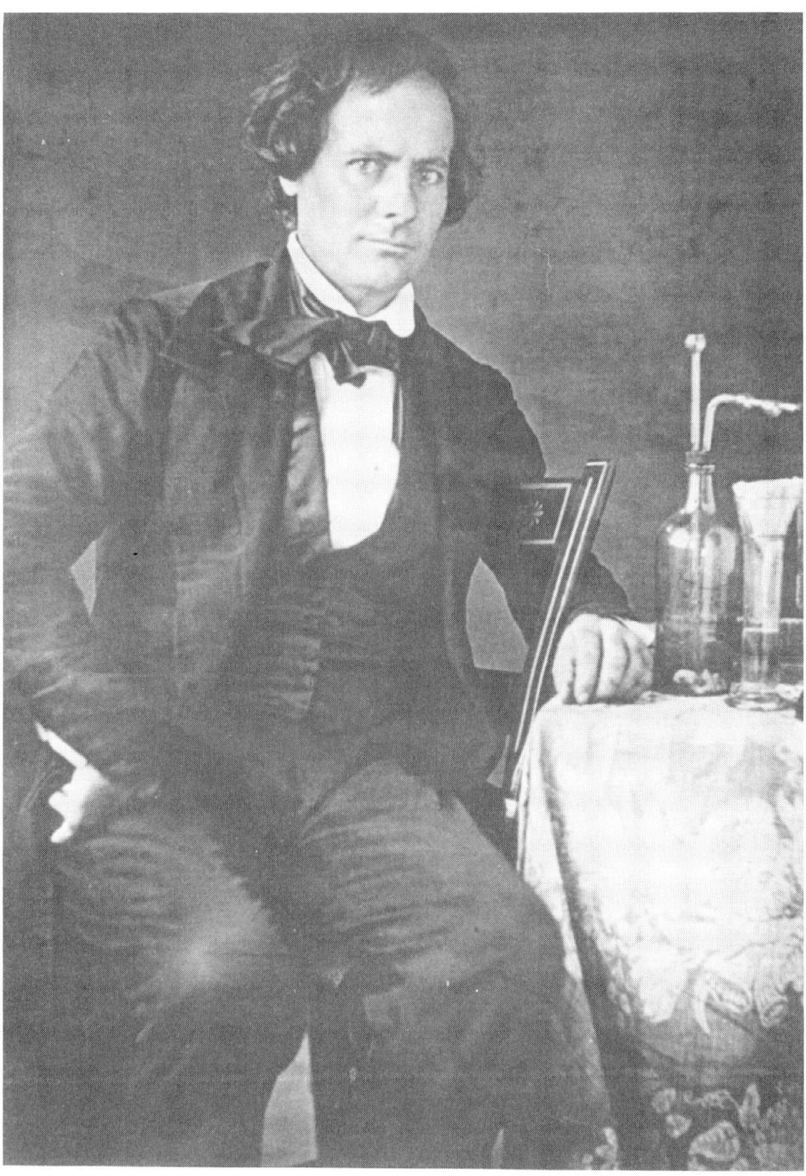

Robert Peter, M.D. (1805-1894)
Last Dean of Medical Department of Transylvania University
Courtesy of Transylvania University Library

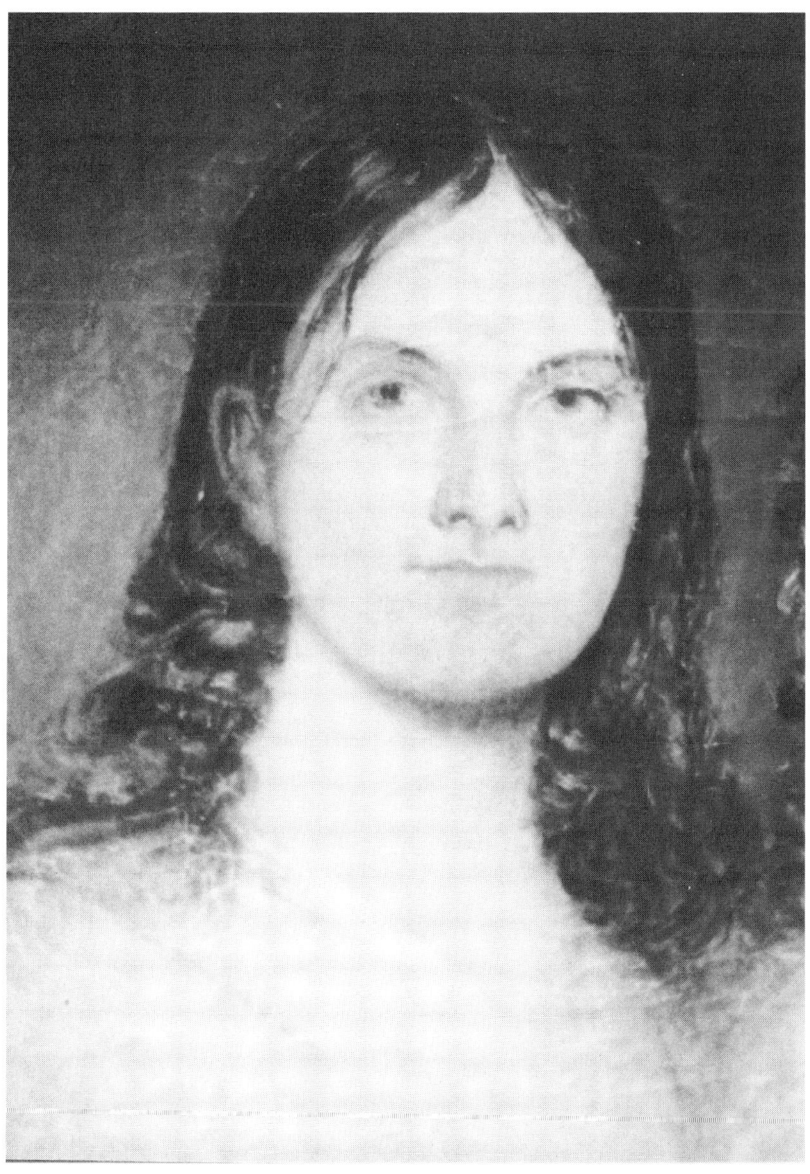

Frances Dallam Peter, daughter of Robert Peter, M.D.
From a portrait of the 1850s by Lewis Morgan (1843-1864)
Courtesy of Special Collections and Archives Service Center, University of Kentucky Libraries

Civil War Diary

Frances Dallam Peter (1843-1864), daughter of Dr. and Mrs. Robert Peter of Lexington, gives in her diary a very sensitive, almost palpable insight into the trappings of wartime Lexington.[393] Sounds and sights come alive as she describes persons and events, divided loyalties, parties and parades, joy and death. She scrutinizes from the security of her doorstep the home of her neighbor and enemy, Mrs. Morgan, an unrepentant secessionist and mother of the feared Confederate General, John Hunt Morgan. Her knowledge is impressive; her perspective slanted. And yet she is most engaging, if not enraging, when bashing the *secesh*. Reflecting her parents' strong allegiance to the Union cause, she is unashamedly biased. Her father, a native of Cornwall, England, enjoyed considerable esteem as a chemist and as Dean of the Medical Department of Transylvania University (1847-1857). In 1862, he was appointed Acting Assistant Surgeon of the U. S. General Hospital, Lexington, Kentucky. Her mother, Frances Paca Dallam, was a Lexingtonian, "a descendant of the famous Henry, Preston, and Breckinridge families of Virginia and Kentucky."[394] Fortunately, Miss Peter describes a few medical situations along with the social, political, and military affairs taking place in wartime Lexington.[395]

> [Thursday] Sept 18th 1862
>
> Pa has been arrested three times the first time Col. Gracie sent for him & wanted him to take an oath to the confederacy; of course Pa refused. The Col. then wanted him to leave the state. Pa represented to him that his family and business were here & he preferred to stay. The Col. then made him give parole and not to give information to the union party & said he might stay here while any of our soldiers were here. The next time the Col. had him arrested (upon what charge

I don't remember) he ordered him not to leave his house except to go to the hospital.

Thursday Feb 26th [1863]

The hospitals have turned out about 200 convalescents to aid in the defense of the city if necessary. There are not more than 800 sick here and none very sick. The rebel raid has been quite beneficial to some of them. One old fellow who had been in Pa's hospital some time and never seemed to get much better, roused himself up the other morning and got his gun. 'Dr.' he said to Pa, 'I'm going out to fight, the news of the rebels being so near has almost cured me!'

Sunday Mar 1st [1863]

Pa said the other day going to the hospital he saw Dr. Payne and several secesh ladies standing at a window of that gentleman's residence which is on the corner of one of the streets near the hospital [Hospital No 1-Masonic Hall] watching the hospital very intently as if they were expecting to see him begin packing up his stores and they were going to watch and see where he put them so they could inform the rebels when they came. Rebel spies are suspected of coming in very often dressed as farmers or union soldiers....

Sunday Dec 13th [1863]

The hospital is full. Some of the sick had to be put on the floor, as there were not enough beds....One old fellow from Camp Nelson had his hand in a kind of a sling and when Dr. Bush came to examine it, held it out with the fingers all cramped up, pretended he could not straighten

> them. Dr. Bush pretended to examine them with a great deal of attention. At last he turned to one of the soldiers near him and told him to bring his dissecting knife, for said he 'I shall have to cut the tendons of this man[']s hand.['] He had no sooner said this than a most wonderful cure was effected. The man's fingers straightened themselves instantly and he became well enough to be sent to his regiment. There have been two cases of this kind in the hospital lately, sneaking fellows who pretend to be disabled, so they may get a discharge, and make money by hiring themselves for substitutes or by reinlisting. But the doctors have seen enough of such tricks to know pretty well how to detect them.

Miss Peter's life ended tragically, as she died suddenly on August 5, 1864, age 21, from seizures with which she was afflicted.

There are no heroic tales of the exploits of Lexington physicians during the Civil War, nor are we left with any sinister legend, or even a myth that would hold us spellbound. Because Lexington was so situated that its people and its goods were alternately subject to the forces of the North and of the South, it is likely that neither side chose to risk large amounts of medical provisions or manpower beyond their immediate needs.

Ethelbert Dudley

One of the most acclaimed Lexington physicians, Ethelbert Dudley (1818-1862), took an active role in the Union Army, but he chose to do so as a general officer and not as a physician. A nephew and student of the famed surgeon Dr. Benjamin Dudley, Ethelbert attended Harvard University and in 1842 graduated from Transylvania Medical School. As a member of the

Transylvania Medical Faculty, he initially filled the position of Demonstrator of Anatomy, advancing to the chair of General and Pathological Anatomy in 1847-48. Other achievements included the editorship of the *Transylvania Medical Journal* (1848-49?). During the 1850s he taught both in the summer sessions of Transylvania University (chair of Surgery) and in the Kentucky School of Medicine in Louisville.[396 397]

With the eruption of the Civil War, Dr. Dudley helped organize a battalion of "Home Guards" of which he was appointed Commandant. Subsequently, he raised a company of volunteers, the 21st Infantry, and with his troops took leave of Lexington for the southern part of the state. His command was short-lived and ironic, for Dudley, who chose the role of field officer rather than that of Medical Director, died not by the sword but by typhoid at Columbia, Kentucky, on February 20, 1862, at the age of forty-four.[398] Miss Peter, in her diary, describes the return of Colonel Dudley's body to Lexington and the burial:[399]

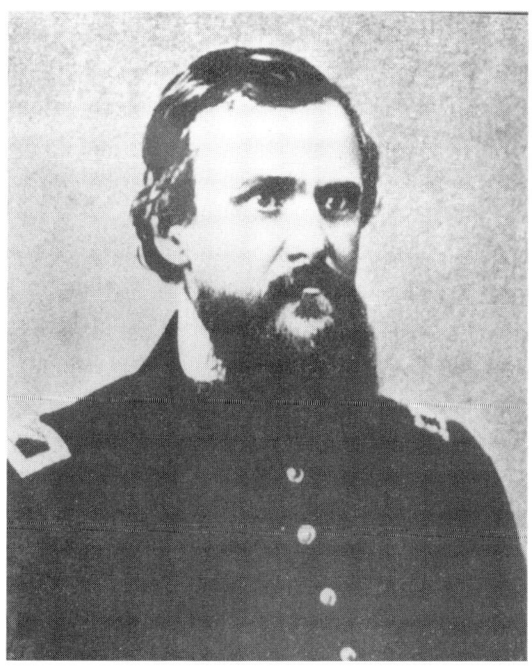

Ethelbert Dudley, M.D.
(1818-1862)
Courtesy of Transylvania University Library

> Last night [February 21, 1862] the bells were tolled for the death of Dr. Ethelbert W. Dudley, Col. of the 21st regiment, Kentucky, who died at Columbia, Adair county, of typhoid fever....[400] [February 25, 1862] Col. E. Dudley's body arrived here Sunday and was attended from the cars to the Odd Fellow's Hall by the Mayor, Councilmen and crowd of citizens. The funeral oration was announced by Mr. Brank today at the Odd Fellow's Hall, where the body lay in state. The 33rd Indiana, Col. Coburn[,] the Lexington Blues[,] Cap. Wilgus, Odd fellows and Masons, with some of the Old infantry and chasseurs, formed part of the procession with some of Dr. Dudley's men who came here with him and a great many carriages. It was the largest funeral ever seen here except Henry Clay's.

Dr. Robert Peter, a friend and colleague of Dr. Dudley's, related the following incident as told by the son-in-law of Dr. Dudley, Union General Joseph C. Breckinridge:[401]

> When, during the Civil War, a struggle was imminent between the secessionists and the Home Guard for possession of a large shipment of arms and ammunition sent into Kentucky by the United States Government for the arming of Union soldiers and citizens, Dudley, fearing the Home Guard at Lexington would be overpowered and the munitions captured on arrival, sent as a trusty messenger to General Nelson, at Camp Dick Robinson, to ask for troops-a midnight journey of twenty miles through a hostile country-his only son, Scott Dudley, a youth scarcely seventeen. He saddled the horse and armed the boy himself, at dead of night, the better to insure secrecy, for in his own household were foes. The mission was successful.

The Breckinridge family and its most prominent member, General John Cabel Breckinridge (1821-1875), are intimately tied to the first president of The Lexington and Fayette County Medical Society (1869), Dr. John Desha. But now we are speaking of another side of the Breckinridge family—Confederates.

The Last Illness of General John C. Breckinridge

One of the most extensive biographies in Collins' *The History of Kentucky* is that of the Confederate General John C. Breckinridge, of Lexington, Kentucky, who was elected Vice President of the United States in 1856, and was a candidate for the presidency of the United States in 1860. Breckinridge was elected to the United States Senate in 1861. While a senator, Breckinridge made every effort to conciliate the North and the South; however, when the war came, he sided with the South. "He quitted the Senate and took up the sword."[402] His biographer, Davis, comments:

> ...that harried flight from Lexington in September, 1861, brought to an end his twenty years as a leading Democrat, the decade he had spent in building his party into the dominant force in Kentucky, and his own unparalleled political career. A simple arrest order brought it all to a head. In an instant his life was totally disrupted, his native state arrayed against him, his family broken up, and his career blasted to nothing at its very peak.[403]

General Breckinridge skillfully and gallantly led his forces, among them the Kentucky Brigade, in many of the bloodiest battles of the Civil War. With the collapse and surrender of the Confederacy (1865), Breckinridge, at the time the Confederate

Secretary of War, escaped to Cuba and, after traveling in Canada and Europe, returned to Lexington about a year later. That much more was expected of the General is vigorously set forth by his contemporary, the historian Collins:[404]

> General Breckinridge has (1873) just turned his 51st year, and is now in the prime of his physical and mental vigor. He entered into the public service in early life, and thus far the promise of his young manhood has been nobly sustained. The unwise policy of the party in power deprives the nation of the safe counsels of men of his stamp. When a more liberal policy obtains, as it must, the eloquent voice of John C. Breckinridge will be heard once more. He was born wise in the council, brave in the field, alike a scholar and statesman. But his history is not yet all written.

Unsuspected by Collins and the General himself, within two years Breckinridge would be dead. His principal physician and close friend, Dr. John Desha, attended the General throughout his illness. His repeated bouts of chest colds and susceptibility to disease caused increasing concern to his family. By early 1875 his condition had worsened. Dr. Desha called into consultation Drs. Louis Sayre, Luke Blackburn, and Samuel Gross of Philadelphia. Once this group of doctors met together at the General's bedside, they "...proceeded to get involved in a rather petty misunderstanding over who was actually *the* attending physician, meanwhile barely concealing their desire to be at the races instead of with the patient. The general, looking on in silence, finally interceded, weary of their professional pedantry. 'Let *me* settle this matter,' he said, 'if I am a sick man. You all want to go to the races, and it is now 12 o'clock. Desha, go with Preston and take your lunch with Gross, and then go to the races; and Blackburn, you go with Sayre, and, after the races, come and overhaul me at 4 o'clock' That finished the controversy." When the physicians examined him later that day, it was apparent that he had a large accumulation of fluid in his right chest, presumably as the result of cirrhosis (brought on by a war injury at Cold Harbor) and a lung abscess. On May 10, with Breckinridge under chloroform anesthesia, a silver tube was inserted into the chest cavity, and the fluid was drained. Although he experienced partial relief for a few days, his condition worsened and he died on May 16, 1875. At his bedside were Dr. and Mrs. Desha and family members.[405]

Medical Practice in the 1860s

In 1916, Dr. Benjamin Prince Earle presented a paper before local Kentucky medical societies, including the Fayette County Medical Society. In it, he affords a first-hand look into the study and practice of medicine in Kentucky during the 1860s.[406]

"I attended my first Course of Lectures at the University of Louisville in 1868-1869 and out of the two hundred and thirty matriculates, not ten had ever seen a [hypodermic] syringe.[407] No one of us had ever heard of a fever thermometer and the first ones that were sent out did not 'self-register.' When you used one you had to look quickly, for the mercury would begin to fall as soon as you removed it from the patient. There was not a microscope in the county (Hopkins) and a stethoscope was a curiosity.[408]

"Then no requirements were exacted as to the preparation of a candidate for the study of medicine. Any one who had the price of tuition could enter Medical School. Now you must have not only a High School Diploma but two years of College work. Then we had two terms in Medical School which was all that was required for graduation.... I was taught that to wound the peritonium was almost certain death....Our Professor of Surgery spent an hour then in teaching us the difference between sanies pus and laudable pus."

The period of time described by Dr. Earle, c. 1868, was twenty years after the birth of the American Medical Association, which was established primarily on the premise of raising the standards of medical education. These twenty years had brought but little gain. In fact, not for an additional twenty to thirty years did any significant changes take place to put American medical schools on a par with their European counterparts.

Earle continues: "Our means of diagnosis consisted often of a poor history of the case given by patient or family. We depended on the pulse, the condition of the tongue, poorly done ascultation, percussion and general inspection."

"All calls for Physicians were by Courier, either on foot or on horseback....Then we used but few remedies as we had to carry all our outfit in our saddle bags. And no matter what the diagnosis was, we gave calomel, quinine, ipecac, morphine, rhubarb, along with a can of cathartical ointment with which to blister skin surfaces. These, with what domestic remedies we could pick up were the principal armament with which we were equipped to fight disease. Then, with many Doctors, Bragging and hectoring over their patients was resorted to. But bluffing and loud-sounding talk is now no longer taken for knowledge but the physician must show by his work that he understands his business."

Although medical practice in rural Kentucky often remained backwards, in the cities, modern advances were quickly adopted. For example, in an 1873 address to the Kentucky State Medical Society, Dr. Lewis Rogers reported on Kentucky's pioneer use of anesthesia.[409] According to Dr. Rogers:

> In October, 1846, ether was first used by inhalation as an anesthesic. In the winter or spring 1847, Dr. Joshua B. Flint administered it for the first time in Kentucky, and possibly in the West, in an amputation of a lower limb performed by him in the presence of a number of professional friends. I was present. The ether was then called "letheon," and administered by the aid of a complicated inhaler.

> Cloroform was first brought forward by Sir James Y. Simpson, as a substitute for ether, in November, 1847. It was used for the first time in midwifery in the city of Louisville, and as far as is known in the state of Kentucky, by Prof. Henry Miller, on the 20th of February, 1848.

Post-Civil War Medical Societies

After the Civil War, a medical society bearing the name *Lexington and Fayette County Medical Society* was organized.[410] The organization of the medical society was given note by the *Lexington Observer and Reporter* on February 13, 1869:

> Medical Society—The physicians of Lexington met at the Court House on Tuesday evening for the purpose of organizing a County Medical Society. There is decided evidence of progress in our midst. Success to the enterprize. We are requested by the Secretary of the Society to say that he was instructed to invite the Physicians of the county to attend and co-operate with the Physicians in Lexington. The next meeting will be held on February 23d at 7 1/2 o'clock, p.m., at the Court House.

The above notice is something of a watershed, as it represents, for the first time, the recognition of a number of physicians outside of Lexington but within the confines of Fayette County. This recognition led to the changing of the name from *Lexington Medical Society* to *Lexington and Fayette County Medical Society.* The original Constitution, By-laws, Amendments, and Minutes are located in the Special Collections, King Library, University of Kentucky. The Constitution consists of ten beautiful hand-written pages. Nineteen physicians pledged themselves to be bound by the Constitution, by-laws, and Code of Ethics. Dr. Jno. R. Desha was elected president; Joseph Smith, senior vice president; H. M. Skillman, junior vice president; W.O. Sweeny, secretary; L. B. Todd, corresponding secretary; and R. R. Wheatley, treasurer. The minutes chronicle seven meetings, the first on March 18, 1869, and the last on July 6, 1869. The society then disappeared without a trace.[411]

Not until 1882 did any further public notice acknowledge the reorganization of a medical society:[412]

> **A Medical Society** has been organized in our city by a number of enterprising and progressive physicians, who desire the benefits that must result from an exchange of views on the subject of medicine and a comparison of experiences in the treatment of disease. It is their purpose to hold weekly meetings, at each of which a paper on some special subject will be read by some member, after which the other members will be at liberty to pick flaws and expose any errors that may have been made by the writer. In this matter our doctors are simply following the example of those in other cities, where similar medical societies have proved to be great.
>
> It is really a matter of surprise that our city has been without an organization of this kind for so many years. Formerly when the Medical College of Transylvania was at the height of its prosperity, there was a Medical Society in Lexington which became famous throughout the medical world. There are at this time quite as many eminent physicians in Lexington who can, if they will, make the new organization rival the rep utation of the old one....

> Our doctors must not depend on the limited experience of a single neighborhood; they should aim at knowing what is going on in other parts of the world, and how disease is treated by other physicians and other schools of medicine....
>
> The public who trust their lives to their physicians have a right to demand that the doctors shall keep fully abreast with all discoveries and improvements in medicine, and in no way can that result be better accomplished than by the cordial and active support of the new Medical Society....

The above account does not specify the name of the society nor does it list the officers. However, in his *Autobiography*, Dr. J. W. Pryor states: "I was of the number active in the organization of the Lexington and Fayette County Medical Society [in 1882]."[413]

Dr. Pryor's Reminiscences

Dr. J. W. Pryor, a native of Palmyra, Missouri, came to Lexington in 1882 to set up his medical practice.[414] He treats us to a few clues about the status of Lexington and its medical practice in the 1880s. "There were no modern improvements in Lexington at that time," he recalled, "....no telephones..., street cars, electric lights, water system or sewers." Although there were many fine residences, "Main Street looked rather dilapidated." Lexington did not make a favorable impression on the young doctor, who curtly summarized his new home as an "overgrown small town." "The best residences in Lexington had cesspools in the backyards and there were hundreds of out-houses without any regard to sanitation. The summer months were redolent with undesirable odors." The choice residential streets were North Broadway and Second

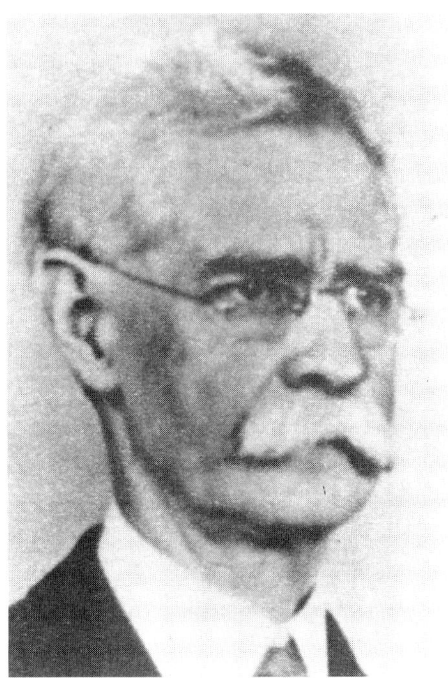

J. W. Pryor, M.D.
(1856-1956)
Courtesy of Special Collections and Archives Service Center, University of Kentucky Libraries

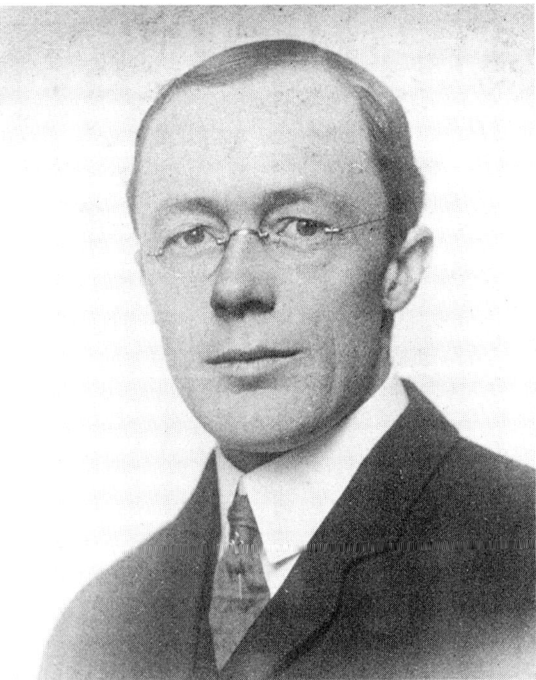

Waller O. Bullock, M.D.
(1875-1953)
Courtesy of Fayette County Medical Society

and Third Streets. His only comment about the courthouse was that it was "worse looking" than the one in his childhood home of Palmyra, Missouri. [The corner stone of the new courthouse was laid on July 4, 1883]. The population of Lexington at this time was about 17,000. Dr. Pryor was much happier once he became acquainted with the physicians of Lexington. He was actively engaged in the affairs of the Medical Society and took a leading role advocating what became the University of Kentucky Medical School. He retired from the University of Kentucky in June,1929, with the title of Professor of Anatomy and Physiology, Emeritus.

Banqueted

The Lexington and Fayette County Medical society played host to the Kentucky State Medical Society in May 1891. *The Kentucky Leader* acclaimed the event on Friday, May 29, with a full-length, two-column, front-page story headed "Banqueted." The writer declared that the banquet "surpassed in brilliancy anything of the sort ever given in this city." Well over three hundred guests were present. A sub-heading trumpeted: "The Menu Comprised Everything That is Good to Eat.":

MENU

Little Neck Clams.
Amontillado Sherry.

Consomme Printannier.

Broiled Spanish Mackerel, a la Colbert.
Potatoes Rosage.
Vine de Graves 1874 Sauterne.

Fried Soft Shell Crabs.
Sliced Cucumbers.
Pommery Sec.

Roast Filet of Beef, with Mushrooms.
Asparagus, Sauce Hollandaise.

Roman Punch.
Cigarettes.

Broiled Spring Chicken on Toast.
Tomatoes Mayonnaise.
Yellow Label.

Strawberries and Ice Cream.
Assorted Cake.
Fruit.
Roquefort Cheese, Bents Biscuits.

French Brandy.
Coffee.
Imported Cigars.

Precisely at ten o'clock the guests were allowed to enter the festive Banquet Room of the Phoenix Hotel to the accompaniment of "an inspiring march by the Opera House orchestra." The entire process took twenty minutes.

A series of toasts were exchanged, but "not until every course of the evening had been served and the guests were half into the luxury of an imported cigar." Lexington received repeated compliments, "....all the more effective because its citizens who were present felt them to be no more than her due." In the same issue and closer to the last page than the first, an "End of the

Meeting" column covered several of the medical papers read at the Society's session on the morning following the banquet and appropriately credited their authors. It was duly noted that "There was a noticeable diminution in the number of doctors present at the meeting of this morning....the banquet had something to do with it, no doubt."

The next notice of the existence of a medical society came with the following account in the *Lexington Leader*, July 10, 1894:

ELECT OFFICERS
Dr. W. B. McClure Chosen President of
the Lexington and Fayette County
Medical Society

> At the annual election of the officers of the Lexington and Fayette County Medical Society, held last evening in the Chamber of Commerce room in the court house, Dr. W.B. McClure was elected president. Dr. McClure is one of the younger members of the society, and his election to the presidency is indeed a high compliment. Under his charge the society will continue its very successful career.
>
> The officials elected last night were as follows: Senior Vice-President, T.L. Patterson; Junior Vice-President, W.L. Elmore; Secretary, R. C. Falconer; Treasurer, David Barrow; Librarian, J.W. Pryor.

The Society had doggedly continued the name of the Lexington Medical Society throughout the nineteenth century while acknowledging the reality of the changing medical topography with the addition of Fayette County in its title. It is unfortunate that Dr. Pryor, in his detailed autobiography, did not mention the names of the officers of the society when it was reorganized in 1882 and that he fails to report the 1894 Lexington and Fayette County Medical Society meeting at which he was named librarian. By the end of the century, the society adopted the name Fayette County Medical Society, and it has remained so since that time.

First Woman Physician in Fayette County

The 1864-1865 Lexington City Directory tabulated the names of Lexington doctors, a total of thirteen. The fourth physician listed was Mrs. Elizabeth Cromwell. We have no record of an active medical society existing in Lexington in 1864-65, but if we did there is little or no possibility that the name of Elizabeth Cromwell would appear in its roster. The membership of a woman in a medical society at that time and for years to come was anathema. No extant records give further listings of a woman either as a member of The Lexington and Fayette County Medical Society or among the physicians listed in the Lexington City Directories (1877-78, 1890, 1902) through the remainder of the nineteenth century. We are treated to the mind set of the times by the following discussion of the place of women in medicine during the 1860s and 1870s. The discussants, for the most part, agreed: *women had their place, but it was not in the medical society.*[415]

Speaking to the State Medical Society in 1874, Dr. J. W. Thompson condemned the "woman movement."[416] Women, he warned, "were demanding permission to descend and enter our legislative halls and command in the senate. They even knock at the door of the temple of medicine, and claim full fellowship with us." "I hold," he continued, "that woman is not adapted physically or mentally to the practice of our profession. Therefore, in keeping with the laws of nature, she cannot succeed as man has hitherto done." He triumphantly concluded: "I am proud to say that

Kentucky's fair women indicate no desire to participate in this ill-advised movement, and that the land so noted for the high character, beauty, and eminent virtue of her women will never be degraded by such unhallowed aspirations."

The first discussion of the admission of women to the American Medical Association came about in 1868 at the annual meeting in Washington, D.C. This meeting is notable primarily because of the salutary effect of the election of a Southern physician, Dr. William O. Baldwin, of Alabama, as President. Dr. H. P. Bowditch,[417] of Boston, made the resolution for recognition of "regularly educated and otherwise well-qualified female physicians." This rather painful issue was thoroughly discussed and then with due consideration "indefinitely postponed." Further discussion on the subject of women in medicine, and in particular as members of the Association, occurred in 1871 at the annual meeting in San Francisco. The discussion, however, turned into something of a tirade against women by the president of the Association, Dr. Alfred Stillé. That he believed such an issue required coverage in his presidential address acknowledges that the battle for acceptance of women into the medical profession would not go away. To that end, Stillé did his utmost to put the "outrage" permanently to rest:[418]

> Certain women seek to rival men in manly sports and occupations, and the "strong-minded" ape them assiduously in all things, even in dress. In doing so, they may command a sort of admiration such as all monstrous productions inspire, especially when they tend towards a higher type than their own. But a man with feminine traits of character, or with the frame and carriage of a female, is despised both by the sex he ostensibly belongs to, and that of which he is at once a caricature and a libel. In every department of active life man excels woman, excels her even in things for which she is esteemed most fit. In the arts of design, in paint-

> ing and sculpture, no woman, albeit the artist's career has always been open to her, has ever risen far above mediocrity; while men have excelled women in not a few employments which are regarded as essentially feminine. In the art of cookery, for example, no woman ever occupied the first rank; and in more than one capital, male hairdressers and dressmakers set the fashions in which court ladies and city dames contend for the palm of beauty.

Stillé continues:

> On the whole then, we believe that all experience teaches that woman is characterized by a combination of distinctive qualities, of which the most striking are uncertainty of rational judgment, capriciousness of sentiment, fickleness of purpose, and indecision of action, which totally unfit her for professional pursuits. Judged by one of her own sex, the verdict is in these words: "The ignorance, the inexactness, the untrustworthiness, the unbusiness-like ways of women are appalling. Men are as bad as they can be, one is sometimes tempted to say; but apparently they can not be so bad as women in these respects. Long ages of experience have, at least, educated them into a consciousness of the difference between yes and no; but women have yet to learn that they are not one and the [s]ame word....They seem to lack a moral sense, or a mental perception, or whatever [t]he faculty is which makes one capable of contracting an engagement. They do not comprehend its nature. It has for them no more binding force than a rope of sand. They break it with a serene unconsciousness that anything is broken, or that there was anything

> to break."
>
> If then, woman is unfitted by nature to become a physician, we should, when we oppose her pretensions, be acquitted of any malicious or even unkindly spirit. We may admit that she is in some sense a perfected man, and was created even a little less lower than the angels; we may admit that, guided by her affections, her judgments sometimes resemble inspirations; but in the business of life, and especially in the practice of a scientific art, it nevertheless may be true, and probably is so, that she usually displays a strange ignorance of the logic of reason, and a profound contempt for the logic of facts.

One year later, at the A.M.A. meeting in 1872 at Philadelphia, Dr. David W. Yandell of Louisville, a graduate of Transylvania University Medical School and president of the Association, took a less confrontational approach to women in medical practice. Indeed he supported their right to practice; however, he cautioned that their nature should be the determinant of their specialty, naturally avoiding surgery. He also advocated that the decision of whether a woman could practice medicine was one to be made by the public. That a public decision would also relieve the A.M.A. of its responsibility went unsaid:[419]

> What the people decree in this matter is a law to which all, we and the women alike, must bow submissively. If they want women doctors, such will be found ready to meet the demand. If those now pressing forward in their studies so eagerly, find their services are not wanted, they will take down their signs, get married-if they can- or turn lecturers, or to some more lucrative employ-

> ment. I hope they will never embarrass us by a personal application for seats in this Association. I could not vote for that.

It was at the meeting in Philadelphia (1876) that the inevitable came to pass: a woman delegate came to the American Medical Association, Dr. Sarah Hackett Stevenson, from the state of Illinois.[420]

Women Admitted into Medical Societies

The admission of women to medical societies in the latter part of the nineteenth century proved to be another hurdle to their acceptance in the mainstream of medical practice. Those men (and women) who had been appalled by the admission of women into regular medical schools earlier in the century were aghast at their request to join the men as members of the closely knit all male domain, the medical society. And just as they had pursued admission to recognized regular medical schools in the forties, fifties and sixties (rejecting the dubious corridors of the proprietary schools), so too, they sought and won admission to the medical societies by the early 1870s and thereafter at an increasing pace.

Lexington's Women Physicians

A report in the *Journal of The Kentucky State Medical Association* (1949) relates that Julia Washburn (1861-1949) was the first woman to practice medicine in Lexington. She graduated from Cleveland Medical College in 1891 and practiced medicine in Lexington for forty-two years. Her name is not listed as a member of the Fayette County Medical Society.[421] The first African-American woman physician to practice medicine in Lexington was Mary E. Britton. Her name first appears in the list of Physicians in the City Directory of 1904. A teacher and an author, she wrote for *Our Women and Children, The American Citizen* and as a regular contributor to the Lexington Herald.[422]

The first woman to become a member of the Fayette County Medical Society was Josephine D. Hunt, a native of Prairie Du Chien, Wisconsin. Dr. Hunt attended Sayre College, graduated from Transylvania University and received her medical education at Johns Hopkins Medical School in Baltimore. Dr. Hunt began her practice of medicine in Lexington in September, 1907, and was active until her retirement in 1956.[423] She was elected to the vice-presidency of the Medical Society in December, 1911, and on February 15, 1912 in a written statement she resigned this office.[424] The minutes do not record a reason for her resignation. Dr. Hunt was the founder of the Lexington Planned Parenthood Clinic.[425]

Lexington's African-American Physicians

Two historic medical events took place at the A.M.A. meeting in Washington, D.C., in 1870. The first dealt with the need for a national medical journal; this need was met in the form of a resolution by Dr. Samuel Gross:[426] "Transactions should be published in a journal to be called The American Medical Association Journal, issued monthly under the supervision of a competent doctor." In his *A History of the American Medical Association*, Fishbein comments: "There was also some disturbance over the number of delegates from the District of Columbia." The disturbance arose over the representation of the National Medical Society (African-American Physicians), the Howard Medical College, Freedman's Hospital and the Smallpox Hospital in the District of Columbia. Charges had been filed against these institutions, effectively banning their admission into the A.M.A. The majority report in favor of the ban was upheld by a vote of 115 to 90. Dr. Davis explained why the Society took such action: "...it had been brought to the attention of the Committee on Ethics that the said National Medical Society recognized and received as members medical men who were not licensed to practice." Howard University delegates were rejected because they were also members of the National Medical Society of the District of Columbia. The session ended with the following resolution:[427]

> Resolved, That inasmuch as it has been distinctly stated and proved that the consideration of race and color has had nothing whatsoever to do with the decision of the question of the reception of the Washington delegates, and inasmuch as charges have been distinctly made in open session today attaching the stigma of dishonor to parties implicated, which charges have not been denied by them, though present, therefore; The report of the majority of the Committee on Ethics be declared, as to all intents and purposes, unanimously adopted by the Association.

The first black doctors to practice medicine in Lexington were Drs. Peter Allison, John E. Hunter and Perry D. Robinson.[428] Dr. Allison is listed under physicians and surgeons in the Lexington City Directory of 1881-82. Dr. Hunter received his medical education at Western Reserve University in Cleveland and began his practice in Lexington in 1890, with Dr. Robinson [Howard University graduate].[429] A Commonwealth of Kentucky historical marker at the intersection of North Broadway and Main Street in Lexington serves to honor and to recall the pioneering exploits of these physicians:

> **African-American Physicians**
>
> Site of office building which housed prominent African-American physicians and pharmacy. Among the doctors who practiced here

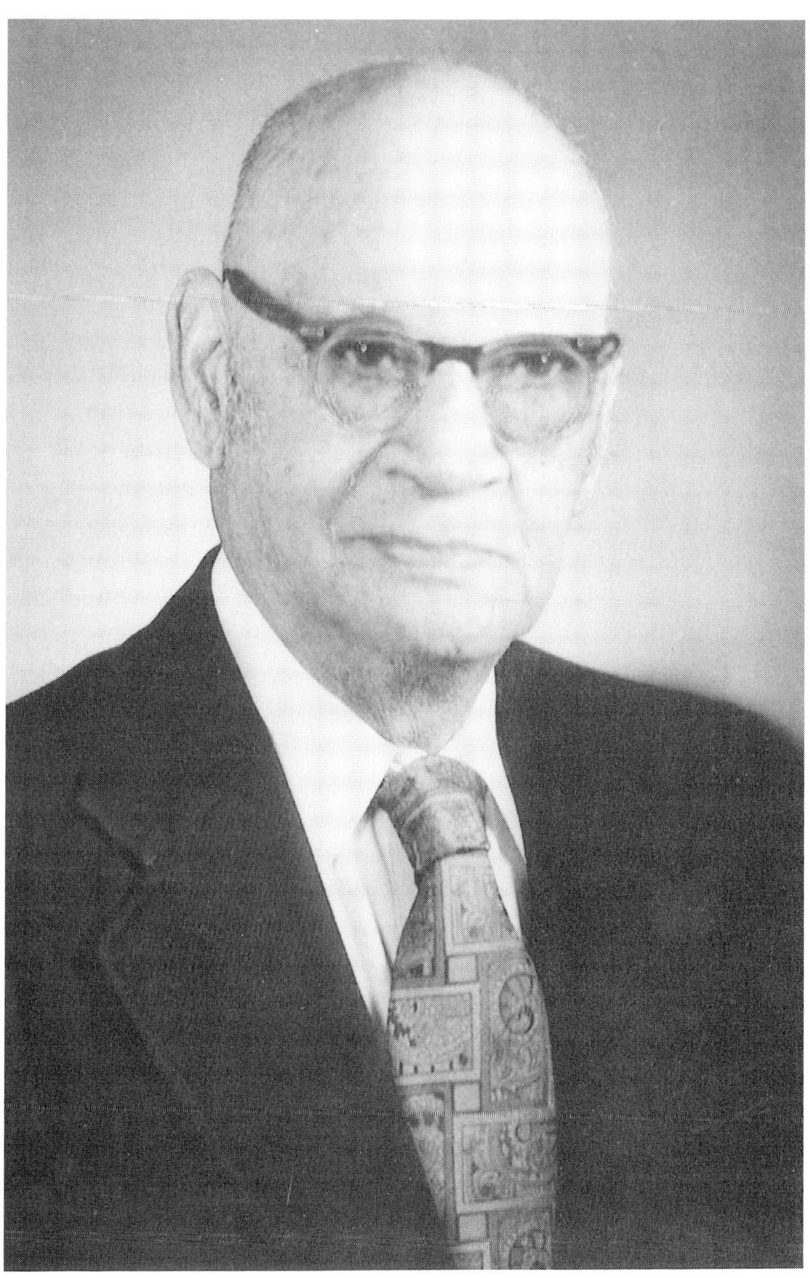

Bush A. Hunter, M.D. (1894-1983)
Courtesy of Fayette County Medical Society

> between 1890 and 1930 were Obed Cooley; Nathaniel J. Ridley; J. C. Coleman; John Hunter, first African-American surgeon at St. Joseph Hospital; and Joseph Laine, who later founded a medical clinic in Louisville.[430]

Without question the most distinguished African-American physician who practiced medicine in Lexington was Dr. Bush Hunter (1894-1983), son of Dr. John E. Hunter. Receiving his M.D. from Howard University, Dr. Hunter entered the practice of medicine in Lexington with his father in 1926. He continued to practice medicine for an additional fifty years, devoting his time and his efforts to the benefit of the community far beyond the confines of his medical practice. He was named the outstanding general practitioner of the year (1970) by the Kentucky State Medical Association, one of but many distinguished acknowledgments. He was the first black physician to become a member of the Fayette County Medical Society in 1963.[431]

Nursing and Hospitals

Nursing was catapulted into prominence in the care of patients by the determined action of Florence Nightingale (1820-1910) during the Crimean War (1854-56). Even so, many years were to pass before measures were taken to initiate an educational system consistent with the expectations and the rewards of professional nursing. In America, the training of nurses was established in the larger cities during the latter quarter of the nineteenth century. Central to this undertaking was the support of the American Medical Association. Such action was initiated by one of the foremost leaders in American Medicine, Dr. Samuel D. Gross. Attending the A.M.A. meeting in Washington in 1868, he said:[432]

> I am not aware that the education of nurses had received any attention from this body; a circumstance the more surprising when we consid-

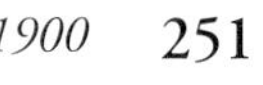

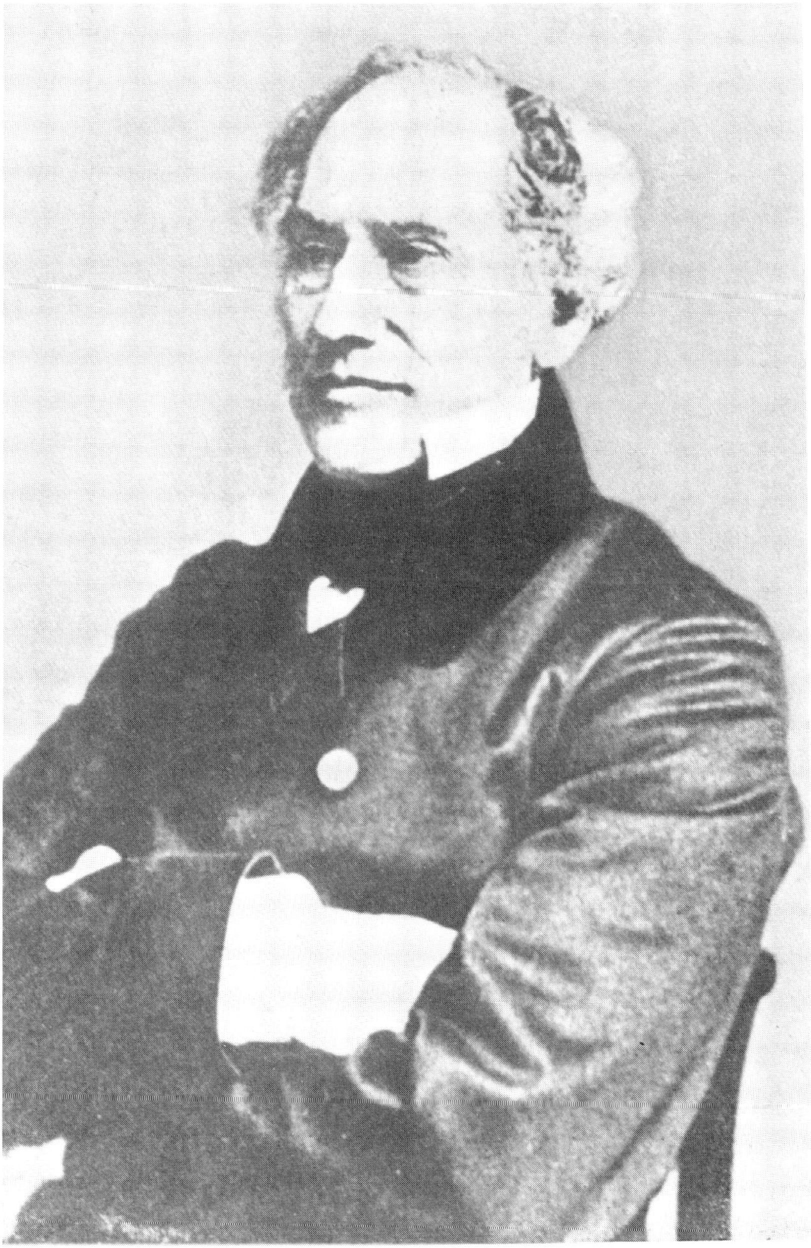

Samuel Gross, M.D.
(1805-1884)
Courtesy of Filson Club
Historical Society,
Louisville, Kentucky

> er the great importance of the subject. It seems to me to be just as necessary to have well-trained, well-instructed nurses as to have intelligent and skillful physicians. I have long been of the opinion that there ought to be, in all the principal towns and cities of the Union, institutions for the education of men and women whose duty it is to take care of the sick, and to carry out the injunction of the medical attendant....We need in this country a million of Florence Nightingales....Myriads of human beings perish annually, in the so-called civilized world, for the want of good nursing.

A new trend was under way in the latter quarter of the nineteenth century, one consistent with the manifold changes in medical care taking place throughout the United States. The large population of American physicians training in Europe and coming home with fresh enthusiasm, skills, and knowledge; the advent of anesthesia, antisepsis, and sterilization; the recognition of the place of nursing in the hospital setting and of the necessity for their training—all of these shaped a new and more receptive attitude toward hospitals. No longer would they serve simply as the refuge of the poor, the vagrants, and the disturbed. A new paradigm of medicine emerged. Now the hospital patient had but one thing in mind: to get well. The modern hospital would house not only the patients in need of medical care but also of surgical therapy, the latter removed after centuries from the makeshift theater of a bedroom or a kitchen. People of all social strata were to gradually accept the new role of the hospitals.

Two hospitals founded in the nineteenth century were destined to fulfill this need for the patients and the medical community of Lexington: St. Joseph Hospital and Good Samaritan Hospital.[433] Not only have the two hospitals faithfully devoted themselves to the care of the patient, but they have also enhanced their ability to do so by introducing schools of nursing. And further, the hospitals have, time and time again, served the needs of physicians, individually and collectively, by making their accommodations and services available to the members of the Medical Society.

St. Joseph Hospital

Founded in 1877, by sisters of the Order of Charity, St. Joseph Hospital was Lexington's first modern hospital. The sisters came to Saint Joseph with only "furniture, a horse, a wagon, a cow and garden implements, also a large supply, nearly 200 dollars worth, of coal" according to the Nazareth annals.[434] The hospital originally occupied a rented space near St. Paul's Catholic Church, but the need for greater space soon prompted a move to the Alford residence on Linden Walk, where initially room was provided for but six patients. Aided by the efforts of Dr. Waller O. Bullock and Father Tom Major, the hospital purchased a 25-room house on West Second Street, west of Jefferson Street, in 1878.[435] Transferring the patients to the Second Street location was not difficult because there were only twelve. "The furniture such as it was, was moved in a wagon covered with black calico drawn by an old lame horse."[436] The cost per day for private patients was $5 or $6 for lodging and care. The city contributed $150 annually "for the privilege of sending temporary paupers there." In 1887, a three-story brick building was raised, and an annex was attached in 1898.[437] Private rooms for patients were available on the first floor, and operating rooms on the third floor. St. Joseph Hospital continued its growth with the addition of an annex by 1908 and the addition of operating rooms and private rooms. A school for nurses was founded in 1918 with the first students graduating in 1921.

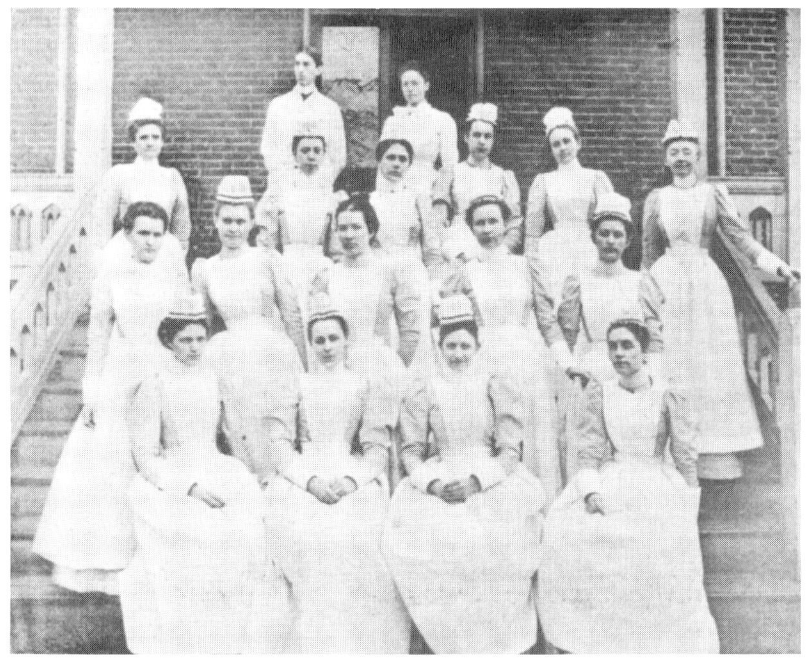

The Training Nurses,
The Good Samaritan Hospital, 1899
Courtesy of Good Samaritan Foundation, Inc.

Good Samaritan Hospital

In 1888, under the leadership of Mary Eliza Harrison,[438] the Protestant Infirmary Organization was "perfected" by the Woman's Guild of Christ Church. In 1889, the Guild provided the "money to purchase...the H. H. Gratz property, including the Farmer Dewees 'White Cottage' on East Short Street, and converted it into a Protestant Infirmary."[439] The Protestant Infirmary adopted a new name in 1899—The Good Samaritan Hospital. As it did for St. Joseph Hospital, the "community at large" contributed to the support of the hospital. Provisions were made for men's and women's wards, with respective bathrooms, an "operating table," and, shortly thereafter, a Negro ward. "Most floors were stained and varnished; some were covered with carpets....each room had almost the appearance of one in a private home....The wards (one male, one female) had iron beds with hair mattresses....occasional donations—-even when combined with the Infirmary charge of $5.00 per week....did not cover the cost of operations."[440] A grand charity ball in 1891, with proceeds of $2000, helped to alleviate the financial strain.

A proposal for establishing a nursing school was put forth in November 1890. Admission to the nursing school was offered to women between the ages of 20 and 35, and only to those qualified to be "examined in reading, penmanship and arithmetic." By January 1891, the school had admitted four student nurses; these four made up the first class to graduate in 1893. In 1905 the hospital acquired property on South Limestone and dedicated its new building on July 3, 1907. The hospital was taken over by the Southern Methodist Church (1925) and subsequently the United Methodist Church. Further construction was initiated in the immediate postwar period, namely, a clinical lab in 1946 and larger projects in the early 1950s.

Medical Transitions

The historian Haber asserts, "Though the medical profession as a whole may not have prospered in the late nineteenth century, clearly it gained respect and influence."[441]Although Lexington had essentially disappeared from leadership in the regional, national, and international medical scene by the mid-nineteenth century and made no further late-century medical contribution of note, the fate of medicine otherwise, nationally and internationally, was one of immense gain. Thanks primarily to the works of French physicians and scientists (Francois-Joseph-Victor Broussais, Philippe Pinel, Marie-Francois Bichat and others) during the first four decades of the nineteenth century, disease was liberated from the humoral theory, for now disease was seen as a local entity residing in specific tissues of organs. Later Rudolph Virchow (1821-1902) conclusively demonstrated that an interruption of cellular function was the basis of disease. The publication of his *Cellular Pathology* in 1858 set the stage for the domination of German medicine through the remainder of the nineteenth century and the first decades of the twentieth century. Not only the perception of disease but also the means by which therapy could be employed changed. Surgery was no longer a last resort but rather found a scientific basis for the removal of localized disease.

Pierre Louis (1787-1872) in France introduced the statistical method into the realm of investigation with emphasis on collection, precise observation, comparison, and interpretation. Specialization was well under way by the 1860s. The generalist of the past grudgingly made room for the specialist, and the specialty was determined to a considerable degree by newly invented instruments, such as the opthalmoscope (Hermann von Helmholtz in 1851) and the laryngoscope (Johann Czermak in 1857). The specialist offered the patient his knowledge, his skill, and his experience-at a price.

Other notable medical achievements of the nineteenth century include anesthesia (Crawford Long, Georgia, 1846) and Listerism (antisepsis). Joseph Lister, (1827-1912) built his theory of wound infection on the suspicion of the great Frenchman, Louis Pasteur, that microbes might cause disease. So revolutionary a discovery was antisepsis that surgery itself has been divided into the pre-Listerian period and the post-Listerian period; other developments included steam sterilization (Ernst von Bergmann, 1886) and the x-ray (William Roentgen, 1894), which led to earlier and more precise diagnosis and treatment and thus secured better care and improved prognosis. The enlightenment of the medical world by Ignaz Philip Semmelweiss (1818-1865) and Oliver Wendell Holmes (1809-94) about the link between childbed fever and the physician's "infected fingernails" helped to reduce the mortality associated with pregnancy. Preventive medicine also played a significant role in the nineteenth century: sanitation, vaccination, pasteurization of milk, sewage disposal, clean water supplies, clean streets, bathtubs and plumbing, all sped the move toward a longer and healthier life.

In the last third of the nineteenth century, thousands of Americans studied medicine in the Germanic nations, returning to the States with a scientific methodology advanced far beyond that of the American schools. Even so, as the nineteenth century came to an end, the American presence in medicine was on the verge of venturing out from beneath the shadow of European dominance. The American century was largely foretold by the proliferation of inventions created by American ingenuity. The steamships and the railroads fostered ever faster, more reliable and more comfortable modes of travel and of moving goods; the telegraph tapped messages from one end of the nation to the other; agriculture, industry, and commerce thrived; military forays into Cuba and the Philippines captivated the American mind and spirit. American power had set the twentieth-century stage, and medicine, in turn, was destined to play its role.

388 D. T. Smith, "Report on Vital Statistics," *Annual Meeting of Kentucky State Medical Society,* (1873) : 119-29.

389 W. L. Sutton, "Annual Address of Dr. W. L. Sutton," *Annual Meeting of the Kentucky State Medical Society* (Louisville: Webb & Levering, 1853), 17-29.

390 Samuel D. Gross, "Report of the Committee on Surgery," *Transactions of the Kentucky State Medical Society* (Louisville: Webb & Levering, 1853), 99-121.

391 Robert S.Peter, *The History of the Medical Department of Transylvania University* (Louisville, Ky.: John P. Morton & Co., 1905), 157. "Notwithstanding the efforts of zealous Trustees and generous citizens, notwithstanding the diligence of an able Faculty, the classes steadily decreased from year to year until, in 1857, with only nine graduates, the Faculty in despair disbanded, and the time-honored Medical Department of Transylvania was no more."

392 C. Vann Woodward, *Origins of the New South 1877-1913* (Baton Rouge: Louisiana State University Press, 1971), 161.

393 *Diary of Frances Dallam Peter,* Special Collections and Archives Service Center, University of Kentucky Libraries, 1863.

394 John David Smith and William Cooper, Jr., eds., *Window on the War, Frances Dallam Peter's Lexington Civil War Diary* (Lexington, Ky.: Lexington-Fayette County Historic Commission, 1976), 1.

395 Ibid., 10, 17, and 43-44.

396 Peter, *The History of the Medical Department of Transylvania University,* 136-38.

397 Mary B. Pratt, comp., *Our Relations, Dudley-Pratt Families* (Indianapolis, Ind.: Pratt Poster Company, 1933), 38-39.

398 Peter, *The History of the Medical Department of Transylvania University,* 136-38.

399 *Civil War Diary of Frances Dallam Peter.*

400 Gordon W. Jones, "The Scourge of Typhoid," *American History Illustrated* I, no. 10 (February 1967) : 23-28. Typhoid was the scourge of the Civil War for both armies, North and South, affecting approximately one hundred thousand men and with a mortality rate of 36 percent.
Courtney R. Hall, "The Lessons of the War between the States," in Felix Marti-Ibañez, ed., *History of American Medicine: A Symposium* (New York: MD Publications, Inc., 1959), 84-85, 91. "In the armies of the North, 4 persons died of sickness for every 1 killed in battle....Typhoid ... was the 'great killer'...disease killed three Confederates to every one who died of battle wounds."

401 Peter, *The History of the Medical Department of Transylvania University,* 137.

402 Lewis Collins, *History of Kentucky* (2 vols.), rev. Richard M. Collins (Louisville: Richard M. Collins, 1877) II, 203.

403 William C. Davis, *Breckinridge: Statesman, Soldier, Symbol* (Baton Rouge: Louisiana State University Press, 1974), 624.

404 Collins, *History of Kentucky*, vol. II, 204.

405 Davis, *Breckinridge: Statesman, Soldier, Symbol*, 616-624. (Davis states that "This account of the operation and Breckinridge's condition is drawn from a letter of Dr. Louis A. Sayre published in the *Louisville Medical Weekly*, June 12, 1875, and from the *Cincinnati Enquirer*, May 18, 1875." Dr. Desha was a member of the Lexington and Fayette County Medical Society

406 The paper by Dr. Benjamin Prince Earle is in the Fayette County Medical Society Archives.

407 In his address to the Kentucky State Medical Society in 1873, Dr. Lewis Rogers reports: "Dr. S. Brandeis, of Louisville, imported the first hypodermic syringe ever used in Kentucky, as he also did, through me, in 1862, the first laryngoscope." Lewis D. Rogers, "Address of the President," *Transactions of the Kentucky State Medical Society* (1873), 25-53.

408 According to Dr. Rogers, in the 1830s, Dr. John P. Harrison of the Louisville Marine Institute imported the first stethoscope brought to Kentucky. "It was of the pattern originally devised and made by Laennec himself...." Ibid.

409 Lewis Rogers, "Address of the President," *Transactions of the Kentucky State Medical Society.*

410 Constitution of Lexington and Fayette County Medical Society, Special Collections, King Library, University of Kentucky, Lexington.

411 Obituaries of several members were perused to gain insight into the sudden collapse of this promising society; however, only the facts of a particular office held give credence to its existence. We can but speculate whether the languishing animosities and the anguish of the Civil War played a role leading to the dissolution of the society.

412 *The Lexington Weekly Press,* 5 July 1882.

413 J. W. Pryor, *Doctor Pryor, An Autobiography* (Cynthiana, Ky.: The Hobson Press, 1943), 124.

414 Ibid., 82-85.

415 The historian Garrison declares that "America, beginning with Elizabeth Blackwell's graduation in 1849, was the pioneer in medical education for women." The total number of women grad uating from medical school in the succeeding years was so small that Garrison saw fit to identify only five additional women graduates. Fielding H. Garrison, *An Introduction to the History of Medicine* (Philadelphia and London: W. B. Saunders Company, 1922), 791. The "English Medical Register of 1858 contains the name of a single lady graduate of Geneva, and a second was examined and qualified in 1865....On the continent, the Swiss Universities took the lead in 1876, the German states followed, one by one, Prussia being the last to open the right of university instruction to women to 1908."

416 J. W. Thompson, "Address of the President," *Transactions of the Kentucky State Medical Society*

(Louisville: John P. Morton and Co., 1874).

417 Morris Fishbein, *A History of the American Medical Association 1847 to 1947* (Philadelphia and London: W. B. Saunders Company, 1947), 77.

418 Ibid., 82-83.

419 Ibid., 85.

420 Dr. Stevenson graduated from the Women's Medical College of Northwestern University and followed this with two years of study in Europe with Thomas Huxley and Charles Darwin. Ibid., 91.

421 *Kentucky Medical Journal*, October, 1949, 421.

422 Marion B. Lucas, *A History of Blacks in Kentucky, Vol. 1* From Slavery to Segregation 1760-1891 (Frankfort, Ky.: Kentucky Historical Society, 1992), 321.

423 *The Lexington Herald*, 20 February 1962.

424 Minutes of the Fayette County Medical Society, 15 February 1912.

425 *The Lexington Herald*, 28 February 1962.

426 Fishbein, *A History of The American Medical Association 1847 to 1947*, 79.

427 Ibid., 80-81.

428 Doris Y. Wilkinson, "Forgotten Pioneers," Kentucky Humanities Council Think Newsletter, October, 1988, 4-5.

429 Marion B. Lucas, *A History of Blacks in Kentucky, Vol. 1*, From Slavery to Segregation 1760-1891, Kentucky Historical Society, Frankfort, Kentucky, 1992, 318

430 Presented by Professor Doris Wilkinson, Historical Sociologist at University of Kentucky, Kentucky Historical Society, Kentucky Department of Transportation.

431 The Fayette County Medical Society Archives, in folder of Dr. Bush Hunter.

432 Fishbein, *A History of The American Medical Association 1847 to 1947*, 77-78.

433 The dedication ceremony for Central Baptist Hospital took place on May 9, 1954. This facilty added 173 beds to the Fayette County medical care system at a cost of $2,600,000.

434 Terri Johnson, Public Relations Specialist, St. Joseph Hospital, Lexington, Ky., to Kathy Fister, 11 September 1991; Archives, St. Joseph Hospital, Lexington, Ky.

435 John D. Wright, Jr., *Lexington Heart of the Bluegrass* (Lexington, Ky.: Lexington-Fayette County Historic Commission, 1983), 134-35.

436 Terri Johnson, to Kathy Fister, 11 September 1991.

437 Wright, *Lexington Heart of the Bluegrass*, 134-35.

438 Phyllis E. Youngerman, *Our First Century of Service, A Tribute to the People of Good Samaritan Hospital 1888-1988* (Lexington, Ky.: Good Samaritan Hospital, 1988), 6-8. "Born in the mid-1830s, she (Mary Eliza Harrison) was one of the lucky ones: Vivacious and bright. No financial worries. A good education. A good family (her mother was a niece of Mrs. Henry Clay; her father was one of Clay's closest friends and a prominent civic leader in his own right)."

439 Wright, *Lexington Heart of the Bluegrass,* 135.

440 Youngerman, *Our First Century of Service, A Tribute to the People of Good Samaritan Hospital 1888-1988,* 12-13.

441 Samuel Haber, *The Quest for Authority and Honor in the American Professions, 1750-1900,* (Chicago: The University of Chicago Press, 1991), 357.

Chapter VI

The Twentieth Century 1901 - 1950

Perhaps nothing tends more to the honor and high estimation of the profession than the organization of State, District and County Medical Associations. These promote the usefulness of the profession in two ways. Men associated for scientific and benevolent purposes must of necessity improve each other.... Again, view the beneficial effect produced on the community. It is impossible that any people can be aware that an association of men meet regularly for mutual improvement, without having an increased respect for them, as a body and as individuals.[442]

W. L. Sutton (1853)
First President of the Kentucky State Medical Society

The Lexington of the Dying Century

The Lexington Herald of Sunday, 30 December 1900 displayed a huge headline entitled "The Lexington of the Dying Century."[443] A subtitle "Prominent Men Write Historical Sketches," confirmed that the editors were looking more to the past than to the future. Among featured topics were articles reminiscing about "Kentucky University," "City Schools," "The City's Progress of the Past One-Hundred Years," "The Chamber of Commerce Plans," "A Spirit of Progressiveness Needed in Lexington," and "The Medical Profession of Lexington." The articles relate the glory of Lexington's past but with an implied confession of the city's present stagnation. The entry by John H. Flood on "A Spirit of Progressiveness Needed in Lexington" reflected the tone of the newspaper headline. He noted that "Lexington is so well situated as not to have been forced by necessity to grasp some of her best opportunities. Surrounded by the richest farming country in the South, one of the richest in the world, her retail stores have been largely supported by a farming population well able to pay for all the comforts, most of the luxuries of life."[444] Cities in the South with far less population, even less adequate railroad facilities and without many of the natural advantages of Lexington, nevertheless sold goods to Lexington's merchants and did so in competition with New York to "say nothing of our bugbears—Cincinnati and Louisville."[445] He then cites Lynchburg, Virginia, as a city similar to Lexington, having no navigable waters, no more and no less railroads, a tobacco district inferior to Lexington's, and yet one of the renowned markets of the world. "Fayette farmers plow with Lynchburg plows, buy shoes from Lynchburg retailers." Indeed, Lynchburg business had, according to the author, "penetrated even to the Pacific…Baltimore, Philadelphia and New York….This should be the case in Lexington."[446]

The Medical Profession article was written by Dr. Lyman Beecher Todd, a prominent member of the Medical Society. He began with the need of the reader to know "the historic and honored past," citing the role of Transylvania University, the accomplishments of the many highly esteemed early physicians, and the courage and the tragedy of the citizens of Lexington during the cholera epidemics. This historical briefing represents about two-thirds of the essay. Next, Dr. Todd described the new medical marvels of the past thirty years: Lister's antisepsis, Roentgen's x-ray, diphtheria toxin and the use of the microscope for blood and urine studies. However, the most important need of the community in Dr. Todd's opinion was the use of preventive measures (clean water, proper sewage, fresh air and proper lighting) to lessen the ravage of infectious disease.[447]

The striking contrast between the Lexington of 1800 and 1900, The Lexington of The Newborn West and The Lexington of the Dying Century, readily explains the humbled countenance of the latter's citizens, the unfavorable analogies drawn between its manufactures and those of cities less endowed with natural riches. That the medical profession of the latter part of the nineteenth century turned the nation's eyes to Lexington is not to be found. For the most part, Lexington's physicians were local men, with local thoughts and local needs. They served the community, a community less demanding of itself than of its past. As the author voiced at the beginning of the book, medicine *follows* in the wake of progress, it does not lead. But once progress is in place, medicine takes its stand and becomes one of the most dynamic forces of society. When and whether and how Lexington would return from its pleasant but placid lassitude to the dynamism of its youth was not apparent in 1900.[448] But when it did so medicine would follow, and it too would excel.

The Good of the Order

Although the physicians of early twentieth century Lexington were not of the stature of Samuel Brown, Daniel Drake or Benjamin Dudley, they were men of merit and foresight. They

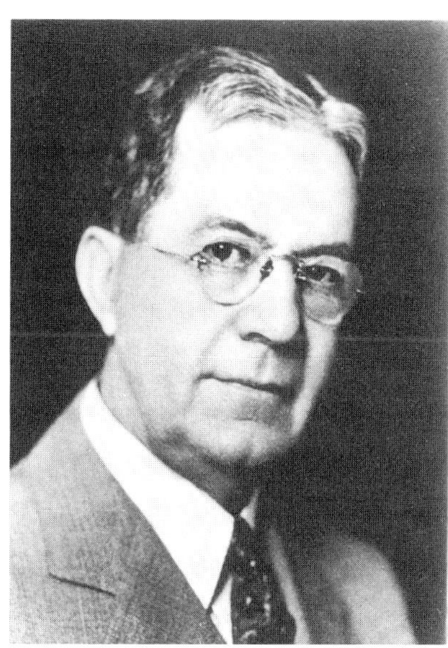

Archibald H. Barkley, M.D.
(1872-1937)
Courtesy of Fayette County Medical Socity

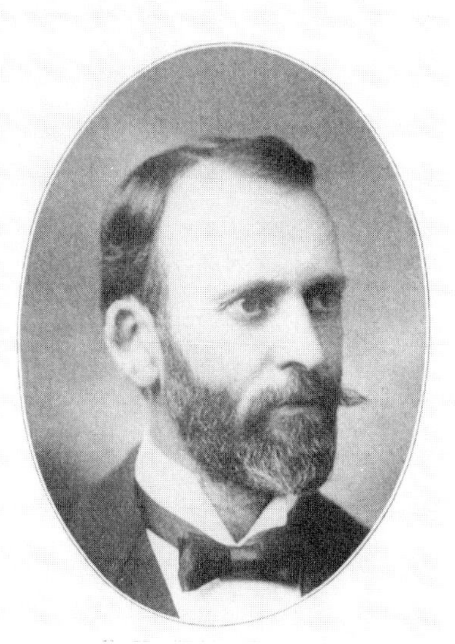

F. H. Clarke, M.D.
Courtesy of Fetter Printing Company (Formerly known as Geo G. Fetter Printing Co.)

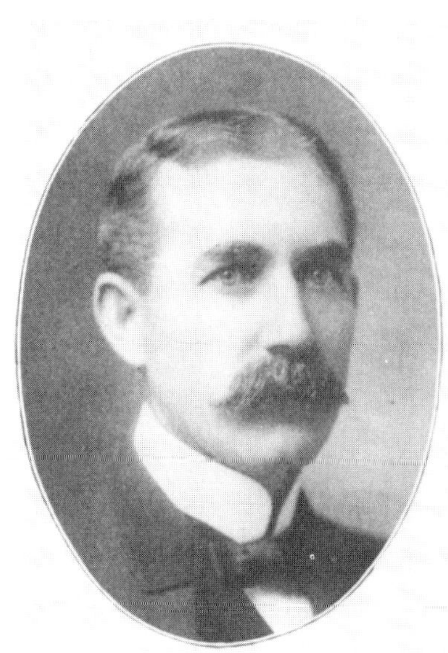

William B. McClure, M.D.
(1858-1947)
Courtesy of Fetter Printing Company (Formerly known as Geo. G. Fetter Printing Co.)

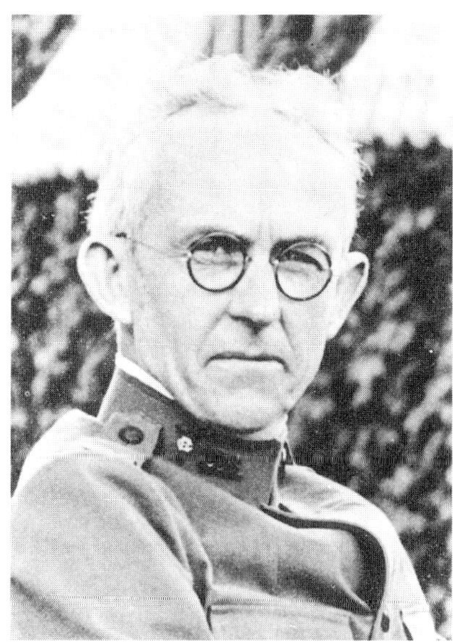

Benjamin F. Van Meter, M.D.
(1873-1934)
Courtesy of Fayette County Medical Society

shared concern for public health and education, the safety of drugs, the care of the poor, the advancement of science, the relationship between general practitioners and consultants, and harmony among physicians. The concerns of Lexington's doctors, and the remedies they proposed, come alive in the pages of the Fayette County Medical Society Minutes Book. The reader is invited to the Society meeting of August 13, 1907, held in the Lexington Public Library.

Note: The secretary's report of the Fayette County Medical Society meeting, August 13, 1907, is transcribed as originally written. The brackets are by the author (WPM).

> August 13th, 1907
>
> The Fayette Co[unty] Med[ical] Society held its regular monthly meeting at the Lex.[ington] Public Library at 8 o'clock p.m. Dr. A.[rchibald] H. Barkley[449] in the chair.
>
> Dr. [William] McClure[450] moved that Dr. A. B. Thrasher of Cincinnati – who will be in Lexington in October – be asked to read a paper before the October Meeting of our Society. Dr. Barkley added an Amendment – that Dr. Wm. Cheatham of Louisville be also asked to read a paper on the same evening – Seconded by Dr. [Benjamin] Van Meter[451] – Motion carried – Secretary instructed to write to these gentlemen.
>
> The subject of admitting Homeopaths to Membership was discussed by Drs. [A.H.] Barkley, [Frank H.] Clark[452] and [Joseph] Stuckey[453] – It was the opinion of the Society that they should be admitted if they dropped the Sectarian name –
>
> This being the meeting set apart for "The

Good of the Order" – The following gentlemen were called upon –

Dr. [George] Sprague[454] "The Relation of The Doctor to the Community" – He said, "This is a trite subject & a very important one[.] The chief object should be the promotion of The Art and Science of Medicine which is the aim of The American Med[ical] Ass[ociation] – But we should go farther than this and have as our Chief Aim – The Good of Mankind and the Glory of God[.] – The legitimate and true relation of the Doctor to his Community is not the treatment of disease, or his business or fraternal relationships – The future true Doctor must be a Sanitarian, Hygienist and Public teacher –

Preventive medicine is more important that the cure & relief of suffering – If we can diminish our death rate by Preventing disease – Small Pox, Tuberculosis etc. – Our accomplishment is much greater than the Cure of the disease when present –

In Germany Small Pox and Typhoid are almost obliterated – In Boston and New York The workers on Tuberculosis say it will be almost obliterated by 1927 – We must not be discouraged – Progress must of necessity be slow – daily discoveries show we know very little about Science.

We should pay more attention to the drugs themselves – for it is a fact that not only are the Patent and Proprietary Medicines unreliable but also that Many of the Tinctures and Extracts in the market are not of Standard Strength & this fact will add to the skepticism concerning the actions of drugs – All drugs must eventually be Standardized by the Amer[ican] Med[ical] Ass[ociatio]n & only in some such way can we depend upon our drugs – We should know more of The Physiological Action of drugs – There is much ignorance along this line among the best doctors – Dosages should not be from memory but by physiological effect –

The Doctor should be connected with Politics as a teacher – and for the general good He can help solve many hard problems –

Our slums here are as bad as elsewhere[.] The Doctor can do much for this class – The Average Doctors are ignoring their most important duties to the community"

Dr. McClure – "Medical Organization" – "Our Organization comprises our National, State & County Societies – Each has its own Constitution & Bylaws, but in spite of all this we yet lack the Harmony among ourselves that should exist – If we only did what we pretend to do we would be elevated in the esteem of ourselves and the Public – Doctors are ostracized in some communities because they have dragged themselves down by eternal fighting among their own ranks – The relations should always be cordial – When not busy they should eat and play together – No Doctor should talk about another Doctor. If these rules were kept there could be no Mal-Practice suits – The Ideal Community with 3 M.D.'s all friends and interchanging ideas constantly – working all together – when one goes away the other 2 look after his interests – In such a condition The Doctors are the Very head of the Community – When a young Doctor comes to such a community the older ones call in a body – welcome him, invite him to their homes and help him start his work – No criticism or sarcasm is heard – Of course this is not real – Only Utopian but the fault is with the Doctors themselves[.] We should practice the Golden Rule. There is no reason why all this should not come to pass in Lexington.

Dr. Clarke – "Medicine must be put on a more Scientific basis – Every Doctor must make the most possible of himself – both personally, professionally and in every other way –

The Physician is a Teacher by reason of his education and position – It is his duty to teach the ignorant[.]

Criticism and differences mean a natural and health growth and if done in the right spirit are for the eventual good or all concerned – discord and strife are results of unworthy and wrong ideas–

American Doctors have not the Law behind them as have the Germans – The German Doctors are officials with the very highest authority to enforce their ideas[.] America should have a "National Department of Health" with Authority to enforce their Laws" –

Dr. [Thomas C.] Holloway[455] – "Every order is dependent upon the enthusiasm of its members – every Doctor must be enthusiastic – a

Doctor gets much encouragement from any interest that another Doctor takes in him and his work – and is discouraged by the reverse attitude – The young practitioner needs the help of older heads – Interchange of Ideas is good for all involved – Doctors should practice harmony every day instead of meeting once a month to talk about it[.] This fellowship would carry on a perpetual clinic and be helpful to all – especially the younger ones – The relationship between the Consultant and practitioner should be well understood and observed[.] A consultation should be called for whenever the condition of the patient indicates it – The Ethics must be rigid and never disregarded – The consultant should not make the Practitioner feel embarrassed and inferior – and he should be very careful not to affect the standing of the practitioner with the family" –

Dr. [Henry H.] Roberts[456] – "It is very important for Doctors to turn their attention to the young – he must watch the growing children – Many subsequent ills may be warded off by this means – deformities may often be prevented by proper care – The Consultant must always be a Help-Mate and not an Antagonistic to the Practitioner.

Doctors must educate the Public up to value the Physician[']s services and by this means can the fee be raised[.] There should be an understanding and schedule for fees" –

Dr. Van Meter – "All that we can say about this subject comes back to the Personality of the

Man himself [.] Every Man must make himself above the other Man's abuse – There are men in this Society that cannot be hurt by any amount of abuse from others – They are above such attacks – Build up your own character and these petty troubles will disappear – The attitude of The Consultant must be modified by the man he is helping [.] If The Family asks for a Consultation then everything should be said in the presence of The Practitioner & Family & there should be no private talk – If The Practitioner calls for the Consultation The talk should be private & to the Practitioner. Stop talking about the other man and investigage yourself and you will be too busy to fight and run down someone else."

Dr. Stucky – "Dr. Van Meter has sounded the key note – Get right yourself and you have solved the matter It is not always what is said that hurts – It is the little Sarcasms, Innuendos and curls of the lip- puff of Smoke & the like – If we had more loyalty to our own profession we could solve all – In Lexington some would rather send 100 miles for a Consultant than get a better one here – Why is This? – No better Talent is looked for –Simply little jealousies We are apt to be over sensitive – We are responsible for our position in the community by the Stand we take – On the subject of fees I think we are fairly well agreed – Should we charge the clergy – Yes – They like you better and give you more respect

There being no further business the Society adjourned –

R. Julian Estill[457] Secy

Medicine In Transition

By the end of the nineteenth century the ability to control pain and avoid infection opened the door for the twentieth century surgeon. He could now elect to operate rather than be forced to do so. Advances in bacteriology, improvement in anesthesia, experience in the use of x-rays, surgical research, and the Halsted revolution in surgical training all had a profound effect on surgery. William Stewart Halsted's (1852-1922) movement derived from his admiration for the German system of surgical training, which he had experienced during three years of study in Europe. When the Johns Hopkins Hospital, Baltimore, opened in 1889, he accepted an appointment as acting surgeon and was named professor of surgery in 1892. Of his many notable contributions to surgery, the most profound and lasting was his establishment of a surgical residency program based on the German system that blended basic science with clinical teaching and full-time professors. Through his surgical disciples, his method of training soon spread throughout the United States.[458]

Within a few years, the Flexner Report (1911) led to the closing of many deficient medical schools and the modernization of the remainder. Following the Flexner Report, the number of medical schools in the United States and Canada declined from 155 to less than 70.[459] The Halsted Revolution and the Flexner Report played major roles in the medical ascendancy of the United States. Reform in medical education also came about through endowments to medical schools by institutions such as the Rockefeller Foundation; full-time professors, modern libraries, clinic facilities, and medical research became the rule.[460] Fewer physicians were being trained, but the caliber of each graduate was significantly improved, and the public became the chief beneficiary. Even so, the plight of the early twentieth century physician was not without financial risk. The cost of rental for a downtown office increased together with the cost of setting up a practice, secretarial assistance, instrumentation and day-to-day expenses.

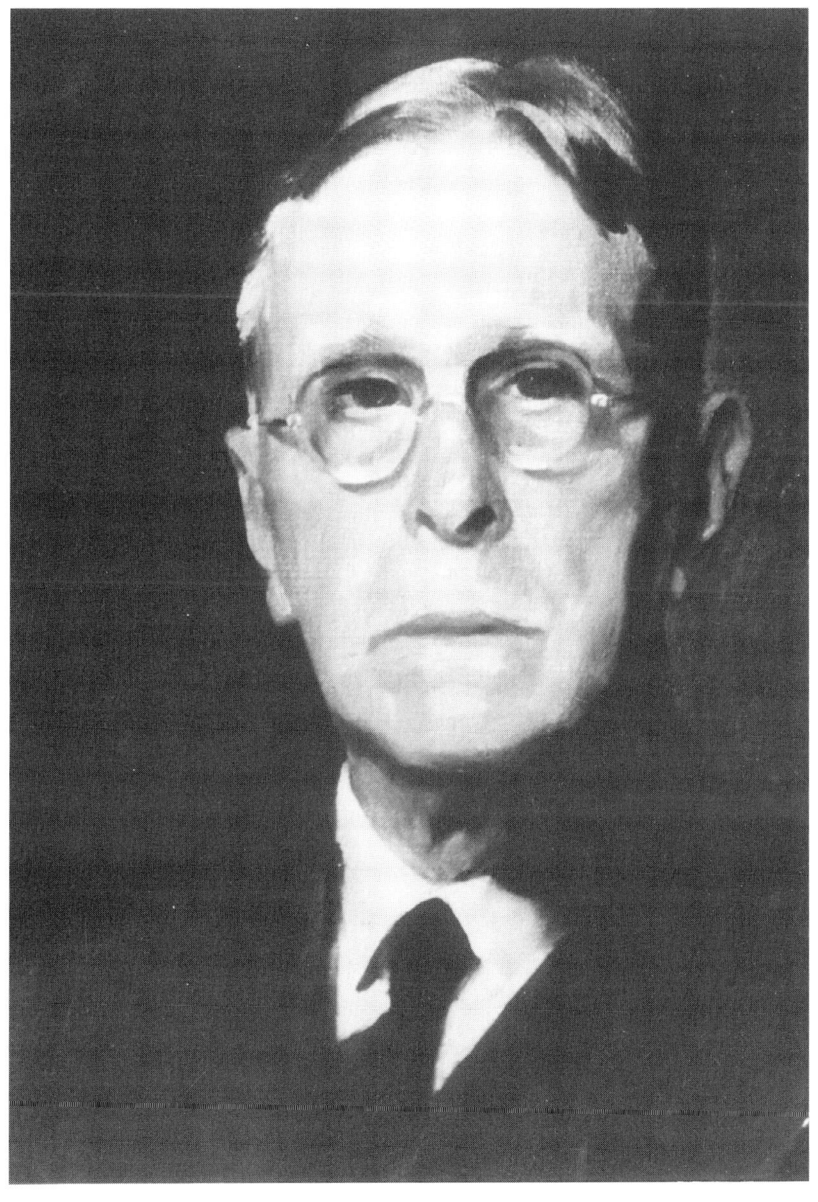

John W. Scott, M.D.
(1875-1966)
Courtesy of Fayette County Medical Society

Minutes from early twentieth century meetings of the Fayette County Medical Society illustrate the comparative poverty of physicians in that era. The April 9, 1907 meeting of the Society took place at the Lexington Public Library.[461] Dr. Roberts reported that the Society could hire a stenographer "to take down discussions – that one could be secured for $5.00 per meeting." The members "decided that the Society could not afford this and the secretary was requested to take the discussions as fully as possible." In 1906, members of the Society were dismayed and sorrowed by the plight of the physicians of San Francisco, following San Francisco's unparalleled destruction by an earthquake. The minutes of the Society of May 15, 1906 read as follows: "A communication from the AMA was read concerning the raising of funds for the relief of the San Francisco physicians in need. Dr. [Waller] Bullock reported some instances of suffering among physicians he had seen while he was there: Dr. [George] Sprague made a motion that the secretary collect contributions from those members of the society who wished to give to this cause and send it on to the AMA...."[462]

Dr. John Scott in his Reminiscences of the "Meeting Places" of the Medical Society relates one incident in the early 1900s that took place in the basement of the Phoenix Hotel "where dinner had been prepared for comparatively few of us. At that time, unwisely, each member paid for his own dinner. The inevitable result was reduced attendance. On the occasion in mind we had a very small attendance and one of our much beloved members, but one who was a little 'close,' rose and left just before the dinner saying that he wouldn't stay to dinner, for obvious reasons. On his way out he picked up a handful of cigars. *Our* cigars!" Dr. Scott also tells the story of when:

> One of the members made a plea that the doctors should not be solicited for funds for charitable enterprises in view of the fact that they did so much charity. I took my favorite line and com-

mented on the fact that if one analyzed this "charity," he would find that extremely little of it is real if need be the only incentive. Dr. Bullock then commented that he had never in his life done anything for nothing. The implication of this was clear. The next morning I visited in the hospital one of the members who had recently had an operation and who had been told about the meeting. He was outraged at the line that Dr. Bullock and I had taken and undertook to tell me how he did a sort of charity that we knew nothing about. He said that recently he had been called to see a patient on Race Street, in the poorer section of town in the middle of the night. When he reached the patient he discovered that the man already owed him $100.[463]

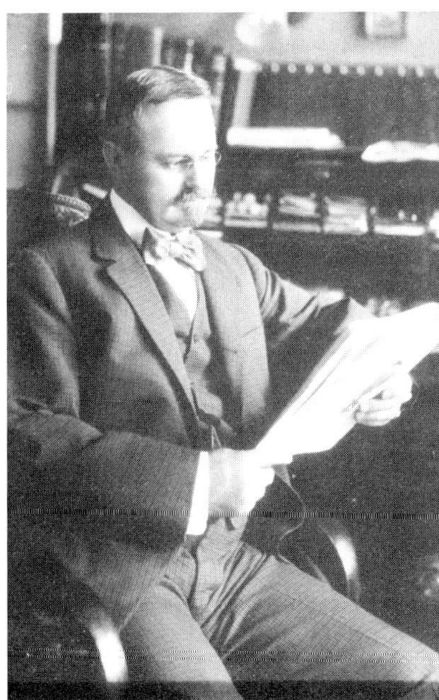

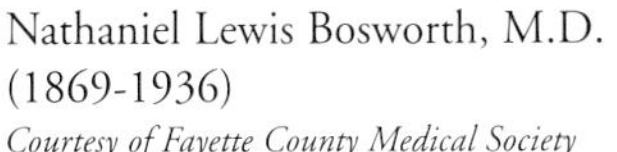

Nathaniel Lewis Bosworth, M.D.
(1869-1936)
Courtesy of Fayette County Medical Society

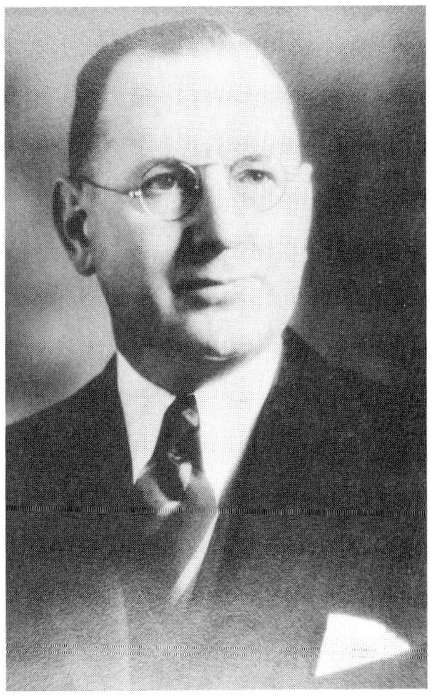

Charles Crain Garr, M.D.
(Died 1957)
Courtesy of Fayette County Medical Society

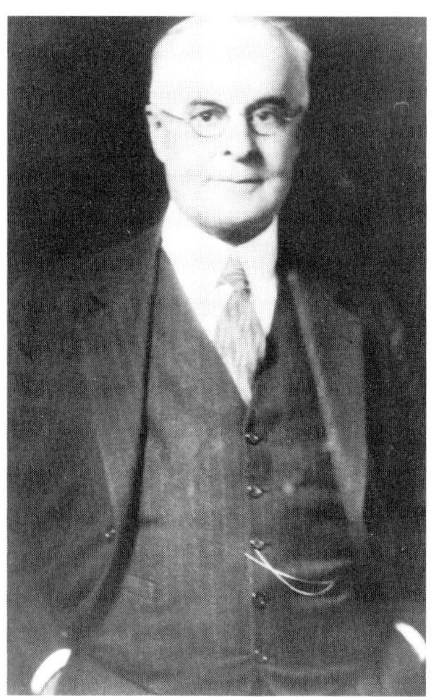

George P. Sprague, M.D.
(1863-1942)
Courtesy of Fayette County Medical Society

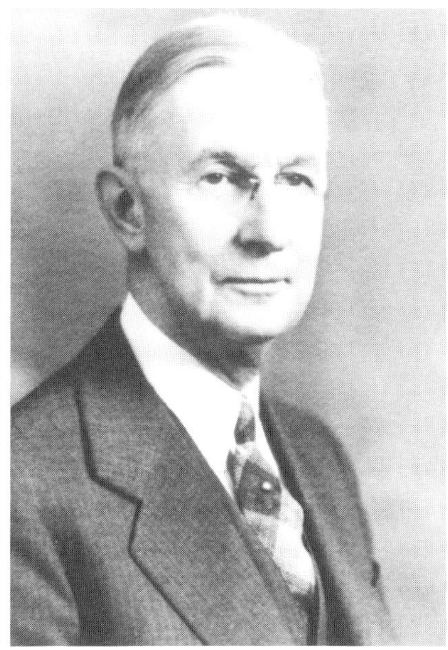

Charles A. Vance, M.D.
(1880-1962)
Courtesy of Fayette County Medical Society

Information about physicians' incomes in the early 1900s "suggests that their average earnings were surprisingly small—About the same as ministers and less than civil servants."[464] The average annual income for American physicians in 1901 was $730 for city practitioners and $1,200 for the country doctor.[465] (In 1999 dollars, the city practitioners' average income was approximately $14,000, and the country doctors' was approximately $20,000.) The relatively low income can, in large measure, be accounted for by the over-abundant supply of physicians. Competition was severe.[466] By 1929 the Physician's average annual income rose to $5,224, but fell with the onset of the Depression.[467]

Social and economic changes also played a major part in defining the physicians' role, not only for the immediate years of concern but for the balance of the century. The advent of the telephone, electric lights, and cars changed social and economic habits. Economic roots were shifting from the soil to the factory floor.

Medical care also was undergoing major changes. Hospitals were no longer simply a haven of last resort. The focus now was on getting well, the return of patients to their homes, their families and community.

As a rule, early twentieth century American men provided the sole family income. Wives customarily stayed home to attend to the many household duties and children. The family was secure. Financial needs were met. Needs were not met, however, when the breadwinner of the house became ill or had an accident. Who would pay his bills? Without an income and with no provision for job-related medical care the worker and his family were soon penniless. The injured worker had but one certain source to turn to: his physician. When and whether physicians were paid seldom had little, if any, direct tie to their time and care, or to the bill submitted. Even so, this one-on-one relationship, physician and patient, was readily accepted by each party, for what would one do without the other? That some alternate provision could benefit both the patient and the physician and in turn society itself soon would be tested.

With the movement of workers from the farm to the factory, injuries rapidly increased and proved costly not only to the individual, but to his employer. Accidents in America became so prevalent during the latter part of the nineteenth century and the first decade of the twentieth century that the states enacted thirty workmen's compensation laws between 1910 and 1915.[468] Such laws were designed to compensate the injured worker for lost wages, but there were no provisions for the injured worker's medical care. Many saw in the workers' illness a national tragedy in the bud, illness of such magnitude as to bring down the social and economic well-being of all Americans, through the loss of productivity of the labor force. Many Americans believed the only remedy to be a national health insurance program similar to that introduced by Bismarck for Germany in 1883 and later by other European nations. According to Paul Starr, "its original function was primarily income stabilization"[469] for the injured worker. However, it was not reformers alone who supported such legislation but also many physicians believed that they could thus gain a reasonable financial return for their services. Likewise, politicians clamored for votes by advocating national health insurance. In 1913, Teddy Roosevelt's Progressive Party advocated: "The protection of home and life against the hazards of sickness, irregular employment and old age through the adoption of a system of social insurance adapted to American use."[470]

One of the more adamant opponents of compulsory health insurance was the president of the American Federation of Labor, Samuel Gompers, who feared that the union's role of providing social benefits for its members would be weakened if usurped by a paternalistic government insurance program.[471] Starr's observation that "the AMA could have initially approved health insurance, while the AFL opposed it," suggests the complexity of the various interests in the national health insurance movement.[472] Among the many reasons for the health insurance failure at this time were the nation's anti-German feelings during World War I, the specter of uncontrollable and unpredictable cost, the opposition of many physicians, and the fact that their incomes rose during the war years. For these reasons the national health insurance movement lay well-nigh dormant through the 1920s.[473]

The consideration of national medical insurance aside, we now turn to the more mundane concerns of time, access and contact. How did the patient get to the doctor? How did the doctor get to the patient? Two relatively new non-medical innovations had an immediate and lasting impact on medical practice—the telephone and the car. Their introduction into Lexington and into the practice of medicine lost little time from their American advent.

The Telephone

The *Lexington Transcript* of January 23, 1880 states that J.

U. Usher was erecting a telephone between his residence and his furniture store. Evidently this was the first telephone to be installed in Lexington and but four years from the pioneering development of the telephone by Alexander Graham Bell (1876). One and a half years later, in May, 1881, the *Lexington Transcript* announced, "The Lexington Exchange has 150 subscribers."[474]

In 1912, in Lexington's first directory, published by The Fayette Home Telephone Company, it had a very succinct message to the citizens of Lexington:

Don't Travel TALK Don't Write

Fifty-seven physicians were listed in the 1912 directory.[475] A few physicians listed two numbers, presumably an office and a home number; however, the directory failed to distinguish between the two. Several names echo to this very day in the Fayette County Medical Society: N. L. Bosworth, C. W. Trapp, John W. Scott, R. C. Faulconer, Thomas C. Holloway, C. Brooks Wilmott, and G. P. Sprague. If you did not want to be burdened by looking up numbers then you could ring # 803 for City Physicians. The directory of 1913 was somewhat more user-friendly. First, the directory reminded: "You Live on a Highway for Talk which reaches millions of out-of-town folks; ASK THE OPERATOR TO OPEN THE GATES; Every Telephone is a Long Distance Station." The directory divided subscribers both numerically and categorically by profession or by trade. Sixty-nine physicians were listed. Once again names such as B. F. Van Meter, T. H. Kinnaird, and John E. Hunter reverberate throughout the Medical Society's twentieth century history. Three companies, namely the Bourbon Remedy Co., the Red Circle Pill Co., and the Viavi Co., all housed on Main Street, were listed in the directory of 1913 under the title Patent Medicine.[476]

At the February 11, 1913, meeting of the Society, members were upset by local telephone charges. The two Lexington telephone companies had combined and were to raise the rate from

$0.50 per month to $1.25 per month.[477] Dr. Garr Moore moved that a committee be appointed to draft a resolution protesting the raise in rates made by the telephone company. Three members of the Society were appointed to act in behalf of the Society, sending resolutions of their objections to both newspapers and to the telephone company. Particulars about the outcome of the Society's objections were not recorded.

The Car

On March 17, 1909 *The Lexington Herald* announced: "Automobile Factory Now Ready For Work. The Lexington Motor Car Company, after putting in all the machinery and parts for the new factory, had all the different parts in motion late yesterday afternoon...."[478] It was to be the first automobile to be manufactured in Lexington. Even so, Lexingtonians had not waited for the output of the home factory to satisfy their desire for the thrill of the motor car. Automobile shows were very popular in Lexington during the first two decades of the twentieth century. An article of October 20, 1904 highlighted the new era: "Fast Time In Motor Car." W.G. Morgan of Lexington had just completed a round trip, Lexington to Cincinnati to Lexington in his Cadillac motor car. The trip began at the Fayette County Courthouse by way of Williamstown to the Michellan Hotel, Cincinnati. The reporter gave the mileage as 370 miles. The run from Lexington to Cincinnati was made in six hours. The purpose of the trip was "purely for pleasure." Perhaps a few Lexington physicians adopted the motor car when it first became available; however, the cost of the car (range $1,000 to $2,800 in 1910), the conditions of the roads, and other considerations of maintenance likely put off their purchase.

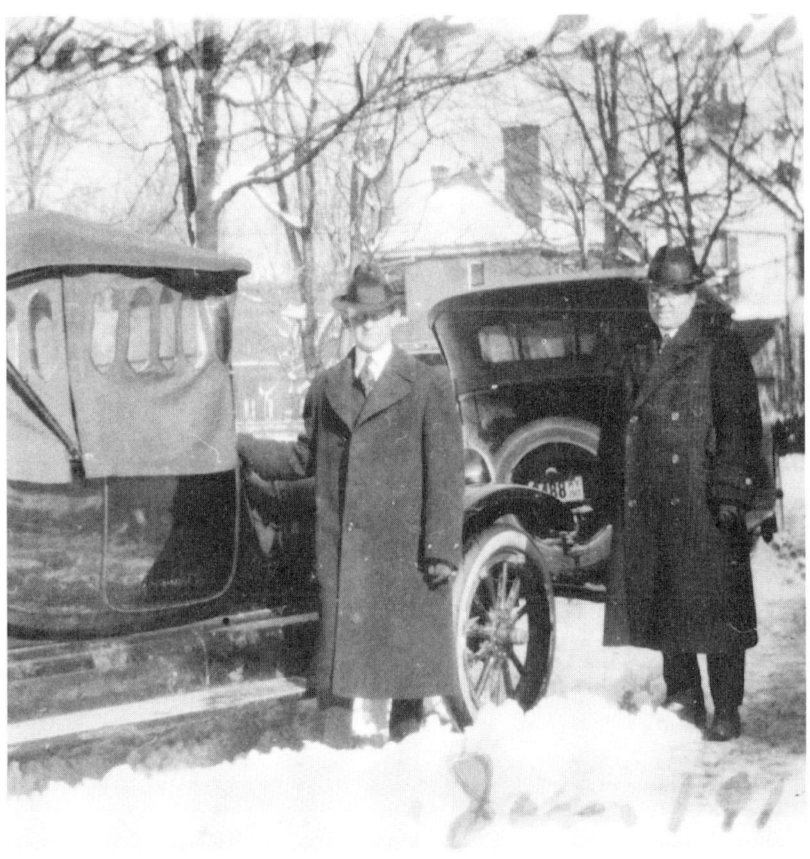

"Button Up Coats and Cars"
Drs. Carrick and Coleman
Courtesy of Fayette County Medical Society

National Medical Meeting in Lexington

Dr. John Scott, one of the most eminent and respected members of the Society and a great admirer of Dr. J. A. Stucky, tells the story of the Laryngo-Oto-Rhinological (the Triological) Society meeting (1903) in Lexington, of which Dr. Stucky "was not only the president, but apparently the bosom friend of each [member of the Triological Society]." It was Lexington's first national medical meeting. "The occasion was a remarkable one with moving demonstrations of the tremendous esteem and affection in which they held Dr. Stucky. I attended the dinner, a remarkable event. Dr. Stucky had a national reputation and was beloved by his fellows, far and wide, in a way that has hardly been equaled by any member of the profession here."[479]

The Prevailing Diseases

For the most part, physicians in the early twentieth century faced the same diseases that had been prevalent during the latter half of the nineteenth century. A newspaper report of January, 1918 indicates that tuberculosis led in the cause of death in Lexington. In 1917, 137 cases of tuberculosis occurred in Lexington, resulting in 120 deaths. Other causes of death included diphtheria (4), scarlet fever (1), measles (1), typhoid fever (16) and pneumonia (11). During the year 1917 there were 40 cases of diphtheria, 32 of scarlet fever, 72 of whooping cough, 91 of chicken pox, 571 of measles, 60 of typhoid, 6 of smallpox and 32 of pneumonia.[480]

Flu Epidemic of 1918 - 1919

On October 4, 1918, in an article titled "Spanish Plague

Threatens City," the *Lexington Herald* reported 31 "Flu" cases now in Lexington. All cases had been quarantined and their residences placarded to warn the public of its presence. Bulletins printed in red were posted in all public places with precautions to take against the disease.[481] By October 29, 797 cases of flu had been recorded with as many as thirty or more new cases per day.[482] An Emergency Flu Hospital was established at the corner of Fourth and Upper Streets staffed by volunteer nurses. The Flu continued its merciless pillage throughout the remainder of October and into November with 31 new cases reported on November 19. Eastern State Hospital was especially hard hit with a total of 415 cases by November 20.[483] Dr. Pryor relates conditions at the University of Kentucky:

> The barracks built on the campus near the corner of Winslow and Rose Streets had not been occupied a great while before we had an outbreak of influenza which proved quite serious. The men's dormitory had been vacated, but was not considered fit for the sick. The milder cases were housed in the gymnasium and Y. M. C. A. rooms. The more serious cases were taken to the Good Samaritan Hospital. There were two medical officers in charge of the soldiers. Captain Fletcher had charge of those at the Good Samaritan when we had forty cases of pneumonia. Captain Fletcher took influenza and I had to take charge of his work. Dr. W. T. Briggs helped me with these cases. Fortunately Captain Fletcher's case was mild and he resumed his work in about ten days. We had a number of fatalities, but I recall that our mortality rate was extremely favorable when compared with other institutions. It was a strenuous year for me.[484]

On November 20, the Health Officer, D. A. Furlong, recorded 1248 cases of flu and pneumonia to date and stated that this number was "comparatively small" compared with other cities. The numerous cases of pneumonia were believed to be caused by the rainy and murky weather. The *Lexington Herald* of December 16 reported that the situation (flu) was under control in Lexington, the ban lifted after 71 days. On December 15 regular services were held in the churches, the first time since the ban against the disease was begun on October 11. Furlong reported that a total of 1513 cases of flu with 69 deaths had occurred in Lexington.

The Lost Records

The minutes of the Fayette County Medical Society meeting of December 13, 1904 opened with the following terse comment: "It was announced that the Secty, Dr. D. J. Healy, had lost all the records of the Society except the charter, and also that he had removed to Washington, D.C." No further comment was made as to the loss of the minutes at that time or in subsequent minutes of the Society. That the announcement on December 13, 1904 of the lost records was given such matter-of-fact commentary is inexplicable, and at odds with the historical consciousness of its members. Possibly Dr. Healy had a very plausible explanation, a reason so obvious and so final as to forever hush inquiry. We probably will never know.[485] The mystery of the lost minutes is further obscured by the fact that the Secretary, Dr. J. D. Healy, under whose guard the minutes were lost, returned to Lexington to practice medicine and in 1924 was elected President of the Medical Society. Dr. Healy obviously remained in the good graces of the Society.

Commenting on the lost records, Dr. J. W. Pryor, in his Medical Society Notes (circa 1930-40), states "*this* book contained the history of the Society up to that date (1904) and the only roster of its members, officers and records of their activities."[486] If Dr.

Pryor is accurate, then all the minutes of the Society beginning in 1882 through 1903 were housed in a single ledger. Although the 1904 minutes stated that the Charter of the Society was not lost, its present location is unknown. The loss of the 1882-1903 records effectively eliminates all knowledge of the society, the members, the officers, and the meeting sites during this period. What information we have is taken from the newspapers and telephone directories. In 1930-40, Dr. Pryor attempted to report the history of the Lexington and Fayette Medical Society stating that he had "assiduously searched the file of the *Lexington Daily and Weekly Press* and the *Lexington Daily Transcript*, however, found comparatively little information," and so, "gave up because of the paucity of information at my command." He asserts that the lack of news coverage about the Medical Society during this period of time was brought about by the profession's being "wary of the press."[487]

Tributes to Ephraim McDowell and Daniel Drake, and the Transylvania Medical Library

On May 9, 1905, the Fayette County Medical Society passed a resolution made by Dr. William McClure "that the statue of Dr. Ephraim McDowell, the greatest of surgeons, should adorn Statuary Hall in our Capitol at Washington." The acceptance and unveiling of the statues of Henry Clay and Dr. Ephraim McDowell took place on March 3, 1929 in Statuary Hall, Capitol of the United States, Washington, D.C. The nomination of these two Kentuckians for such an honor came about with the offer in 1925 by Isaac W. Bernheim, formerly of Louisville, "to give to the State of Kentucky statues of two of the most notable men of the state if the legislature would appoint a commission to designate its wishes in the matter."[488] The legislature in 1926 passed an act appointing a commission and requesting that the committee report its findings to the next legislature. The commission concluded that the state should be represented "by two exponents of the State's attitude of mind." Clay and McDowell were the leading contenders and the unanimous choices of the commission.

The April 14, 1931 meeting of the Fayette County Medical Society took place at McVey Hall, University of Kentucky. An important announcement was made by the highly regarded Dr. J. A. Stucky:[489]

> At this point Dr. Stucky asked for the floor and stated that it was suggested to him by a member of the society that a gavel be procured. After considerable thought and inquiry and through the kindness of President Turck of Old Centre College and President Braden of Transylvania University, I was able to obtain a piece of cherry from a tree planted by Dr. Ephraim McDowell on his lawn and a piece of yellow pine from the window of his office, where the first ovariotomy was performed, also through President Braden's effort a piece of white oak rafter from Old Morris Chapel of Transylvania University. Our Society has grown and flourished among the glorious traditions of our pioneer medical men of national renown and it seems especially fitting to me that this gavel composed of woods from these historic spots be presented to our society.
>
> It gives me great pleasure to present this [gavel] to the Fayette County Medical Society with the hope that it will stimulate our members to greater deeds in their profession.[490]

In a meeting of the Society held on June 4, 1926, the Society objected to the rumored sale of the Transylvania Medical Library.[491] President George Wilson explained the purpose of the meeting which was followed by a general discussion. "Dr. Barkley moved that the Society send a letter to the Curators of Transylvania stating that the Society deplored the losing from this State so valuable and rare a collection of books, and earnestly request the Board of Curators to hold for the posterity of this State that which has added so much to the luster of its past. The motion was unanimously adopted."

In 1937 the Fayette County Medical Society had the good fortune to acquire an oil portrait of Dr. Daniel Drake, its most celebrated member and an early president of the Society. The portrait, a work by Chester Harding, one of the most acclaimed artists in the era after Gilbert Stuart, was acquired by the Medical Society from the descendants of Dr. Joseph C. Carter of Versailles, Kentucky, physician and intimate friend of Dr. Drake. The portrait which had hung for some 100 years in the Carter home in Versailles now hangs in the board room of the Medical Society.[492] The noted nineteenth century physician, Dr. Samuel Gross, of Louisville and Philadelphia, described Drake: "His features, remarkably regular, were indicative of manly beauty, and were lighted up and improved by blue eyes of wonderful power and penetration."[493] In 1984 the portrait of Drake was exhibited by the National Portrait Gallery with other works by Chester Harding.

A Medical College in Lexington?

From the time of the closing of Transylvania's Medical Department in 1857, two preliminary steps were essential before the dream of re-establishing a medical school in Lexington could become a reality. First was the establishment of a state university and second was the encouragement of the AMA.

The Morrill Act of 1862, provided the states with federal support in the form of land grants for the encouragement of colleges of agriculture and the mechanic arts.[494] The Kentucky Legislature gave the land grants to "Kentucky University," located in Harrodsburg. In 1865, Transylvania merged with Kentucky

University, and "the state charged the new university with the responsibility of providing medical education in Kentucky."[495] However, Kentucky University did not gain the support necessary to re-open the medical school. In 1878 the Legislature acted to separate the Agricultural and Mechanical Colleges from Kentucky University and located "State College" in Lexington on land donated by the city of Lexington. Kentucky University then resumed the name of Transylvania University. By an act of the state legislature, State College on March 16, 1908 became known as State University.[496] The act dedicated the institution to "teaching and original research," and specified the introduction of courses of instruction leading to degrees in medicine and law.[497]

Unfortunately, Kentucky had eight medical schools in the 1890s, many being proprietary schools.[498] A number of these schools made attempts to ally with State University; however, the University Board did not desire to proceed with anything less than a school under the "control of the president of the University and the Board of Trustees."[499] Even so, the founding of a medical school was considered to be much more complex and though studied no action was taken.[500]

For its meeting of June 13, 1905, the Fayette County Medical Society met in the County Court House. The guest speaker of the evening was President Patterson of State College (later the University of Kentucky). He spoke of "the desirability of having a medical college at Lexington in connection with State College." The Society responded by approving a lengthy resolution offered by Dr. J.W. Pryor, supporting Dr. Patterson. After noting that "the population of Lexington has now increased far beyond that which it had sixty years ago, when the Medical College of Transylvania was in its prime," the resolution touted the construction of railways and interurban electrical buses, the establishment of hospitals and infirmaries, plus the excellent preliminary secular education offered by State College. It was as Pryor said, "an opportune time to establish a medical college of high character in the city of Lexington." Lexington, he suggested, should appropriate funds to erect suitable buildings.[501]

It was the "consensus of the society" to establish a medical school in Lexington. A meeting was held at the Public Library[502] on May 12, 1908, to discuss the organization of a medical department in State College. A week later, on May 19, Dr. Pryor used the century-old rivalry between Lexington and Louisville to rally the troops. "Louisville is also trying to get the medical college." By 1910, an attempt to begin a Medical Department at the State University was underway. The plan was to have a two-year program at the University and presumably complete the second two years in a university medical center having clinical credentials. Dr. J. W. Pryor tells the story in his *Autobiography*:[503]

> It had long been my ambition to have a Medical Department at the University. The medical schools in Kentucky were not in high favor with the American Medical Association on account of their low requirements for entrance. Our pre-medical work was overlapping the freshmen year of the medical schools, and I thought it would require very little additional expense to establish the first two years as a number of the universities had done, and that we could make these years equal to the best.

In January 1910, a bill was introduced in the Kentucky Senate similar to those enacted in several other states providing for two years at the university to be followed by two years at a recognized medical school having clinical instruction.[504] The bill was endorsed by the Kentucky State Medical Society and numerous county medical societies throughout the state. Initially the bill was favorably received and its passage all but assured; however, through machinations in the Rules Committee, the bill was defeated in the Senate and did not come up for consideration in the House.[505]

Even though the Bill was defeated, the effort to establish a medical school in Lexington did not die. In 1928 Dr. Frank J. McVey, President of the University of Kentucky, summoned Dr. J. S. Chambers, head of the Department of Hygiene and Public Health, to his office. Dr. McVey instructed Dr. Chambers to appraise the need of medical education in Kentucky. The 1929 report by Chambers urged the location of a medical school in Lexington. The onset of the Depression and the entry into World War II delayed any significant action until 1951 at which time the second and essential factor in the establishment of a medical school in Lexington came into play; the American Medical Association Council on Medical Education recommended the establishment of a medical school at the University of Kentucky.[506] The Fayette County Medical Society announced its support of the medical school, and three of its most prominent members, Francis Massie, Edward Ray, and Coleman Johnston, presented the case for the Lexington location before the Board of Trustees of the Kentucky Medical Association.[507]

Two Imminent Dangers: Coca-Cola and Tuberculosis

In the meeting of April 9, 1907, the members tackled an immediate concern. "Dr. Stucky suggested that the Large Sale of Coca-Cola be investigated."[508] Dr. Sprague moved that the "secretary secure an analysis of Coca-Cola and report at next meeting."[509] The motion was carried but no further entries on Coca-Cola were made.

On June 18, 1909 the Society discussed the dangers of meat and milk contamination by TB (Tubercle bacilli) and passed a resolution to require inspection of all meat, milk and animals for TB and elimination of infected animals.[510] The discussion was likely prompted by the publication of Upton Sinclair's *The Jungle.* The book "went out to the world in February, 1906."[511] Depicting the atrocious conditions in the meat packing industry in Chicago, Sinclair's book aroused the revulsion of the nation; it became a best seller within a few months.

The meeting of October 12, 1909 was held at the Lexington Public Library. A guest of the Society, Mr. R. M. Allen of the Kentucky Experiment Station, spoke to the Society:[512]

> The Pure Food Commission desires the Medical Society to aid in the Local Meat inspection. The work has already begun. The same plan will be used as was used in Louisville in working the Milk Commission. Three Doctors gave time & interest to the Commission. This inspection has been the greatest factor in good milk in Kentucky all due to those Doctors co-operation.

The Minutes then note:

> Mr. Allen has just completed a preliminary inspection of Slaughtering houses in Kentucky and finds the usual problems of the uninspected. He wants to take up in Lexington Effective & Continuous local inspection following the plan of the Louisville Milk Inspection Commission. He wants to make Lex[ington] the starting place.

Commenting on the subject of meat inspection, Dr. G. P. Sprague said that inspection of local cattle for tuberculosis in the previous year showed a very large number to be positive. Drs. Estill, Robert, and Bradley were appointed to a Committee to work with Mr. Allen.

Criminal Abortion

On May 11, 1909 the Medical Society met at the Lexington Public

Library. A report on the practice of "Criminal Abortion" in Lexington by Drs. Sprague, Holloway and Stucky was read by the secretary and subsequently forwarded to Dr. J. M. McCormick, Secretary of the State Board of Health.[513] At the September 13 meeting Dr. Charles Vance read a resolution acknowledging the State Board of Health's thorough investigation against two Lexington doctors accused of practicing criminal abortion, and "respectfully demanding a fair, square, and complete investigation of those charges of criminal abortion." In the prosecution of the case, the Fayette County Medical Society was embarrassed by the fact that "more than twenty of the best physicians in Lexington and Fayette County had written letters on behalf of the Doctors charged with committing abortions, requesting that the State Board of Health be lenient and that the investigation be stopped." Dr. Vance acknowledged that criminal abortion had been "notoriously prevalent in this city and County for many years, though heartily condemned by all honest, upright and law abiding physicians."[514]

The State Board of Health met in Louisville September 17, 1909 to hear evidence for and against the accused, Dr. F. O. Young. The hearing was very emotional. Four members of the Board voted to revocate the accused physician's license, however, four other members voted against revocation "upon the ground of a reasonable doubt as to whether the charges were technically or legally sanctioned by the proof, but expressed themselves as being convinced that he was an abortionist." Even so, they "voted against revocation of his Certificate out of consideration for his family, and in the hope that the painful ordeal through which he had passed since these charges were made and during this trial would be sufficient to deter him and others from such practice in the future."[515] The accused physician was not convicted, however, and the Board sought additional evidence.

The hearing was open to the public, and newspaper reporters were present at every session. The decision of the State Board of Health was published in the *Lexington Leader* of

September 19, 1909. The report stated that the charges against Dr. Young were dropped and that he had been permitted to resume the practice of his profession. *Charges preferred* was the single term appearing in this account of the Board's decision. The word "abortion" did not appear in the write-up. Coverage of the hearing as related by the newspapers, namely: *The Lexington Herald, The Lexington Leader, The Kentucky Evening Gazette,* the *Courier Journal* and the *Cincinnati Enquirer* dated September 19, 1909 were, according to the minutes of the Medical Society, "materially and radically different" from the report by the State Board of Health.[516] The reports as published by the newspapers were at odds with impressions held by several members of the Society and did not correctly or truly represent the attitude of the State Board of Health or its actions on the charges.[517]

The verdict of the State Board of Health did not sit well with many members. Dr. G. P. Sprague, in particular, was appalled by the verdict and stated "in the Committee's investigation he has come to feel that [the accused] is a cold-blooded abortionist and murderer and thinks that if there is any way for the society to prosecute further and rid the Community and State of this practice, it is our solemn duty to do so." Dr. Sprague believed that the letters by the Lexington and Fayette County physicians had allowed their sympathy for the accused and his wife to over-run the safety of his victims. The letters [by members of the Fayette County Medical Society], he relates, made the decision for the Board of Health ever more difficult and hurt the "standard of morals."[518] Dr. T. C. Holloway emphasized the prompt need for remedial laws pertaining to criminal abortion. He challenged the members to let the committee know whether the matter should be dropped or "go on and accomplish something."[519] Dr. Holloway also acknowledged that the young members of the Society had taken their stand "on the right side."[520] The older members, he said, were hampered by former associations with the accused. Dr. J. A. Stucky, the third member of the Committee, spoke quite bluntly: "It is necessary for the Committee to unload the tension under which it has been laboring. The profession is bigger than any one man." He was especially chagrined that one-third of the members of the Society wrote letters "pleading for the man they had asked the Committee to investigate, pleading for a cold-blooded murderer."[521] Even though the State Board had rendered its decision in the instance of Dr. Young, the outcome of charges against the second accused physician, Dr. Melvin Rhorer, were delayed, and there is no further entry in the Society minutes regarding Dr. Rhorer.

The affair came to an uneasy rest when Dr. Charles Vance moved that "The same Committee be set to work for new evidence and present same to the Board of Health." Dr. Sprague's comment: "accept the verdict in good faith and not mistrust the Board" caused Dr. B. L Van Meter to retort: "This is the first time he ever heard Dr. Sprague say what he did not mean." He continues "Dr. Sprague knows perfectly well that the Board of Health did not act in good faith."[522] Dr. W. O. Bullock moved that the investigation of the accused physicians should not stop but that the Society should abandon the idea of publishing a statement. His Resolution passed, 36 to3.[523]

The Lexington Clinic

After World War I there was a movement towards group practice by American physicians and among the earliest of such was the Lexington Clinic; formally initiated on July 1, 1920 by the signing of the first partnership agreement by nine members: David Barrow, Woolfolk Barrow, W. O. Bullock, Ernest B. Bradley, F. H. Clarke, W. T. Briggs, J. T. McClymonds, W. S. Wyatt, and Charles C. Garr. Six of these partners were former or future presidents of the Medical Society. The Clinic was housed in a two-story building at Second and Upper Streets. The 1920s proved to be a very trying time for the struggling Clinic. The tragic death of Woolfolk Barrow in a car accident in 1923, together with retirements and departures, tested the will and the wisdom of the energetic group.

Even so, the partners moved immediately to fill the vacancies by the appointment of such stalwarts as Dr. Fred Rankin (surgery), Dr. C. N. Kavanaugh (cardiology), and Dr. Carrol Yates (otolaryngology). It was during this decade that the Clinic introduced the use of the x-ray to Lexington, first by Dr. Herring, who founded the Radiology Department at the Lexington Clinic,[524] The Good Samaritan Hospital and St. Joseph Hospital. A bold move by the Clinic in 1920 inaugurated the first clinical laboratory in the city. The addition of Dr. Elmer S. Maxwell, the first pathologist in Lexington, led to the establishment of tissue diagnosis at both hospitals provided by Dr. Maxwell and his technicians. He also initiated a more aggressive role in the performance of autopsies. By the early 1930s the Clinic had secured its role in the medical community, and though the members suffered financially during the Depression, the need to move ahead never died. Two outstanding young physicians joined the Clinic in the early 1930s, William H. Pennington in surgery and Carl H. Fortune in internal medicine.

The Clinic partners, as were most Americans, were severely tested during World War II. Those partners who served in the armed forces and those who stayed behind acted in concert to hold the closely knit group together. By 1953 there were 21 members of the professional staff (14 partners). Having outgrown its building, even the three-story addition, plans were underway as early as 1942 to prepare for the post-war day when its housing would merit the strength of its members.[525]

Specialization

From the onset of medical practice in America the physician was the medical doctor, the surgeon, and the pharmacist; ready and sometimes able to meet all his patient's needs. The very thought of specialization was repugnant to the regular physician. This all-in-one general practice dominance was seldom successfully challenged and, so, held sway throughout the latter part of the nineteenth century and well into the twentieth. Even so, throughout the nineteenth and into the twentieth century this self-serving ideology did not prevent patients and doctors alike from calling on those physicians known by reputation to be the most skilled specialist.

The generalist was fearful that the specialist would charge higher fees, downplay the ability of the generalist, perform medical acts other than those he professed, and that he would advertise. That the American Medical Association members were predominantly generalists had much to do in delaying the emergence of specialties in the nineteenth century.

But specialists were not to be denied. In 1874, Dr. J. W. Thompson, president of the Kentucky State Medical Society, commented: "The subject of specialties is receiving considerable notice by our profession, especially in large and growing cities. Experience in the division of practice in this country and in Europe is decidedly in favor of specialties."[526] By the 1870s national organizations were underway, with specialties first in ophthalmology, The American Opthalmological Society (1864), followed by the American Otological Society (1867), and several others by the end of the century. Other organizations, namely regional medical societies, also came on stage during the last quarter of the century. The AMA had always looked favorably on the organization of county, district, and state organizations but feared that the regional societies would undermine their influence.[527]

What evidence would support a professional split existing among Lexington physicians? If we were to look for public criticism of one or the other, generalist or specialist, the search would be in vain, for physicians had suffered through the self-destruction of mid-nineteenth century accusations and knew the ill consequences all too well. This is not to imply that all was serene between the two adversaries or that in private conversation differences were not hotly contested. The American Medical Association made the point again and again that physicians must refrain from personal assaults and derogatory accusations.

"Nothing weakened the medical profession more than the bitter feuds and divisions that plagued doctors through the nineteenth century....Professional tradition insisted that doctors present a unified front to the public."[528] Even though we lack personal memoirs or other tangible evidence of rift among Fayette County Medical Society members we have one undisputed record of generalist/specialist divergence, if not discord—the telephone directory.

The *Fayette Home Telephone Company Directory of 1912* listed physicians in the numerically ordered white pages alongside other citizens without reference to their practice or other suggestion of advertising. The directory of 1913 introduced a new section, *Classified Business,* in which one heading identified *Physicians and Surgeons.* Even so, the individual physician was not identified as one or the other. There was no change in the form of the 1915 directory other than that the classified business section now was made up of yellow pages. A change took place in the 1926 directory; the title in the Classified Section now read *Physicians, Surgeons and Specialists.* But even then there was no differentiation in the listing. Word of mouth was the only means accessible to the public should they seek special care short of referral by the generalist. Not until 1947 did this facade end. And yet, even in the 1947 telephone directory, the first to list specialties, several physicians chose not to do so. Why? The failure of the specialist to list himself as such in the directory can best be explained by a prevailing unwritten code that forbade advertising, a breach of professionalism which would have been leveled against any physician choosing to identify his expertise. To deviate from what was considered acceptable, specialists likely would have experienced the sudden loss of referrals and other less quantifiable inconveniences. Professional ethics would come unglued in the absence of professional unity. As recently as 1935, two-thirds of the doctors in the United States were general practitioners.[529] It is noteworthy that the change in listing the identification by specialty came in 1947 consistent with one of many economic, social, and professional changes brought about by World War II.

The lack of telephone listings identifying the specialist as such is even more puzzling in the context of the Lexington Clinic. The Clinic (1920), as such, was not listed in the physician section of the Classified Business pages for 1922-23. Even so, individual members of the Clinic were so listed but in no way identified with the Lexington Clinic. However, the Lexington Clinic was listed in the white pages with address and telephone number but without particulars such as the name of physicians. On the second line of the white page listing was the following: "Private Branch Exchange Connecting all Offices." Even in 1947 when several physicians first were listed as specialists, the Lexington Clinic did not appear in the yellow page directory of physicians.

This half-century absence of telephone listings by specialty can only be explained by the fear and implicit dread of advertising—whatever its form. To list one's specialty was to advertise. To advertise was to attract patients, patients that may or may not have gone through the generalists' domain. And yet all physicians, generalist or specialist, apparently accepted this unwritten code of ethics. The AMA strongly urged physicians to face the public with a united front. That the withholding of such information was not in the public's interest apparently fell on deaf ears.

Unfair Competition

The Society meeting of April 9, 1935 faced the members with a dilemma not previously entertained: the ethical or unethical practice of the Lexington Clinic to supply medical services for post-office employees and their families. The post-office employees initially approached the Clinic stating that they could pay yearly dues, a fixed amount for such service. The Clinic sought the opinion of the Medical Society as to whether "such a plan would be unethical or unfair to other doctors."[530] Because a similar program already was in force between the Clinic and the Railroad

Hospital Association to provide office examinations and medical and surgical care to its members when hospitalized in one of the local hospitals, the extension was believed to be ethical by the Clinic. For the plan to be cost effective, at least one-hundred employees were necessary to form their own organization, collect dues, and compensate the Clinic monthly in advance. Even so, the minutes stated that some members of the Medical Society had raised objections to "any such form of practice…unfair competition." The recording secretary continues, "…it was made plain to them [the Lexington Clinic] that only the employees themselves and not their families, would be taken care of." The secretary then records: "These men [presumably Lexington Clinic physicians] have been reading the newspapers and medical journals concerning these plans for medical insurance and are anxious to put some such scheme into operation." The proposal by the post-office employees was later "voluntarily cancelled" by the Lexington Clinic.

Other than "unfair competition" no other specific complaint was raised by the Society members. Quite likely the phrase "unfair competition" embraced any and all competitive threats by one doctor or group of doctors to other physicians, and so the need to state further cause was redundant. Unfair competition was deemed unethical, nothing less, nothing more. To permit employees to enter into a contractual relationship with the physician or physician group was evidently acceptable, but to include employee family members was considered by most physicians as nothing less than a break with the principles of medical practice, a surrender of physician rights, unfair competition. Practicing physicians during the thirties were predominantly opposed to third party or national insurance intervention in the patient-physician relationship. And too, the fact that almost all Lexington Clinic members were specialists would not have been lost on the members of the Society. Even with this difference of opinion there is evidence only of the greatest respect between the Clinic members and the non-Clinic members of the Society.

To suggest that there was serious discord between members

of the Society would be a mistake. Generalists appealed to the oneness of the physician. Specialists too were anxious to avoid provocative acts; they were in the minority. Even more so, they were equally familiar with the disturbing, if not the threatening, menace of divisiveness in the ranks. This contention is supported by a report to the House of Delegates, Kentucky Medical Association, by Dr. A. H. Barkley, Delegate of the Fayette County Medical Society, 1923: "One thing that I am particularly proud of is the absence of constant criticism of one doctor by another. Those of us who look back twenty-five or thirty years remember the conditions and can see the material change then and now." Dr. Barkley continues, "We are very grateful and very proud indeed to report to this body the entire absence of bad feeling. I don't know of a more harmonious society anywhere than Fayette County...Every man [physician] in Fayette County is a member of the Fayette County Medical Society."[531]

High Mortality Rate

At the January 14, 1930 meeting at McVey Hall, University of Kentucky, "Dr. [Waller] Bullock discussed a recent editorial [in the January 1930 issue of the *Spectator*], in which it was stated that the mortality in appendicitis [1928] is larger here in Lexington than in any other city in the U.S.A." The Society appointed a committee on appendicitis death rate. The committee reported that it had looked into the subject "not with the idea of clearing its skirts but of finding out, if possible, just how bad we are and what may be done to improve our status."[532] The committee secured the names of all persons dying of appendicitis in 1928 together with those patients dying of peritonitis, sub-phrenic abscess, intestinal obstruction and pulmonary embolus. The committee made its Report June 10, 1930, refuting the assertions of the previously quoted statistics. The committee concluded that the figures and percentage rate presented by Dr. Hoffman in the

Spectator were incorrect.

Depression

The Great Depression (1931-39) fell upon the nation with such force that there were few indeed who escaped the ravages of pain and suffering. The pain and suffering of the Depression were of a different kind than those customarily inflicted by disease. And yet not too different, for the pain of need, of hunger, of leaking roofs, of relentless cold and heat, and of hopelessness were just as real and how they hurt. Jobs were scarce, and incomes shrunk. And yet disease and misfortune took no holiday. Even so, a review of the minutes of the Medical Society through the 1930s fails to divulge any sense of despair. We can, however, sense the times through their minute book entries.

Society members attending the meeting of June 13, 1933 weighed the status of those members of the Society who had been "constant in their interest and attendance for years and now find the payment of dues a burden, should have their membership continued by the society for this year."[533] A constitutional amendment was proposed for this purpose.

Federal Subsidies to Medicine!

At the meeting of December 14, 1937, Dr. Charles Kavanaugh read "certain" proposals by the American Foundation of Medicine advocating medical care for indigent patients and the role to be played by governmental agencies in such care. Other related articles read by Dr. Kavanaugh were from the *AMA Journal* of October 16, 1937, and the *New England Journal of Medicine* of November 11, 1937 and November 18, 1937. The *JAMA* editorial critiqued the report of 1937 by the American Foundation. The American Foundation's proposals were based on the belief that "certain deficiencies in the medical scheme were clearly apparent and that concrete proposals should be made which would have the approval of the medical profession and which might lead to governmental action."[534] The proposals were far-reaching, encompassing not only the provision of federal funds for indigent care but among others recommendations, the use of federal subsidies for medical schools. The *JAMA* editorial suggested that many of the 450 persons who signed the American Foundation's proposals signed because "it looked like a good list."[535] The editorial chastised the "careless participation in propaganda and requested prompt disclaimers by the signers."[536] The Society endorsed the *JAMA* editorial and sent copies of the endorsement to the State Medical Association and to the AMA.

Women's Auxiliary

The Society met at the Good Samaritan Hospital on January 14, 1936 on which occasion a letter from Mrs. F. E. Fallis was read contemplating the formation of a Women's Auxiliary. No action was taken. At the April 14, 1942 meeting the subject was again discussed at the request of the President of the Kentucky Medical Association. A committee was appointed to "canvas the attitude of the women concerned." The report of the canvas was aired on May 12, 1942 stating that "letters to women concerning a Medical Auxiliary showed opposition at the rate of 7 to 1. However, of those opposed, most expressed a willingness to do their part should an Auxiliary be felt necessary."[537] Six years later the ladies prevailed upon their husbands to act. On July 13, 1948, the Fayette County Medical Society passed a motion to form a Women's Auxiliary if they so wished (described by the women as "a minor miracle or the consummate wisdom of doctors").[538] The organizational meeting of the Women's Auxiliary was held June 3, 1948. Mrs. Halbert Leet was named the first President. The first major undertaking by the Auxiliary, in concert with the Fayette County Medical Society, was the furnishing of a bedroom in the

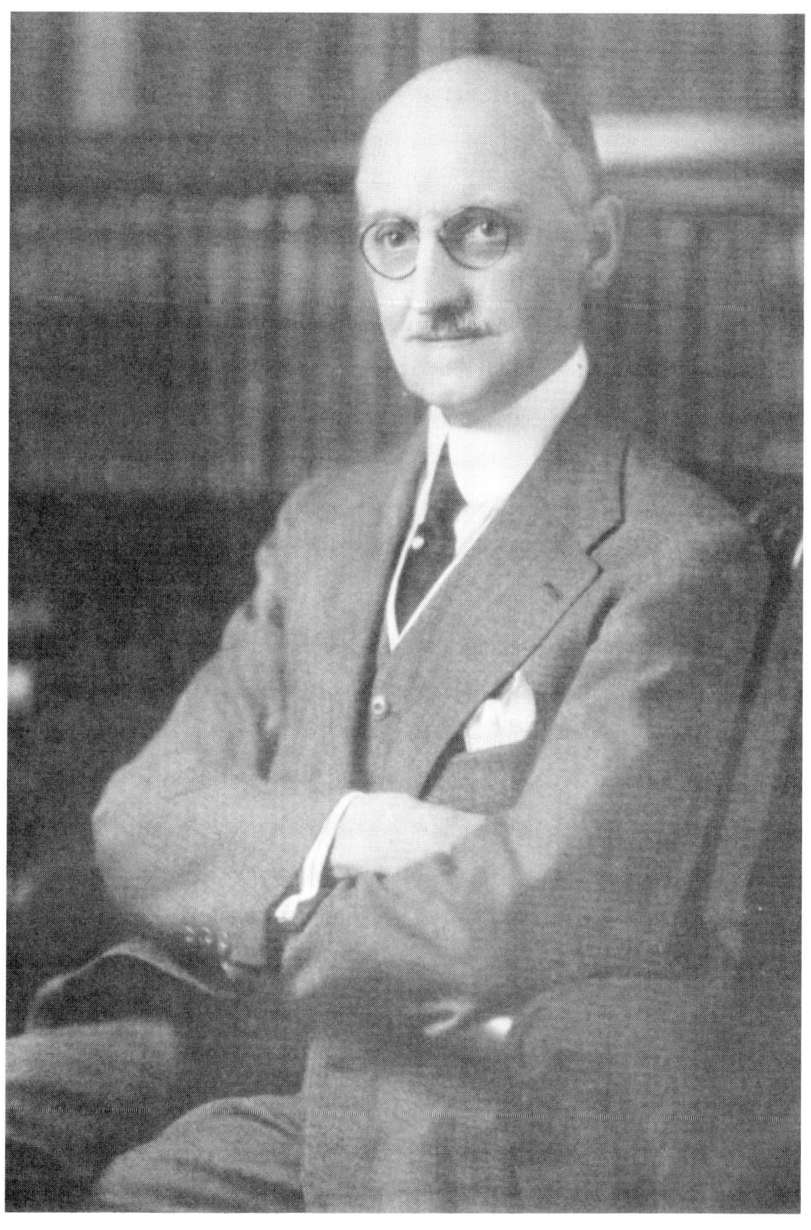

Joseph A. Stucky, M.D.
(1857-1931)
Courtesy of Fayette County Medical Society

McDowell House, Danville, Kentucky.[539]

African-Americans

On March 12, 1946 the meeting of the Society took place at Good Samaritan Hospital. Among the issues discussed was "whether colored members of medical profession [were] to be allowed privileges in proposed new hospital" [Central Baptist Hospital, founded in 1954]. Dr. Francis Massie also reported the "colored physicians desired to attend scientific meetings of county Society and various hospital staffs." Dr. John Scott moved that colored physicians be invited to attend the scientific meetings of the Society. However, Dr. Carl Fortune moved that Dr. Scott's motion not be voted on until the next meeting, and Dr. Fortune's motion passed.[540] The following month Dr. Scott's motion regarding colored physicians was amended to read: "Fayette County Medical Society scientific sessions" instead of "scientific meetings."[541] Not until seventeen years later, 1963, did the admission of an African-American, Dr. Bush Hunter, to the Fayette County Medical Society come about.

Twentieth Century Specialty Institutions

During the first thirty years of the twentieth century several outstanding medical institutions were founded in Lexington. Many Fayette County Medical Society members participated in their development. The need for such institutions arose from the peculiar needs of patients having medical conditions requiring special skills, accommodations and atmosphere. Among these conditions were tuberculosis, crippled children, children with orthopedic handicaps and afflictions affecting veterans.

Julius Marks Sanatorium for the treatment of victims of tuberculosis began with a civic meeting November 20, 1905 when the "foundation of a dual campaign—local and state—against the white plague was laid."[542] The opening of the sanatorium took place in 1917 through the efforts of Mrs. Desha Breckinridge and Thomas A. Combs. In 1924, an unexpected gift of $125,000 from Leo J. Marks of New York City as a memorial to his father, Julius Marks, was earmarked for a sixty bed hospital. Known thereafter as the Julius Marks Sanatorium, the hospital, under the guidance of its capable medical director, Dr. Edward J. Murray, faithfully and competently administered to the needs of those persons afflicted with tuberculosis. From 1917 to 1952, some 5000 patients were treated at the sanatorium. By the 1960s, outpatient medical care of patients having tuberculosis eliminated the need for the sanatorium.

The Oleika Temple founded the **Shriners Hospital for Children** in 1925. When first opened the hospital was located at the corner of East Maxwell Street and Highland Avenue and connected with the children's ward of Good Samaritan Hospital. "Oleika Temple was the first temple to build a hospital with its own funds and turn it over to the Imperial Council to maintain."[543] Highly successful, the twenty-bed unit outgrew its initial boundaries and moved to a new hospital in 1955 on 27.8 acres of land, formerly a part of Henry Clay's estate, *"Ashland."*

In 1943, **Cardinal Hill Hospital** had its beginning in the minds of members of the Kentucky Society for Crippled Children (Kentucky Easter Seal Society). Their experience had led them to the concept of a convalescent hospital for crippled children to be built in Lexington. Because of the war-time economy construction was not begun until 1948. The cost of the land and building was approximately $700,000. The hospital opened August 1, 1950. The need for such an institution was well justified, for within a few months the 49 beds were far too few. The overflow was, in part, caused by the numerous victims of the polio epidemic of the 1940s and 1950s. Once again, the need for such specialized care and the admirable management of the administrative and medical components gave rise to a "full-service rehabilitation center specializing in severe physical disabilities in children and adults."[544]

The Departments of Veterans Affairs Medical Center (Lexington Veteran's Administration Hospital) began with the purchase of 291 acres, three miles west of the city of Lexington, by the United States Government in 1929. Construction of the hospital began in 1929 with completion in 1931 at an estimated cost of two and one-half million dollars. A dedication ceremony was held May 31, 1931 with more than 2000 people in attendance including many dignitaries such as Governor Flem D. Sampson and United States Senator Alben W. Barkley. The hospital opened as a General Medical and General Surgical Hospital, having a bed capacity of 350. New additions began almost immediately, the first in 1932 followed by further construction in 1938, 1945, 1947 and 1951. By 1947 the bed capacity had increased to 1216.[545]

Second Term Movement

The Society met in the basement of the "Ott Building" in December, 1940. Dr. Scott relates "there was a stirring scene."

> It was just after the nation had been afflicted with the election of a president to a third term and our president at that time, Dr. Wyatt was very sensitive to any sort of re-election. He had been such a good president, however, that there was a distinct movement, at least an inclination, to break down the precedent of a hundred years or more and elect him for the second time. He realized that something of the sort was going on and, determined not to be the instrument of such sacrilege, armed himself before going to the meeting. When nominations were called for, the nominations as well as the election at that time being by secret ballot, there came a flood of nominations for Dr. Wyatt. So much so that he became greatly dis-

turbed, and determined not to be re-elected, "quelled forcibly," in the words of the secretary, Dr. Douglas Scott, "the rising tide of second term sentiment by drawing two large caliber revolvers." It was a tense moment. He desisted however, and bloodshed was avoided.[546]

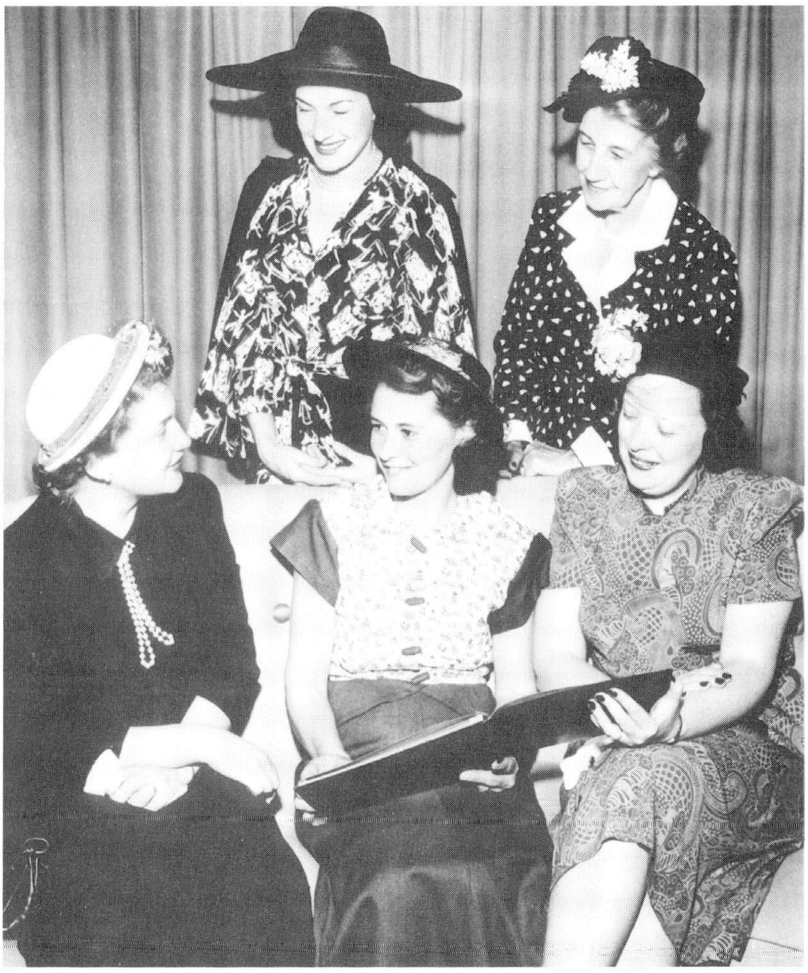

Inauguration of the Fayette County Medical Society Women's Auxiliary – 1948
Seated: Mrs. Harvey Chenault, Mrs. Halbert Leet, First President and Mrs. Harold Nickell Standing: Mrs. Warren Sergeant and Mrs. Jefferson Overstreet
Courtesy of Fayette County Medical Society Auxiliary.

The Spanish-American War, World War I and II

Physicians have always been in the battlefield alongside soldiers. Indeed, physicians for hundreds of years, especially those who practiced surgery, often learned their craft through the study of body parts torn asunder. As often as they could, the battlefield healer gave care and comfort to the wounded and to the dying. The purpose remains the same today; we are little changed. However rapid the pace of research and application of medicine to mankind, the advantage always goes to the weapons of war, for here man is at his best and his worst.

During the Spanish-American War and the two world wars of this century, members of the Fayette County Medical Society responded admirably both at home and overseas, with or without a uniform. The desire to aid their fellow Americans led to the rapid deployment of physician-volunteers and to the establishment of medical units representing the Society and their affiliated hospitals, Good Samaritan and St. Joseph. One of the most noted events in Lexington of World War I was the formation of the Barrow Base Hospital Unit No. 40. Dr. David Barrow founded the unit in the summer of 1917 for services on the French front.

With the outbreak of World War II in Europe (1939) Americans edged slowly but inexorably toward military preparation. The Fayette County Medical Society, as did others, considered means by which those members called to military service could be aided. Although desirable, members were not able to design a reasonable plan to retain patients for those men called into service and even less able to "fairly apportion any income." In the absence of any concrete means of aiding their colleagues, members sought to assure the seniority and prestige of men in the service. Press notices of those going into and coming from the military were believed to be appropriate "if these could be worded with good taste." A proposal to pay Society dues for members of the Society called into active service in the military forces passed in February 1941.[547] Dr. William E. Bannister, a former president of

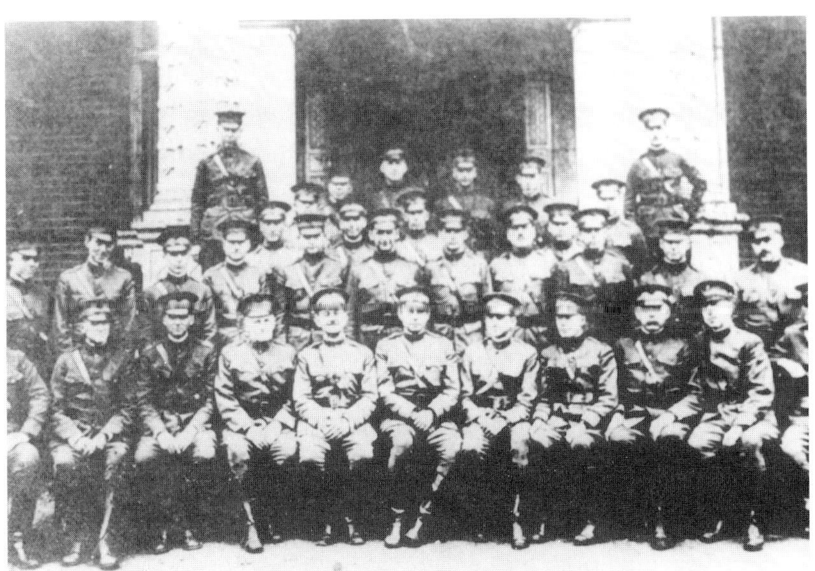

World War I – Barrow Unit
Good Samaritan Base Hospital, Unit No. 40
Courtesy of Good Samaritan Foundation, Inc.

DAVID BARROW, M. D.
Physician and Surgeon, Lexington, Ky.

David Barrow, M.D.
(1858-1932)
Courtesy of Fetter Printing Company (Formerly known as Geo G. Fetter Printing Co.)

the Fayette County Medical Society (1921), came out of retirement during World War II, as did others, to provide medical care for the community.

To the members of the Fayette County Medical Society and to those nurses and others who served with them during both World Wars we echo *Well Done; Well Done.* Their deeds excel their number. Although there were many members whose services were well beyond the line of duty, I have chosen to highlight two members, Dr. Matthew Darnell, one of the younger members who served in the front-line, and Dr. Fred Rankin, Chief Consulting Surgeon to the office of the Surgeon General.

Matthew Cotton Darnell

Matthew Cotton Darnell (1913-1992), a native of Ducker's Station, Woodford County Kentucky, and a graduate of Boston University Medical School (1943), volunteered for active naval service in 1944 after an internship in Boston.[548] Serving as medical officer of the destroyer U.S.S. Laffey, Dr. Darnell saw action in several theaters of war—the D-Day Normandy invasion, the Philippine and Iwo Jima invasions and the battle near Okinawa. Thirty-two members of The Laffey were killed and seventy-one injured by the Kamikaze attack at Okinawa (April 15, 1945). Dr. Darnell was among the wounded; "fragments of metal cut the tips of two of Dr. Darnell's fingers, but they were bandaged and he kept going." In recognition of Matt Darnell's distinguished service to his country he received two awards: the Bronze Star and the Purple Heart.[549]

Following the war Dr. Darnell interned at St. Joseph Hospital, Lexington, Kentucky. A Diplomate of the American Board of Medicine, he practiced in Lexington from 1947 through 1985. Among his many accomplishments, he served as Chief of Medical Service, both at Good Samaritan and St. Joseph Hospitals, and Chief of Intermediate Medicine at Veterans Administration

Our Fayette County Physicians In The Service
Brig. Gen. Fred W. Rankin
Lt. Col. Wm. H. Pennington
Lt. Com. Thornton Scott
Maj. Coleman C. Johnston
Maj. A. J. Alexander
Maj. Rufus C. Alley
Maj. Arthur B. Barrett
Maj. Rankin C. Blount
Lt. Com. Arnold B. Combs
Lt. Col. Richard G. Elliott
Lt. Col. Carl H. Fortune
Lt. Col. John Harvey
Lt. Col. Wm. R. Thompson
Capt. Robert B. Warfield
Com. Stanley S. Parks
Maj. Robert C. Riggs
Maj. Halbert H. Leet
Capt. Excum Lionel Moore
Lt. Col. William L. Heizer
Maj. Kenneth R. Andrews
Maj. Lawrence E. Hurt
Maj. I. F. Kanner
Capt. Wm. C. Robinson
Maj. Theodore L. Adams
Maj. C. G. McLean
Capt. Samuel E. Williams
Capt. Nathaniel L. Bosworth
Lt. Col. David W. Barrow
Maj. Daniel V. Sublette
Lt. Wm. T. Maxson
Maj. Wm. N. Lipscomb
Capt. Ernest A. Welch
Capt. Carl L. Wheeler
Lt. Col. Robert J. Griffin
Capt. R. V. Stevenson
Capt. Robert E. Downing
Lt. Col. J. B. Romph

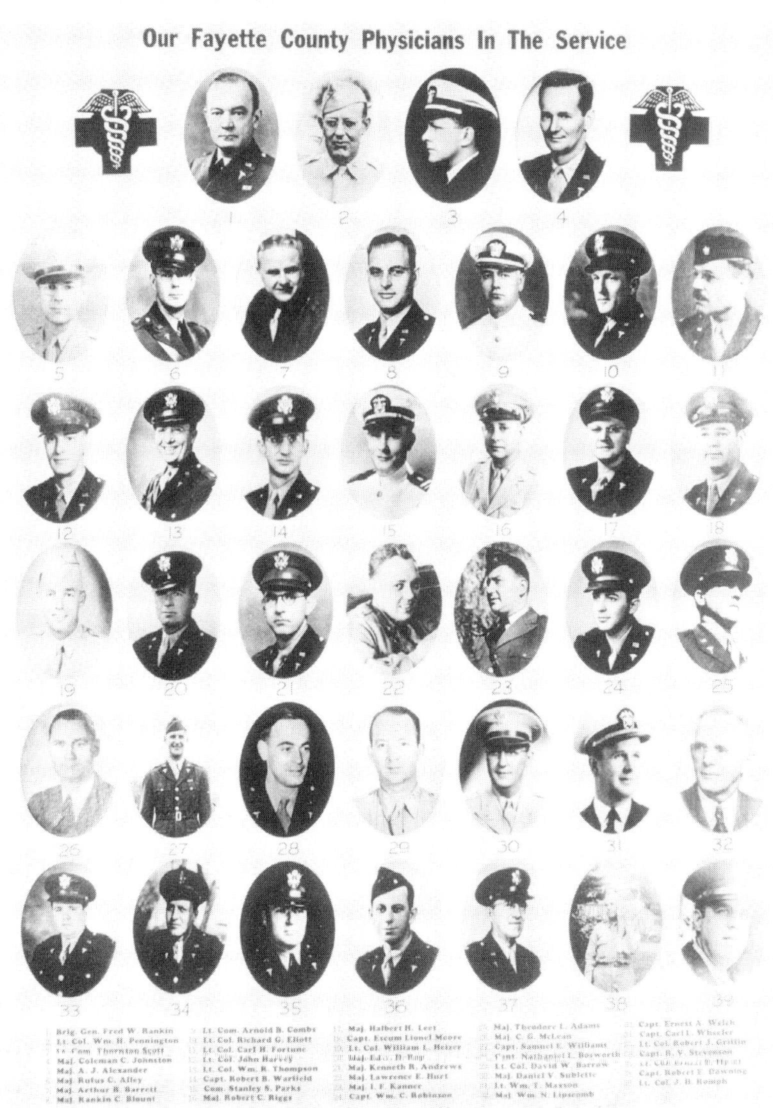

Fayette County physicians in service WW II
Courtesy of Fayette County Medical Society

Medical Center of Lexington. He also founded the Hospice of the Bluegrass. In 1960 Dr. Darnell served as president of the Fayette County Medical Society. Death came to Dr. Darnell May 17, 1992.[550] Twelve association members of the Laffey "saw to the lowering of the colors in his honor."[551]

Fred Wharton Rankin

Fred Wharton Rankin, a native of Mooresville, North Carolina, graduated from the University of Maryland Medical School in 1909. From 1909 to 1912 he served as a resident surgeon at the University Hospital in Baltimore and later (1913-1916) as an associate in surgery at the same institution. His first move from Baltimore took him to the Mayo Clinic, Rochester, Minnesota, where he became an assistant surgeon and continued serving in this capacity from 1916 to 1923. Further recognition of his surgical leadership was acknowledged by his appointment as surgeon to the Mayo Clinic and associate professor in the Graduate Medical School University of Minnesota and the Mayo Foundation (1926-33).

In 1933 Dr. Rankin moved to Lexington, Kentucky. His surgical skills were already widely known in Lexington not only through his tenure at the Mayo Clinic but also by his association with the Lexington Clinic from 1924-26.[552] While in Lexington for the practice of surgery, Dr. Rankin continued his alliance with medical education through his affiliation as professor of clinical surgery with the University of Louisville. (He had served as professor of surgery at the University of Louisville for one year: 1922-23).

Dr. Rankin served his country in both World Wars, as a major in the medical corp in France during World War I and as Chief Consulting Surgeon to the office of the Surgeon General in World War II. In 1945, for his "meritorious services" General Rankin was awarded the Distinguished Service Medal. A founding

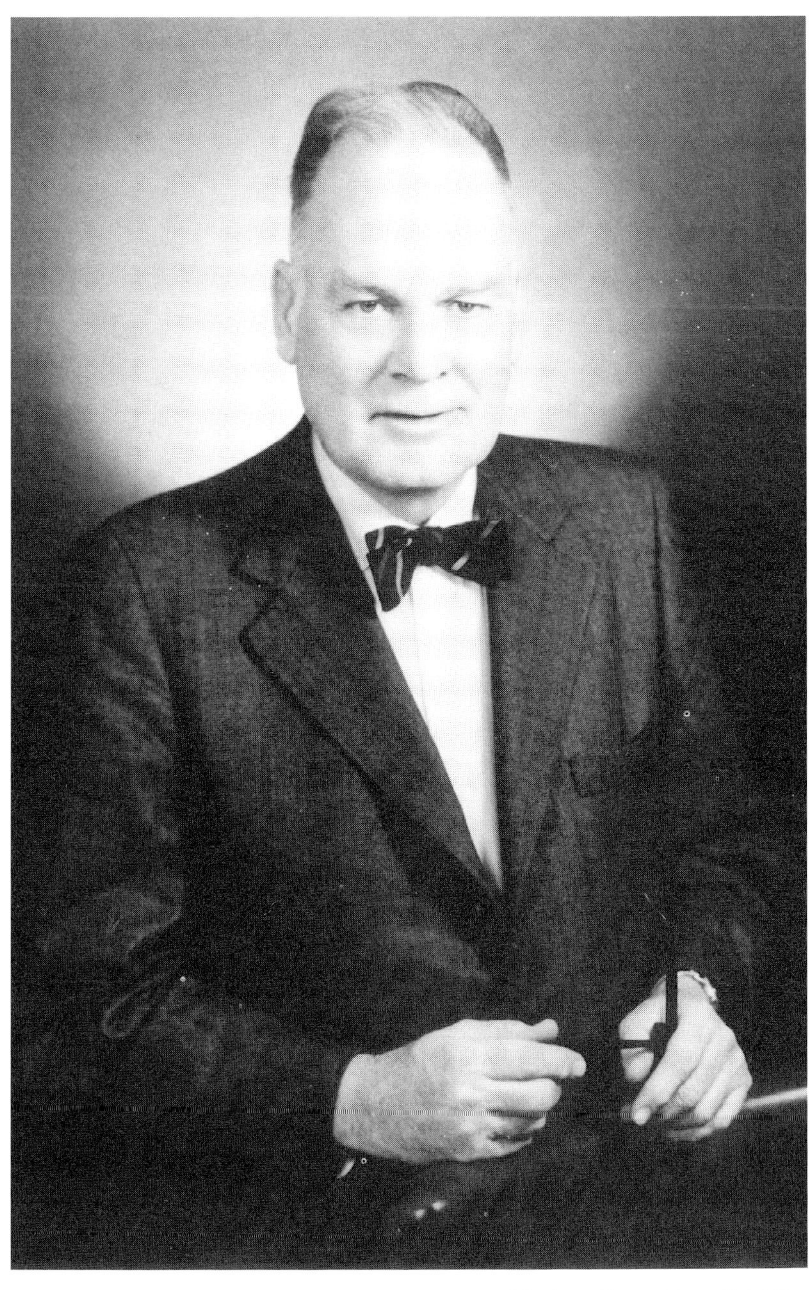

Matthew Cotton Darnell, M.D.
(1913-1992)
Courtesy of Fayette County Medical Society

member of the American Board of Surgery, in 1942 he became the second member of the Lexington-Fayette County Medical Society to preside as President of the American Medical Association.[553]

Why Belong?

> It has been said by someone that associated action constitutes the mainspring, the controlling motive power, and whoever surveys with the eye of intelligence the present aspect and tendencies of civilization, will readily acknowledge the truth of this remark.
>
> N. S. Davis
> Founder of the American Medical Association[554]

There is no denial of hospital privileges in Fayette County, Kentucky for those physicians who do not belong to the Medical Society. Indeed, there is no impediment whatever in Kentucky to the practice of medicine by a licensed physician in good standing, member or not, of the Society. Then why belong? If one expects immediate or extended financial gratification through membership he or she will be disappointed. This is not the purpose of a medical society; this is not its aim.

The practice of medicine has a higher purpose; the prevention of illness and the care of those in need of medical service. Even so, a lone physician cannot fulfill this dual role for his patient no matter how devoted his care, no matter how skilled his application. Each prescribed act of today's physician increasingly represents a complex interaction, and one not solely limited to the discretion of the physician. There are other associates; allied health providers, pharmaceutical companies, the hospitals, the state legislature, the federal agencies are but a few of the many participants. This is not necessarily an indictment of such limitations imposed

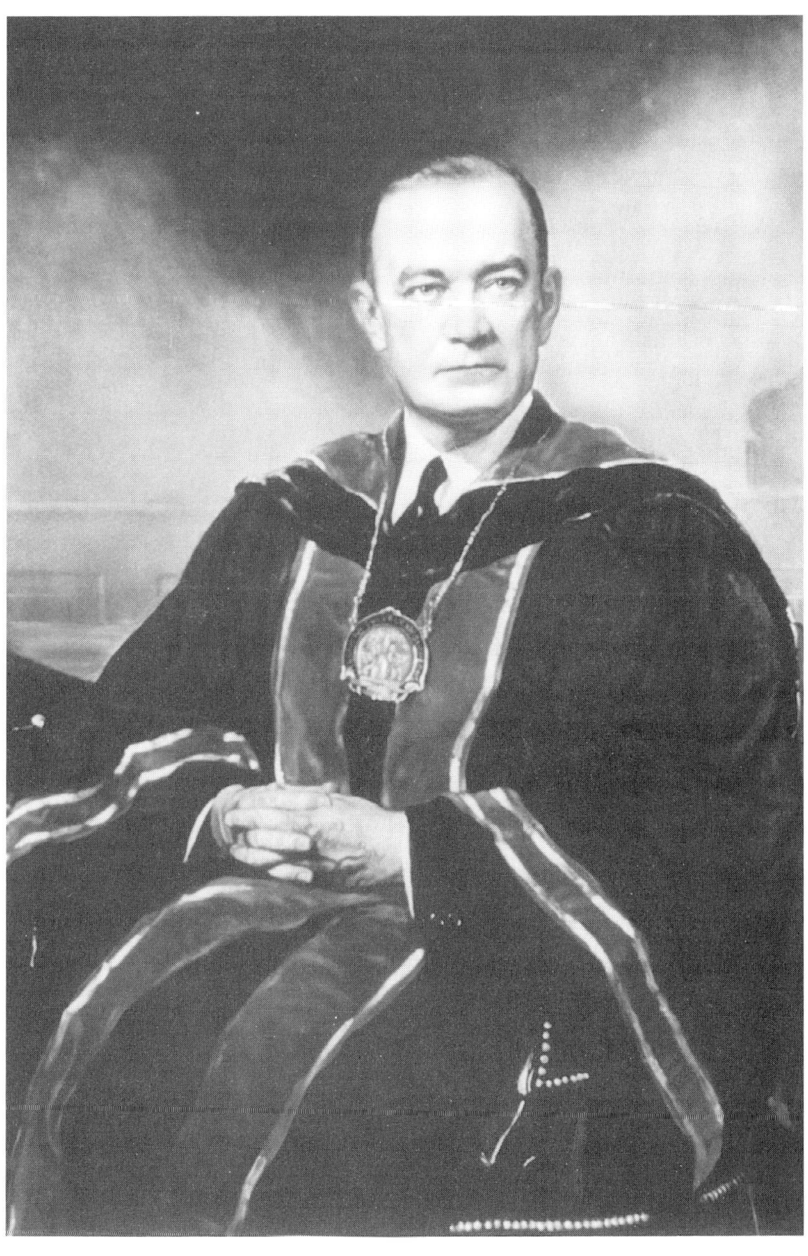

Fred Wharton Rankin, M.D.
(1886-1954)
Courtesy of Fayette County Medical Society

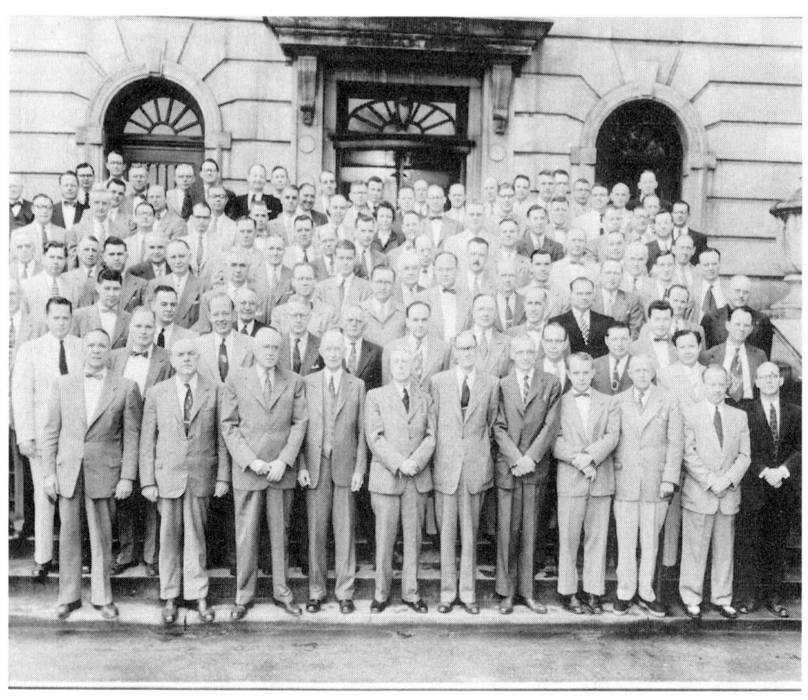

Medical Staff – St. Joseph Hospital, Lexington, Kentucky
(Early 1950s)
Courtesy of St. Joseph Hospital, Lexington, Kentucky

on the physician but simply an awareness of the socioeconomic turf on which we play.

What to do? What role can I play? What can I do as an individual physician? Will I have a greater impact as a member of a medical society? Why? We Americans almost worship the individual, and we admonish each other of the importance of each life, each vote. Yet we are increasingly infatuated with teams and especially the togetherness of teams that win. May we never downplay the individual and yet may we never forget that the individual is simply one who can stand alone—*with help.* We never act alone. Previously, we said that the physician spent the better part of the nineteenth century in search of respect. Not only has that respect been gained, it has been earned. It came about through individual effort fused together through the trials and tribulations of dedicated men and women acting together through their respective societies. Physicians join their medical societies both to share the honor and the burden of responsibility to the individual, their patients, and to the society itself. Better health for all people will come not by wishing but by action. For physicians, opportunity of concerted and informed societal input is to champion their patients' rights and those of their profession.

> This Society was instituted and is sustained, as I construe it, not to subserve the selfish interests of a class or of a profession. Not for this, but to melt the gold out of the past, rejecting the dross of error, to save all the old treasures of knowledge and to mine diligently for new, to cultivate the mutual respect of which outward courtesy is the sign; to work together, to feel together, to take counsel together, and to stand together for the truth, now and always, here and everywhere.
>
> H. B. Brown, M.D.[555] 1892
> President of Kentucky State Medical Society

442 W. L. Sutton, "Annual Address of the President of the Society," *Transactions of the Kentucky State Medical Society* (Louisville: Webb and Levering, 1853), 17-29. President of the Kentucky State Medical Society 1851-51, Sutton is the father of vital statistics in Kentucky, the first state West of the Alleghenies to pass a law requiring the registration of marriages, births, and deaths.

443 *The Lexington Herald,* 30 December 1900.

444 Ibid.

445 Ibid.

446 Ibid.

447 Ibid.

448 John D. Wright, "Lexington," in *The Kentucky Encyclopedia,* editor-in-chief, John E. Kleber (Lexington: The University Press of Kentucky, 1992), 549-551. Dates of Lexington construction in early- and mid-twentieth century: Union Station, Main Street, 1907; Fayette National Bank, 1913-14; Lafayette Hotel, 1921; Keeneland, 1930s; Blue Grass Airport, 1942; IBM Corporation, 1956; Chandler Medical Center, 1962.

449 *Lexington Herald,* 2 June 1937. **Dr. Archibald Henry Barkley**: (1872-1937). A native of Georgetown, Kentucky, Dr. Barkley graduated from Transylvania University following which he took his medical training at Columbia University. He began his medical practice in New York but after a number of years returned to Lexington where he practiced as a physician and surgeon for more than 30 years. Dr. Barkley served in the medical corps during both the Spanish American War and World War I. He was the author of several books among them "Miscellany" and "Kentucky Pioneer Lithotomists." He was a member of the AMA, KSMA, and the FCMS.

450 *Lexington Herald,* 11 June 1947. **Dr. William B. McClure**: Born in Louisa, Kentucky in 1858, Dr. McClure graduated from the University of Louisville Medical College in 1883 and later took post-graduate training in New York and London. In the 1890s he came to Lexington to practice his specialty, surgery of the ear, nose, and throat and continued to do so until his retirement in 1937. He served as treasurer of the Kentucky State Medical Association for 25 years and later became president of the Association. Honored throughout the state by his medical colleagues, McClure also took an active role in community affairs supporting the Humane Society and for several years was a vestryman at Christ Episcopal Church. Dr. McClure was one of the early members of the Lexington-Fayette County Medical Society at the time of its reorganization in 1882.

451 *Lexington Herald,* 1934. **Dr. Benjamin F. Van Meter**: A native of Clark County, Dr. Van Meter served as an Army surgeon during the Spanish-American War and World War I. A graduate of Bellevue Hospital Medical College in 1899, he served as president of the Fayette County Medical Society in 1911 and as attending surgeon at both the Good Samaritan and St. Joseph Hospitals.

452 *Lexington Herald,* 28 October 1942. **Dr. Frank H. Clarke**: Born in New Orleans, Dr. Clarke attended medical school at Evansville, Indiana and did post-graduate studies in Vienna, London, and Bellevue Hospital, New York City. He came to Lexington to become superintendent of Eastern State Hospital and later was associated with Dr. David Barrow taking part in the organization of the Lexington Clinic where he remained for several years. Dr. Clarke was an elder in the First Presbyterian Church and served the Bethel Presbyterian Church as Superintendent of the Sunday

School. At the time of his death, Dr. Clarke, age 88, was a member of the FCMS and the oldest member of the Kentucky State Medical Society.

453 Minutes of the Fayette County Medical Society, 12 May 1931. **Dr. Joseph A. Stucky**: Born in Louisville in 1857, Dr. Stucky became the most prominent of Lexington Physicians during the nineteen-twenties until the time of his sudden death in 1931. A graduate of the University of Louisville Medical School in 1878 he became the leading specialist on disease of the eye, ear, nose and throat, and was elected president of eight different medical associations including the American Laryngological, Rhinological and Otological Society, KSMA, and FCMS. A prolific writer he also lectured on Social Welfare and Public Health. An active member of the Masonic Fraternity, YMCA and Kiwanis Club he also served his church, Central Christian Church, as an elder.

454 *Lexington Herald*, 19 January 1942. **Dr. George Sprague**: A native of Philadelphia, Dr. Sprague left his medical practice in Massachusetts in 1890 to become the superintendent of the High Oaks Sanatorium in Lexington, Kentucky. He served in this capacity for 42 years. Dr. Sprague graduated from the Jefferson Medical College, Philadelphia, following which he did his post-graduate training in the New York Psychological Institute. This distinguished physician was a life member of the American Psychiatric Association and also a member of the AMA, KSMA, and the FCMS. Through his writing of an anonymous letter to the Lexington Optimist Club he started the yearly presentation of the Lexington Optimist Cup and for the first two years donated the cup.

455 *Lexington Herald*, 17 March 1925. **Dr. Thomas C. Holloway**: Dr. Holloway's obituary is long on the event of his death but short in the details of his life. A surgeon, he reportedly was very popular with the members of the medical profession and the laity. Dr. Holloway, age 51, took his own life and the commentary dwells at length on the pistol used and his activities on the day of his death by suicide. He was a member of the KSMA and the FCMS. There were no further specifics.

456 **Dr. Henry H. Roberts**: Unable to gain information of his person or his medical practice. [Author]

457 *Lexington Herald*, 11 October 1952. **Dr. Robert Julian Estill**: Born in Fayette County, Kentucky in 1877, Dr. Estill graduated from Kentucky University (Transylvania University) in 1897 and completed his medical training at Columbia University Physicians and Surgeons School, New York, in 1902. A pediatrician, he was one of the first Lexington doctors associated with the Baby Milk Supply. During his practice lifetime, Dr. Estill served as president of the Kentucky State Medical Association in 1927-28 and was a dedicated member of the AMA, KSMA, and the FCMS.

458 William Stewart Halsted, "The Training of the Surgeon," *Surgery in America,* ed. A. Scott Earle (New York: Praeger Publishers, 1983), 369-390.

459 Mason G. Robertson, "Abraham Flexner: Patron of American Medical Education," *Southern Medical Bulletin*, vol. 59, No.4, 1971; 49-53.

460 Paul Starr, *The Social Transformation of American Medicine* (New York: Basic Books Inc., 1949), 118.

461 Minutes of the Fayette County Medical Society, 9 April 1907. The Minutes for the years 1904-1913 and 1919 to the present are located in the Fayette County Medical Society Archives.

462 Minutes of the Fayette County Medical Society, 15 May 1906.

463 John W. Scott, "Reminiscences of the Fayette County Medical Society," a speech delivered before the Society on December 12, 1950, Fayette County Medical Society Archives.

464 Samuel Haber, *The Quest for Authority and Honor in the American Professions,* 1750-1900 (Chicago: The University of Chicago Press, 1991), 357.

465 C.R. Mabee, *The Physician's Business and Financial Advisor,* 5th ed. (Cleveland: Continental Publishing, 1901), 170.

466 Starr, *The Social Transformation of American Medicine,* 85.

467 Ibid., 142-143.

468 "Workmen's Compensation," *Encyclopedia Britannica* (Chicago, 1973), vol. 23, 675.

469 Starr, *The Social Transformation of American Medicine,* 238.

470 Donald Bruce Johnson and Kirk H. Porter, *National Party Platforms 1840-1972,* 5th ed. (Chicago: University of Illinois Press, 1975), 178.

471 Starr, *The Social Transformation of American Medicine,* 249.

472 Ibid., 255.

473 Ibid., 252-255.

474 *Lexington Transcript,* 20 May 1881.

475 *The Fayette Home Telephone Company Exchange Directory,* Lexington, Kentucky, June 1912.

476 *The Fayette Home Telephone Company Exchange Directory,* 1913.

477 Minutes of the Fayette County Medical Society, 11 February 1913.

478 *Lexington Herald,* 17 March 1909.

479 Dr. Scott's Reminiscences.

480 *Lexington Herald,* 20 January 1918, page 1, col.3 "Board Rules to Force Law On Contagion."

481 *Lexington Herald,* 4 October 1918, page 1.

482 *Lexington Herald,* 29 October 1918, page 6, column 2.

483 Ibid., 20 November 1918, page 12, column 1.

484 J. W. Pryor, *Doctor Pryor, An Autobiography* (Cynthiana, Ky.: The Hobson Press, 1943), 302-303.

485 Dr. John Scott (1875-1966), a member of the Society in 1904, offered no clue to the mystery of the lost minute book in his historical review (1950) of the meeting places of the Society. "Reminiscences of the Fayette County Medical Society."

486 Notes by Dr. J. W. Pryor housed in the Archives of The Fayette County Medical Society, circa 1930s, 1.

487 Ibid.

488 *Acceptance and Unveiling of the Statues of Henry Clay and Dr. Ephraim McDowell Presented by the State of Kentucky, Proceedings in the Congress and in Statuary Hall, United States Capitol.* (Washington: United States Government Printing Office, 1929).

489 Minutes of the Fayette County Medical Society, 14 April 1931.

490 Fayette County Medical Archives. The gavel given by Dr. Stucky was not as described made up of three woods but one. The mistake was realized and the gavel as described by Dr. Stucky was later given to the Society.

491 Minutes of the Fayette County Medical Society, 4 June 1926.

492 Frederick Jackson, "Physicians Will Exhibit Newly-Acquired Picture of Pioneer in Medicine who Declined to Fight Except in His Own Field." *Lexington Leader,* April 11, 1937.

493 Samuel D. Gross, "Daniel Drake, 1785-1852," *Lives of Eminent American Physicians and Surgeons of the Nineteenth Century,* Samuel D. Gross, ed. (Philadelphia: Lindsay & Blakistan, 1861), 660.

494 David F. Noble, *America By Design* (Oxford: Oxford University Press, 1977), 24.

495 Carl Moreland, "New Era in State Medicine Signified by the University of Kentucky Center," *Lexington Herald-Leader,* University of Kentucky Medical Center Section, April 22, 1962.

496 Carl B. Cone, *The University of Kentucky, A Pictorial History* (Lexington: The University of Kentucky Press, 1989), 38. State University became the University of Kentucky in 1916.

497 Ibid.

498 Hampden C. Lawson, "The Early Medical Schools of Kentucky," *Bulletin of the History of Medicine* 24 (May-June, 1950) : 168-173. "Between 1200 and 1500 medical students populated Louisville in the 1890s."

499 Pryor, *Autobiography,* 294.

500 Cone, *The University of Kentucky, A Pictorial History.*

501 Minutes of the Fayette County Medical Society, 13 June 1904.

502 Ibid., 12 May 1908.

503 Ibid., 19 May 1908.

504 *Journal of the Regular Session of the Senate of the Commonwealth of Kentucky* (Louisville: The Continental Printing Co., 1910), 153-54.

505 Pryor, *Autobiography,* 296-297.

506 *Lexington Herald-Leader,* University of Kentucky Medical Center Section (Lexington, Ky.), 22 April 1962.

507 Branham B. Bauman, "The Beginning of the Medical School of the University of Kentucky – the Political and Scientific Background," *Journal of the Kentucky State Medical Association,* October, 1979.

508 Minutes of the Fayette County Medical Society, 9 April 1907.

509 Ibid.

510 Minutes of the Fayette County Medical Society, 18 June 1909.

511 Upton Sinclair, *The Jungle* (Norwalk, Conn.: The Hermitage Press, 1965), Foreward, vii.

512 Minutes of the Fayette County Medical Society, 12 October 1909.

513 Minutes of the Fayette County Medical Society, 11 May 1909.

514 Minutes of the Fayette County Medical Society, 13 September 1909.

515 Minutes of the Fayette County Medical Society, 21 September 1909.

516 Ibid.

517 Ibid.

518 Ibid., 18 September 1909.

519 Ibid.

520 Ibid.

521 Ibid.

522 Ibid.

523 Ibid., 21 September 1909.

524 Dr. J. W. Pryor in his *Autobiography* states that he had been doing x-ray work at his home in 1907 and that in 1916 he took an x-ray course with Dr. James Thomas Case at St. Lukes Hospital, Chicago. Dr. Pryor joined the Lexington Clinic. During his six year tenure with the Clinic he provided both diagnostic and therapeutic services.

Pryor, *Autobiography*, 187-89.

525 Carl H. Fortune, *The Lexington Clinic 1920 to 1980* (Lexington, Ky.: The Lexington Clinic, 1981), 1-29. The author drew liberally from the work by Dr. Fortune.

526 J. W. Thompson, "Address of the President," *Transactions of the Kentucky State Medical Society* (Louisville: John P. Morton and Co., 1874), 23.

527 James G. Burrow, *Voice of American Medicine* (Baltimore: The John Hopkins Press, 1963), 7.

528 Starr, *The Social Transformation of American Medicine*, 93-94.

529 Russell V. Lee and Sarah Eimerl, *The Physician* (New York: Life Sciences Library, Time, 1967), 101.

530 Minutes of the Fayette County Medical Society, 9 April 1935.

531 A. H. Barkley, Minutes of the House of Delegates, Kentucky Medical Association, 1923.

532 "Report of Committee From Fayette County Medical Society on Appendicitis Death Rate for Lexington, Ky. For 1928."

533 Minutes of the Fayette County Medical Society, 13 June 1933.

534 Editor, *Journal of the American Medical Association*, 108 (Oct-Dec, 1937); Ibid.

535 Ibid.

536 Ibid.

537 Ibid., 12 May 1942.

538 *Women's Auxiliary Twenty-fifth Anniversary Booklet*, Forward, (1973).

539 Ibid.

540 Minutes of the Fayette County Medical Society, 12 March 1946.

541 Ibid., 9 April 1946.

542 Andrew Eckdahl, "Julius Marks Sanatorium in 35thYear Serving Victims of Tuberculosis,"

Lexington Herald, 3 February 1952.

[543] *Lexington Hospital History*, a three page publication by the Shriners Hospital first written in March, 1989 and revised in January 1991, and September 1998.

[544] *Cardinal Hill Rehabilitation Hospital History*, a one page summary of Cardinal Hill. (Undated and unsigned FAX. Received February 24, 1999 from Cardinal Hill)

[545] *History of the VAMC*, Lexington, KY., a seven page compendium of the history of The Department of Veterans Affairs VA Medical Center, with an attached copy of the Title page of the 1931 Dedication. (Undated and unsigned FAX. Received February 25, 1999).

[546] Dr. Scott's Reminiscences.

[547] Minutes of the Fayette County Medical Society, 11 February 1941.

[548] *Lexington Herald-Leader* (Lexington, Ky.) 21 May 1992. Joseph Saunders and Robert D. Shepard, Memorial Resolution of Matthew Cotton Darnell, Minutes of the Fayette County Medical Society, June 1992.

[549] *Laffey News*, U.S.S. Laffey Association, April/ May/ June 1992, #49.

[550] *Lexington Herald-Leader* (Lexington, Ky.) 18 May 1992.

[551] *Laffey News*, U.S.S. Laffey Association, April/ May/ June 1992, #49.

[552] Carl H. Fortune, *The Lexington Clinic 1920 to1980* (Lexington, Ky.: The Lexington Clinic, 1981), 15.

[553] Morris Fishbein, *A History of The American Medical Association* 1847-1947 (New York: W.B. Saunders & Company, 1969), 816-18.

[554] N. S. Davis, *History of the American Medical Association* (Philadelphia: Lippincott & Company, 1855), 17-18.

[555] H. B. Brown, M.D., The President's Annual Address, "The Use and Abuse of Medicines," Transactions of the Kentucky Stat Medical Society, new series, Vol. I (Louisville: John P. Morton & Co, 1892), 33-34.

Chronology of The City of Lexington, Kentucky, The Lexington-Fayette County Medical Society, and Related National and International Events

During the years 1750-1775, while the Atlantic Coast Colonists were busy developing their own institutions and on the threshold of separating from England, the wilderness of the eastern and middle Kentucky territory was first explored in 1750 by the physician and surveyor Thomas Walker (1715-1794) of Virginia.[1] Other expeditions into Kentucky, an extension of Fincastle County, Virginia, were made by a fur trader, John Finley, in 1752 as he traveled along the Ohio River near present-day Louisville.[2] Daniel Boone (1731-1820) and a party of hunters from Yadkin Valley, North Carolina, explored Kentucky in 1769.[3] Boone made an abortive attempt to return to Kentucky in March 1773. Presumably, no permanent establishment in Kentucky occurred until that of Ft. Harrod by James Harrod and his party in 1775. Fort Boonesborough also was founded in 1775. Reportedly, in June 1775, a band of settlers from Ft. Harrod camped at the site of what is now Lexington. It was at this time and place that these settlers first heard of the Revolutionary War Battle of Lexington, Massachusetts, (April 1775). Thus this small group of men chose the name Lexington for their campsite to honor the courage and the valor of those who first fought for American freedom.[4] In 1775 the first legislative assembly west of the Alleghenies took place at Ft. Boonesborough. This assembly, headed by Colonel Richard Henderson, was convened for the purpose of establishing "a separate and independent government under the sovereignty of Great Britain, resembling the proprietary colonies then existing."[5] *Transylvania was* the name given to this enterprise, and it included the country between the Ohio, Cumberland, and Kentucky Rivers.[6] The Colony of Virginia, however, took exception to this venture. Although the land had been acquired by the Transylvania Company from the Cherokee Indians, Virginia claimed sovereignty and so annulled the proprietor's covenant with the Indians.

1 Thomas Walker, *Journal First Explorations of Kentucky (Louisville, Ky.: Morton & Co., Filson Club Publication No. 13, 1898), 1-75.*

2 Schlesinger, Arthur M:, *The Almanac of American History (New York: G. P. Putnam's Sons, 1983), 91.*

3 Michael R. Lefaro, *The Life and Adventures of Daniel Boone (Lexington, Ky.: University of Kentucky Press, 1973), 26-40.*

4 Lewis Collins and Richard Collins, *Collins History of Kentucky, Vol. II (Frankfort, Ky.: Kentucky Historical Society, 1966), 179.*

5 Robert Peter and Johanna Peter, *Transylvania University, Its Origin, Rise, Decline, and Fall (Louisville, Ky.: John P. Morton & Co., Filson Club Publication No. 11, 1896), 14.*

6 Ibid.

1775 - 1800

The city of Lexington and the Lexington-Fayette County Medical Society	Important National and International Medical Events	National Social and Political Events
• In June 1775, a small group of settlers from Ft Harrod camped in the vicinity of what is now Lexington (near the Lexington Cemetery). They named the new settlement Lexington to commemorate the Revolutionary battle at Lexington, Massachusetts (April, 1775)	• First hospital in North America, Philadelphia (1751) by Dr. Thomas Bond, supported by Benjamin Franklin • John Morgan (1735-1789), a medical graduate of Edinburgh founds the first medical school in North America, The College of Philadelphia (University of Pennsylvania), (1765) • University of Edinburgh Medical Faculty attracts many American students during the last half of the eighteenth century	• Declaration of Independence, penned by Thomas Jefferson, age 33, adopted by Congress on July 4, 1776 • Four physicians sign the Declaration of Independence: Josiah Bartlett, Matthew Thornton, Benjamin Hall, and Benjamin Rush • George Washington (1732-99) appointed Commander in Chief of the Continental Armies (1775)
• First schoolhouse built in Lexington (1782) • Lexingtonians move out of fort (1783)	• Disease specificity, championed by the English Hippocrates, Thomas Sydenham (1621-1689), is de-emphasized by the doctrine of theorists, namely William Cullen, John Brown, and others. Purgatives, bleeding, emetic, and sweating predominate therapy	• French alliance with freedom-seeking American Colonies (1778) • French navy comes to aid the Americans (1780)
• First Constitutional Convention for statehood (separation of Kentucky from Virginia) held at Danville, December 27, 1784	• About 90 percent of the deaths that occurred during the Revolutionary War were not caused by battle injuries but were the direct result of disease	• Peace of Paris (1783). Britain recognizes independence of American colonies
	• Smallpox, at its peak in the 18th century, kills 60 million Europeans, most of them children	• Philadelphia Convention drafts Constitution (1787) • George Washington, president (1789-1797)
• Lexington physician, Frederick Ridgely joins the forces of "Mad" Anthony Wayne in Battle of Fallen Timbers (August 30,1794). • Lexington Library founded (1795) • Ten physicians practice medicine in Lexington (1790s) • Samuel Brown begins practice of medicine in Lexington, (September 1797)	• William Withering (1741-1799) introduces digitalis (foxglove), (1785) • John Hunter, England, (1728-1793), a pioneer of physiological surgery promotes surgery as a branch of scientific medicine • Congress passes the first National Quarantine Act (1799)	• Whiskey Rebellion (1794) • Antione Lavoisier (1743-1794) "Father of Modern Chemistry" executed by the guillotine (1794) • John Adams elected as the second president (1797-1801) • Quasi War with France (1797-1801) • Congress passes the Sedition Act (1798)

• Lexington Medical Society founded (1799) • The Board of Transylvania University, Lexington, appoints a medical faculty (1799). • Samuel Brown is the first named professor (Anatomy, Chemistry, and Surgery). •Frederick Ridgely is also appointed professor of Materia Medica (1799) • Honorary Members (physicians) and their medical apprentices, Ordinary Members, attend weekly meetings of the Lexington Medical Society (1799) • Population of Lexington: 2,400 (1800)	• New York *Medical Repository*, the first medical journal published in America (1797) • Yellow Fever strikes citizens of Philadelphia (1797-99) • Edward Jenner (1749-1823) discovers vaccination for smallpox (1798) •Alessandro Volta invents an apparatus to cause a continuous flow of electricity an electric battery (1799) •Five American Medical Schools operative by 1800 (University of Pennsylvania, Columbia, Harvard , Dartmouth and College of Philadelphia) • Eighteenth century surgical methods differ little from the sixteenth century	• Population of USA 5.3 million (1799) • Population of Kentucky, 220,955 (1800) • French Revolution (1789-1797) • Napoleon seizes power in France (1799) • George Washington dies (1799) • President John Adams and his wife move to new capitol city (Washington) and to a new house. (1800)

1801 - 1825

The city of Lexington and the Lexington-Fayette County Medical Society	Important National and International Medical Events	National Social and Political Events
• S. L. Mitchell (estimated age: 16 to 18), medical apprentice, first known President of the Lexington Medical Society (1803) • Samuel Brown vaccinates 500 citizens of Lexington (smallpox) (1800-01) • Lexington trustees forbid citizens from keeping pet panthers (1805) • F. A. Michaux, famous French biologist, visits Lexington and meets with Samuel Brown (1802) • Benjamin Dudley (Lexington) goes to Philadelphia to attend University of Pennsylvania Medical School. William Richardson (Lexington) and Daniel Drake (Maysville) also are class members (Fall of 1804)	• Marie Francois Bichat (1771-1802), "Father of Descriptive Anatomy." To Bichat the ultimate unit of physiology was not the organ, as it had been for Morgagni (1682-1771), but the tissue, of which he described twenty-one kinds • Sir Humphrey Davy (1788-1829) suggests the use of ether and nitrous oxide as anesthetics (1800) • Ephraim McDowell (1771-1830) surgically removes a large ovarian tumor from Jane Todd Crawford at his home in Danville, Kentucky (1809) • Paris is the undisputed leader of medicine in the world during the first half of the nineteenth century	• Thomas Jefferson (1743-1826) president (1801-1809) defeats Aaron Burr (1801) (Thirty-six ballots required) • Jefferson dispatches Naval ships to quell piracy along the North-African Coast (1803) • Alexander Hamilton/Aaron Burr duel; Hamilton dies (1803) • United States purchases province of Louisiana from France ($14,500,000) (May 1803)

• James Fishback appointed professor of Theory and Practice, Transylvania Medical Faculty (1805) • First City Directory of Lexington (1806) • Lexington contains 104 brick, 10 stone and 187 frame and log houses (1806) • Frederick Ridgely leaves Lexington to settle in Richmond, Kentucky (1806) • Samuel Brown leaves Lexington to join his brother James in New Orleans (1807) • An effort to resurrect the Transylvania Medical Department fails (1809)		• Twelfth amendment (1804) • Lewis and Clark expedition, "Across the Great Divide" (1804-06) • Aaron Burr plans to establish a nation separate from USA (1805) • Robert Fulton invents the steamboat (1806) • Steamboats plying the major rivers. River cities of Louisville, St. Louis, and Cincinnati increase in population (1812) • Embargo Act (1807)
• Benjamin Dudley, Lexington physician, (1810) leaves for Paris and London for surgery training. Returns to Lexington in summer of 1814	• Guillame Dupuytren (1777-1834) Eminent French surgeon (Dupuytren's contracture) first to successfully remove the lower jaw. His most famous quote, "Nothing should be feared so much for a man as mediocrity." • Dominique Larrey (1776-1842) friend and surgeon to Napoleon invents "flying ambulances" to pick up soldiers when wounded in battle instead of waiting until end of battle.	• William Henry Harrison defeats Indians in Battle of Tippecanoe (1811) • James Madison president (1809-1817) • United States declares war on Great Britain (1812) • Napoleon enters Moscow September 14, 1812 to find it set on fire by the fleeing inhabitants • First canned goods (1812) • *Pride and Prejudice* by Jane Austin (1813)
• Transylvania University Medical Department reorganizes (1817) • Horace Holley appointed as President of Transylvania (1818) • Daniel Drake (1785-1852) joins medical faculty, Transylvania University (1817) • Dudley-Richardson [Drake] duel (August 1818) • Twenty students enroll in the medical school session of 1817-18. (Transylvania Medical Department)	• William Beaumont (1785-1853) American physiologist, treats Alexis St. Martin, performs experiments on gastric juice (1822) • An increasing interest in diagnosis evident in the early eighteen hundreds • Percussion, developed by Leopold Auenbrugger (1722-1809) in 1761 but "lost," rediscovered by Napoleon's physician Jean Nicholas Corvisart (1755-1821); restored and popularized by him to its rightful place in physical diagnosis (1808).	• New states in Union: Kentucky (1792); Tennessee (1796); Ohio (1803); Louisiana (1812); Indiana (1816); Mississippi (1817); Illinois (1818); and Alabama (1819). • The Creek Indians cede 23 million acres of land to U.S. (Parts of Georgia and Alabama) (1814) • Napoleon defeated at the Battle of Waterloo (Belgium) (1815)

• Benjamin Dudley elected president of the Lexington Medical Society (1818) • Samuel Brown rejoins medical faculty, Transylvania University (1819)	• Parkinson's disease, the "shaking palsy" described by English surgeon James Parkinson (1817) • Stethoscope "To look at the chest" invented by Rene Theophile Laennec, France (1819)	
• Charles Caldwell (1772-1853) of Philadelphia joins the Transylvania University Medical Faculty (1819) • The first graduate of the Transylvania Medical School: John Lawson McCullough of Lexington, Kentucky (1818)	• Sir Astley Cooper (London) ligates the abdominal aorta (1817) • Purkinje investigates fingerprints (1823).	• Sir Humphrey Davy invents safety lamp for coal miners (1815) • James Monroe elected president (1817-1825). "Monroe Doctrine" and "Era of Good Feeling." • Purchase of Florida from King Ferdinand of Spain (1819) • Steamship crosses the Atlantic Ocean (1819) • Economic depression, Panic of 1819 • George III, Britain's mad king dies (1820) • John Quincy Adams president (1825-1829)
• President James Monroe and General Andrew Jackson visit Lexington (July 3, 1819) • The first national medical society, Kappa Lambda Society, founded in 1819-20 by Samuel Brown • Board, lodging, fire, washing, and candles: three dollars a week for Transylvania Medical students (1820) • Lexington in financial distress (1821) • Two hundred students in Transylvania Medical Department (1823-24) • Daniel Drake, President of the Lexington Medical Society (1824) • Kentucky opens a state mental hospital in Lexington (1824) • General Lafayette visits Lexington (1825)	• William Gerhardt of Philadelphia differentiates between typhoid and typhus (1824) • Speed and daring were considered among the qualifications for brilliance in surgery during the first half of the Nineteenth Century	• The Westward movement of American settlers • Missouri Compromise (1820); Maine admitted to the union as a free state, Missouri as a slave state • Electric motor built by James Faraday (1821) • University of Virginia founded (1825)

1826 - 1850

The city of Lexington and the Lexington-Fayette County Medical Society	Important National and International Medical Events	National Social and Political Events
• *North American Medical and Surgical Journal*, the first national medical journal, published under the auspices of Kappa Lambda Society, Philadelphia (January 1826-October 1831, Vol. 1-12) • Dr. Horace Holley forced to resign as president of Transylvania University (1827) • Daniel Drake offered the Chair of Theory and Practice of Medicine, Jefferson Medical School, Philadelphia, the first western physician to be offered a professorship in an eastern medical school (1830) • *The Transylvania Journal of Medicine and the Associated Sciences* (February 1828-March 1839)	• Louis Braille introduces printing for the blind (1829) • Pierre Louis (France, 1787-1872), founder of medical statistics. Proves statistically that bloodletting is of no value in the treatment of pneumonia (1830-1840) • Theodore Schwann an early proponent of the cell theory (1834-37) • James Syme amputates a leg through the hip joint in just over one minute (1834) • Robert Graves (1797-1853) describes an affection of the thyroid gland in females (1835) • University of Louisville Medical School founded (1837) • London becomes the world's leading surgical center between 1840 and 1870, supplanting Paris • William Stokes (1804-1878) publishes a description of heart block (1846) • Founding of American Medical Association, (1846-47) Nathaniel Chapman of Philadelphia elected first president (1847) • Leopold Semmelweiss discovers the cause of puerperal fever (1847)	• Thomas Jefferson and John Adams die July 4, 1826 • First photograph (1826) • Jackson-Clay Campaign. Andrew Jackson president (1829-37) • Edgar Allen Poe dismissed from West Point Military Academy because of gross neglect of duty (1830) • President Jackson vetoes a bill authorizing the federal government to subscribe to the stock of the Maysville (Ky) to Lexington (Ky) turnpike (1830) • First all-steam railway (1830) • Britain's teenagers work hours reduced to 12 hours per day (1833) • Slavery abolished in the British Empire (1833) • Ralph Waldo Emerson publishes *Nature* (1835) • Land speculation and financial panic of 1837
• Population of Lexington (1830) 5,000; Louisville 10,000; Cincinnati 24,000 • Cholera epidemic strikes Lexington (1833). Hundreds of people in and near Lexington die. The myth of Lexington as a paradise of health dies • The Lexington Medical Society ceases to exist (1834)	• Morphine and hypodermic needle introduced into medical practice (1840s) • Jacob Henle (1809-1885) proclaimed the idea that epidemic diseases were transmitted by contagion and carried by micro-organisms (1840), a theory set forth by Fracastorius in the sixteenth century	• For the first time in the USA women are given legal control over their property (Mississippi 1839) • Martin Van Buren president (1837-1841) • Development of railroads (1840s & 1850s) • William Henry Harrison president (March-April 1841). First president to die in office

• Formation of the Lexington College of Physicians and Surgeons (1835) • Lexington incorporated (1832). Charleton Hunt is the first mayor	• Oliver Wendell Homes (1809-1894) Professor of Anatomy and Physiology at Harvard, published "The contagiousness of puerperal fever." New England Quarterly-1842-1843 • Crawford Long uses ether for anesthesia (1842)	• John Tyler president (1841-1845), "Tippecanoe and Tyler too" • Telegraph goes on line in 1844 in Washington, D.C. to Baltimore (Samuel F.B.Morse • James K. Polk president (1845-49). His platform: Re-annexation of Texas and re-occupation of Oregon • Elias Howe patents the sewing machine (1846)
• Charles Caldwell,, Esten Cooke, and Lunsford Yandell of the Transylvania Medical Department resign (transfer to Louisville in 1837-38) to become professors in the new medical school (Louisville Medical Institute) • Citizens of Lexington resolve that an anti-slavery newspaper (Cassius M. Clay, *The True American*) should be sent beyond the confines of the state (1845*)* • A telegraph line is established between Lexington and Louisville (1848) • Cholera reappears in Lexington causing a number of deaths (1849)	• Homeopathy finds a niche in medical practice (1844) • William Morton (1819-1868) gives ether anesthesia to patient undergoing surgical removal of tumor of jaw by Dr. John Warren in Boston, (October 16, 1846) • John Hutchinson uses spirometer to measure vital functions (1846)	• Mexican War (1846-47). Mexican forces defeated. Rio Grande River identifies Texas border. Mexico cedes New Mexico and California to United States • Smithsonian Institution (Washington, DC) founded (1846) • Brigham Young settles Mormons in Utah (1847)
• Daniel Drake: Publication of his now famous *A Treatise, Historical, Etiological, and Practical, On the Principal Diseases of the Interior Valley of North America (1850)*	• Sir James Young Simpson, Scotland (1811-1870), introduces the use of chloroform as an anesthetic (1847) • Vaginal fistula successfully repaired by J. Marion Sims (1809-1882) (1849)	• New Orleans becomes a major commercial center in Antebellum South • Frederic Chopin, great Polish composer died from consumption at the age of 38, (October, 1849) • Speed of light measured (186,000 miles a second), Armand H. L. Fizeau (1849) • Zachary Taylor, Mexican War hero, president of the United States (1849-1850) • California Gold Rush (1849) • Edgar Allen Poe dies at age of 40 impoverished and addicted (1849)

• Lexington Cemetery dedicated June 25, 1850 • Population of Lexington 7,000 (1850)	• Recording of temperature becomes an important guide for therapy (1840-1860)	• Millard Fillmore president (1850-1853)

1851 - 1875

The city of Lexington and the Lexington-Fayette County Medical Society	**Important National and International Medical Events**	**National Social and Political Events**
• Lexington lighted with gas lamps (July 27, 1853) • Transylvania Medical School closes (1857). Robert Peter, author of *The History of The Medical Department of Transylvania University*, serves as the last Dean of the medical school	• Medical specialization well on its way 1850-70 • Hermann Ludwig Ferdinand von Helmholtz invents the opthalmoscope (1851) • First sanitarium established for treatment of tuberculosis by Hermann Behrman (1854) • Florence Nightingale; Crimean War; revolution in nursing, (November 1854) • Laryngoscope invented (1855) • The English physician, John Snow, traces an outbreak of cholera to a pump near a river (1854). The filtration of drinking water (plus the use of chlorine) is probably the most significant public health advance of the millennium	• YMCA founded in 1851 • Eleven thousand people die in the Yellow Fever epidemic in New Orleans (1853) • Franklin Pierce president (1853-1857) • Charles Darwin publishes *Origin of Species* (1854) • Walt Whitman publishes *Leaves of Grass* (1855)
• Francis Dallam Peter, daughter of Robert Peter of Transylvania University, busy writing her Civil War Diary, (1861-1864), dies of seizures • Medical Hall of Transylvania University burns (1865) • Transylvania University consolidated with Kentucky University (Feb.28, 1865) • The Lexington-Fayette County Medical Society (January-July 1869) The demise of the society remains unexplained. No further records of a city or county medical society until 1882	• Louis Pasteur, France (1822-1895) demonstrates organisms are introduced by air and not spontaneously generated. Germ theory of disease solidly based (1865) • Heroic medical practice declines in 1860s • Medical Licensing Law (Kentucky) (1861) • Joseph Lister (1822-1884) uses carbolic acid spray as an antiseptic (1864-65) • Basic law of heredity (1866) advanced by Gregor Mendel (1822-1884)	• James Buchanan president (1857-1861) • Abraham Lincoln sixteenth president of the United States (1861-1865) • Civil War (1861-65) • Stonewall Jackson dies in battle (1863) • Battle of Gettysburg (1863) • Union troops destroy Richmond,Va, the Confederate Capitol (1865) • General Robert E. Lee surrenders to General Ulysses S. Grant, April 9, 1865 • President Lincoln assassinated, April 15, 1865

	• Thermometers introduced into English hospitals (1866-67) • President Charles Eliot of Harvard lengthens medical school curriculum to three years • The USA has but 178 hospitals in 1873 • American students flock to Paris and to London to study medicine in the 18th and 19th centuries. An estimated 15,000 Americans went abroad, principally to Germany, for this purpose between 1875-1914	• Andrew Johnson president (1865-1869) • General Ulysses S. Grant president (1869-1877) • Suez Canal completed (1869)

1876 - 1900

The city of Lexington and the Lexington-Fayette County Medical Society	**Important National and International Medical Events**	**National Social and Political Events**
• Re-establishment of the Lexington-Fayette County Medical Society (1882) • Saint Joseph Hospital (1877); Good Samaritan Hospital (1889) • *The Lexington Herald* challenges local physicians to revive medical excellence in the manner of their Lexington forbears (1882) • Peter Allison, First African-American physician practicing medicine in Lexington (1881) • Twelve hundred to fourteen hundred medical students enroll in eight medical schools in Louisville (1890s)	• Center of medical training moves from Paris to Berlin and Vienna in later part of the nineteenth century • Founding of the *Journal of the American Medical Association* (1882-1883) • Robert Koch discovers tubercle bacillus (1882) and cholera bacillus (1884) • Ernst Von Bergmann (1836-1907) Professor of Surgery, Berlin, introduces steam sterilization in surgery (1886) • Paul Ehrlich discovers Salvarsan for use against Syphilis (1891) • William Osler (1849-1920) becomes Professor of Medicine, John Hopkins Hospital (1889). Publishes *Principles and Practice of Medicine* (1892) • John Hopkins University Medical School (Baltimore) founded after a model adopted from the European, particularly the German influence (1893)	• The National Association of Professional Baseball Players is founded (1871) • John Hopkins University founded (1876) • Alexander Graham Bell introduces and patents the telephone (1876) • Rutherford B. Hayes president (1877-1881) • James Garfield president (March 1881-September 1881); Garfield assassinated (September 20, 1881) • Chester A. Arthur president (1881-1885) • Brooklyn Bridge opened (1883) • Grover Cleveland president (1885-1889)

• Lexington and Fayette County Medical Society host the Kentucky State Medical Association (1891) • Four nurses make up the first class to graduate from the School of Nursing, Good Samaritan Hospital (1893) • Julia Washburn, first woman physician, to practice in Lexington (1893). If confirmed, Elizabeth Cromwell possibly had claims to such distinction (1864-65) • *The Lexington and Fayette County Medical Society* named the *Fayette County Medical Society* (Between 1894 and 1898)	• William S. Halsted (1852-1922) first to use surgical gloves (1890) • Beginning of modern-day psychiatry in 1890s: Sigmund Freud (1856-1939) • Karl Wilhelm Roentgen (1845-1922) discovers x-rays (1895). "A New Kind of Ray" published January 8, 1896 • Sigmund Freud publishes *The Interpretation of Dreams* (1900) • Walter Reed, US Army Medical Corp., discovers the viral cause of Yellow Fever and confirms that the infection is transmitted by mosquitoes (1900)	• Benjamin Harrison president (1889-1893) • Grover Cleveland president (1893-1897) • Introduction of Hershey Bar (1894); Pepsi Cola (1898) • *Jude the Obscure* by Thomas Hardy (1895) • *The Red Badge of Courage* by Stephen Crane (1896)

1901 - 1925

The city of Lexington and the Lexington-Fayette County Medical Society	**Important National and International Medical Events**	**National Social and Political Events**
• Fayette County Medical Society members contribute to fund for suffering physicians of San Francisco, following the earthquake (1906) • Society investigates the sale of "Coca Cola" (1907). A resolution is passed for inspection of all meat, milk, and animals for tuberculosis (1907) • Mary Britton, First African-American woman MD, to practice medicine in 20th century Lexington	• All local and state medical societies become constituent parts of the AMA (1901) • Council on medical education established by AMA (1904) Medical education reform supported by Carnegie and Rockefeller foundations (1909) • Ivan Petrovich Pavlov (1849-1936) expounds on conditioned reflexes • Edward VII of England successfully operated upon for appendiceal abscess (1902) • Fritz Shaudinn (1871-1906) discovers cause of syphilis, the spirocheta pallida (1905) • Abraham Flexner report on medical education reform (1910)	• Leon Czolgosz assassinates President William McKinley (September 1901) • Morse code crosses Atlantic Ocean, Guglielmo Marconi, age 27, (December 11, 1901) • Theodore Roosevelt (age 42) becomes president (1901-1909) • Orville and Wilbur Wright accomplish the first powered airplane flight at Kitty Hawk, North Carolina (1903). It lasted but 12 seconds, rose ten feet above the ground for a distance of 120 feet. • Upton Sinclair's novel *The Jungle* exposes the filthy conditions in the Chicago slaughterhouses (1906) • Congress passes a Pure Food and Drug Act (1906) • Henry Ford introduces the Model T Ford (1908)

• Fayette County Medical Society passes a resolution for inspection of all milk, meat, and animals for tuberculosis (1909) • Bill 66, to establish a medical school (as part of Kentucky State University) dies in the Senate Rules Committee, Frankfort, Kentucky (1910) • The Kentucky State legislature changes the name of State University to the University of Kentucky (1916) • Frank LeRond McVey, president of University of Kentucky August 15, 1917	• Confirmation of measles as a virus infection by C. Hermann (1914) • First decade of 20th century known as "Golden Age of German Medicine"	• President Theodore Roosevelt supports federal income and estate taxes • Woodrow Wilson president (1913-1921) • National income tax with a maximum fixed rate of 7% passed in 1913 • Federal Reserve Act (1913); Federal Trade Commission established by Congress (1914)
• Josephine Hunt elected to the office of vice-presidency of the Medical Society, (December, 1911) • First telephone directory for Lexington (1912) • Fayette County Medical Society minutes of meetings (1913-1916) lost • Members of the Fayette County Medical Society enlist in World Ward I effort • Barrow's Unit organized (1917) • Lexington Clinic forms (1920) • Elmer Maxwell, first pathologist in Lexington (October 1, 1920) • Members of the Fayette County Medical Society number 90 (1924) • Fayette County Medical Society meets at the City Hall, the Lexington Cemetery, Good Samaritan, St. Joseph Hospital, the Lexington Brewery, LaFayette Hotel, Walter Cox's residence, and Phoenix Hotel (1924)	• Two years of college required to enter medical school • Worldwide flu epidemic (1917-1919) • Frederick Grant Banning (1891-1941) and Herbert Best (1899-1978 discover Insulin (1922) • Margaret Sanger founds the Birth Control Clinic Research Bureau, the first doctor-staffed birth control clinic (1923)	• World War I, "The Great War" (1914-1918) • Britain and France borrow $2 billion plus from United States Banks (1917) • USA enters war (1917) • Women's rights to vote in USA (1918) • National prohibition (1920) Bootlegger's heyday • Ku Klux Klan experiences a major revival in the early 1920's • League of Nations established but America does not join (1920) • Warren G. Harding, president (March 1921-August 1923) scandals (Teapot Dome, 1924) • Calvin Coolidge president (1923-29) • F. Scott Fitzgerald: *The Great Gatsby* (1925)

1926 - 1950

The city of Lexington and the Lexington-Fayette County Medical Society	Important National and International Medical Events	National Social and Political Events
• Medical Society dues raised from $7.50 to $10.00 per year (1926) • Woolfolk Barrow, Lexington physician killed in car accident (1927) • Mortality in cases of appendicitis in Lexington, Kentucky, reportedly greater than in any other city in the USA (1928)	• Sir Alexander Fleming identifies penicillin (1928) • Seventy-four medical schools in America in 1928 compared to 154 twenty years earlier. • Tetanus antidotes given to wounded in WWI and an effective vaccine was produced against tetanus in the 1930s • Mass immunization of children with diphtheria toxoid (1930-40s) • Pentothal, an intravenous anesthetic, introduced by John Lundy (1935)	• Sinclair Lewis: *Main Street* (1920); *Babbit* (1922); Arrowsmith (1925); and *Elmer Gantry* (1927) • Ernest Hemingway: *A Farewell to Arms* (1929)
• J. A. Stucky, prominent Lexington physician killed in a car accident (1931) • Medical Society resumes meeting at Good Samaritan Hospital (1932) • Medical Society appoints a Public Relations Committee (1939) • Medical Society turns down request to found a Medical Auxiliary (1942)	• Gerhard Domagk discovers first sulfa drug (mid 1930s) • Blue Cross Health Insurance • Congress passes Food, Drug, and Cosmetic Act calling for detailed disclosure of the ingredients of food, drugs, and cosmetics on their labels (1938)	• Herbert Hoover president (1929-1933) • Stock market crash (1929) • The great Depression begins (1930) • Fascist dictatorial threat evident early in the 1930s • Franklin Roosevelt, president (1933-1945) • "New Deal" underway (1930s) • Robert Watson-Watt (1892-1973) discovers radar waves (circa 1935)
• Portrait of Daniel Drake purchased by the Fayette County Medical Society (1937) Cost:$400.00) • First woman member of the Society, Josephine Hunt, retires (1947)	• Samuel A. Waksman isolates streptomycin (1944) • Vaccine for influenza (1945) • Claude Beck performs the first successful electrical defibrillation of the heart in a man (1947) • Dwight Harken, Boston, treats mitral valvular stenosis. He dilated the valve with his finger and cut the calcified valve (1948).	• Social Security Act (1935) • Father Charles Coughlin the radical "Radio Priest" (1930s) • Huey P. Long, Senator (Louisiana) (1930-1935) • Germans invade Poland. World War II begins (1939)

• 156 members of the Fayette County Medical Society (1948) • Fayette County Medical Society Auxiliary established (1948) • The first president of the Medical Auxiliary, Dorothy Leet • Office space at a premium as physicians return from WWII to practice medicine in Lexington (1947-50)	• Alfred Blalock (John Hopkins University) performs first successful operation for the congenital heart defect, Tetralogy of Fallot. Helen Taussig (John Hopkins University) had previously defined the basic concept for surgical repair of the defect. Blalock-Taussig operation (1945)	• Pearl Harbor (December, 7, 1941) • Germany surrenders (May 8, 1945) • Atomic bomb flattens Hiroshima (August 6, 1945); Nagasaki (August 9, 1945) • World War II ends (August 10, 1945) • The GI Bill; veterans return to school (1945) • Cold War underway (1946) Soviet Union versus Allies • Transistor age begins (1947) • Harry Truman, president (1945-53)

References:

Ackernecht, Erwin H. *A Short History of Medicine.* Baltimore: The John Hopkins University Press, 1982.

Boerhaave, E. Ashworth. *Men; At Leyden and After, Underwood.* Edinburgh: Edinburgh University Press, 1977.

Clark, Thomas C. *A History of Kentucky.* Lexington, Ky.: The John Bradford Press, 1960.

Encyclopedia Britannica. 1973.

Garraty, John A. *A Short History of the American Nation.* New York: Harper & Row, 1974.

Garrison, Fielding H. *An Introduction to the History of Medicine.* Philadelphia: W.B. Saunders Company, 1922.

Green, John. *Medical History for Students.* Springfield, Ill.: Charles C. Thomas Publisher, 1968.

Grun, Bernard. *Timetables of History.* Based upon Werner Stein's *Kulturfahrplan.* New York: Simon and Shuster, 1982.

Jerome, Edward, ed. *Chronicle of the World.* Paris: J. L. International Publications, 1989.

Krout, John A. *United States to 1877.* San Francisco: Harper & Row, 1971.

McGrew, Robert E. *Encyclopedia of Medical History.* New York: McGraw-Hill Book Company, 1985.

Mettler, Cecilia C. *History of Medicine.* Birmingham, Ala.: The Classics of Medicine Library, Division of Gryphon Editions, Ltd., 1986.

Ranck, George W. *History of Lexington.* Cincinnati: Robert Clark and Company, 1872.

Reiser, Joel. *Medicine and the Reign of Technology.* Cambridge, England: Stanley Cambridge University Press, 1978.

Rhodes, Philip. *An Outline of History of Medicine.* London: Butterworths, 1985.

Roemol Henry, Director (HEW grant). *Catalogue of Transylvania University Medical Library.* Lexington, Ky.: Transylvania University Press, 1987.

Rothstein, William G. *American Medical Schools and the Practice of Medicine.* Oxford. Oxford University Press, 1987.

Singer, Charles. *A Short History of Medicine.* New York: Oxford University Press, 1928.

Born in Prestonsburg, Kentucky September 20, 1922, Dr. Porter Mayo attended Eastern Kentucky University and Vanderbilt University. A 1946 graduate of the University of Louisville Medical School, he interned at Parkland Hospital, Dallas, Texas. Dr. Mayo then served two years in the U.S. Navy followed by a year of respiratory physiology research at the University of Michigan School of Medicine receiving the M.S. degree in physiology in 1950. Next he took a general surgery residency in the Veteran's Administration Hospital, Louisville, Kentucky and a thoracic surgery residency at the University of Michigan, Ann Arbor, Michigan. His surgery practice in Lexington extended from 1954 to 1984. In January, 1984 Dr. Mayo began a second career, enrolling in the doctorate program, Department of History, University of Kentucky, and receiving his Ph.D. degree in 1988. From 1989 to 1995 he served as Clinical Professor of Surgery and Director of the Problem-Based-Learning Program in the Department of Surgery, University of Kentucky Medical Center. Professor Emeritus, School of Medicine, University of Kentucky, Dr. Mayo is certified by the American Board of Surgery and the Board of Thoracic Surgery. He is a Founding Member of both the Southern Thoracic Surgical Society and the Society of Thoracic Surgery. Author and co-author of eighty scientific publications, Dr. Mayo now devotes his writing to the history of medicine.

Walker Mayo is a lawyer and historian residing in Lexington, Kentucky. He is a graduate of Washington & Lee University, Duke University Law School, and the University of Oxford in England, where he earned a doctorate in history. He is a partner in the law firm of Getty, Keyser & Mayo, LLP in Lexington, Kentucky.

Camille Mayo Jernigan was born and raised in Lexington, Kentucky. She attended Hollins College in Roanoke, VA for two years before transferring to the University of Kentucky. She graduated from UK in 1979 with a BA in Journalism.

Ms. Jernigan began her career as a medical writer in Lexington. After moving to Huntsville, AL, she worked as a NASA sub-contractor and as a software documentation manager with Intergraph Corporation. Ms. Jernigan currently resides in Nashville, TN and is employed by Square D Company as a senior technical writer.

Ms. Jernigan has won awards for writing and illustration by the Society of Technical Communication and has been recognized by NASA for her contributions to the Launch Vehicle X and Space Station proposals.

Florence M. Witte has master's degrees in English and German from the University of Southern Mississippi and in International Business from the University of Kentucky. For nearly eight years she was director of the Publications Office of the Department of Surgery at the UK College of Medicine. She is now the director of the Scientific Editing Department at St. Jude Children's Research Hospital, Memphis.

Flo is a board-certified medical editor, having passed the certification examination offered by the Board of Editors in the Life Sciences. She is also active in the Council of Biology Editors and the American Medical Writers Association. She was recently named a Fellow of AMWA and will receive the Golden Apple Award for workshop leadership at AMWA's annual conference in October, 1999. She is a member of AMWA's Executive Committee and is the administrator of publications for the organization.

Past Presidents of Lexington and Fayette County Medical Societies

Lexington Medical Society

Samuel Venable, Student	1803
S. L. Mitchell, Student	1803
John R. Bedford, Student	1804
Benjamin W. Dudley, M.D.	1818
Henry Miller, M.D.	1822
Daniel Drake, M.D.	1824
Charles Caldwell, M.D.	1828

Lexington and Fayette County Medical Society

Jno. Desha, M.D.	1869
Edward Maxwell Wiley, M.D.	Unknown
Lyman Beecher Todd, M.D.	1890
F. M. Greene, M.D.	1891
Benjamin Lindsey Coleman, M.D.	Unknown
W. B. McClure, M.D.	1894
H. M. Skillman, M.D.	Unknown
William S. Stucky, M.D.	Unknown

Lexington College of Physicians and Surgeons

Charles Caldwell, M.D.	1835
Benjamin W. Dudley, M.D.	1838

Fayette County Medical Society

Nathaniel L. Bosworth, M.D.	1904
Waller O. Bullock, M.D.	1905
John W. Scott, M.D.	1906
Archibald H. Barkley, M.D.	1907
W. J. Foley, M.D.	1908
E. M. Wiley, M.D.	1909
Julian T. McClymonds, M.D.	1910
Benjamin F. Van Meter, M.D.	1911
Claude W. Trapp, M.D.	1912
George P. Sprague, M.D.	1913
Charles A. Vance, M.D.	1914
J. C. Lewis, M.D.	1916
Charles A. Vance, M.D.	1917
Ernest B. Bradley, M.D.	1918
D. Woolfolk Barrow, M.D.	1919
Lee C. Redmon, M.D.	1920
William E. Bannister, M.D.	1921
Jesse P. Warren, M.D.	1922
Samuel B. Marks, M.D.	1923

D. J. Healy, M.D.	1924
Charles C. Garr, M.D.	1925
George H. Wilson, M.D.	1926
William S. Stucky, M.D.	1927
William T. Briggs, M.D.	1928
Scott D. Breckinridge, M.D.	1929
W. Dandridge Reddish, M.D.	1930
Thomas J. Ray, M.D.	1931
Elmer S. Maxwell, M.D.	1932
Edward J. Murray, M.D.	1933
G. Bedford Brown, M.D.	1934
Harry G. Herring, M.D.	1935
Thomas M. Marks, M.D.	1936
Charles N. Kavanaugh, M.D.	1937
Francis M. Massie, M.D.	1938
John Harvey, M.D.	1939
W. Simrall Wyatt, M.D.	1940
Charles M. McKinlay, M.D.	1941
J. Farra Van Meter, M.D.	1942
Donnan B. Harding, M.D.	1943
Amplias O. Sisk, M.D.	1944
Joseph A. Stoeckinger, M.D.	1945
Earl C. Yates, M.D.	1946
Douglas E. Scott, M.D.	1947
Edward H. Ray, M.D.	1948
Carl H. Fortune, M.D.	1949
Theodore L. Adams, M.D.	1950
William H. Pennington, M.D.	1951
Richard G. Elliott, M.D.	1952
Coleman C. Johnson, M.D.	1953
Rankin C. Blount, M.D.	1954
N. Lewis Bosworth, M.D.	1955
John S. Sprague, M.D.	1956
Arthur B. Barrett, M.D.	1957
Robert B. Warfield, M.D.	1958
William O. Preston, M.D.	1959
Matthew C. Darnell, M.D.	1960
Joseph H. Saunders, M.D.	1961
Harvey Chenault, M.D.	1962
M. Randolph Gilliam, M.D.	1963
Andrew M. Moore, M.D.	1964
Thomson R. Bryant, Jr., M.D.	1965
Irving F. Kanner, M.D.	1966
John F. Berry, M.D.	1967
David B. Stevens, M.D.	1968
David A. Hull, M.D.	1969
Richard B. McElvein, M.D.	1970

Leslie W. Blakey, M.D.	1971
James B. Holloway, M.D.	1972
James G. Wilhite, M.D.	1973
Glenn U. Dorroh, M.D.	1974
Colby N. Cowherd, M.D.	1975
Melvin L. Dean, M.D.	1976
P. Raphael Caffrey, M.D.	1977
Allen E. Grimes, Jr., M.D.	1978
Franklin B. Moosnick, M.D.	1979
Peter P. Bosomworth, M.D.	1980
Thomas M. Jarboe, M.D.	1981
John W. Garden, M.D.	1982
Edwin J. Nighbert, M.D.	1983
Preston P. Nunnelley, M.D.	1984
Robert P. Belin, M.D.	1985
Dennis B. Kelly, M.D.	1986
Sally S. Mattingly, M.D.	1987
Harold T. Faulconer, M.D.	1987
John E. Trevey, M.D.	1988
William F. Gee, M.D.	1989
Thomas K. Slabaugh, M.D.	1990
Gary R. Wallace, M.D.	1991
Andrew M. Moore, II, M.D.	1992
Andrew R. Pulito, M.D.	1993
John W. Collins, M.D.	1994
John R. White, M.D.	1995
Daniel E. Kenady, M.D.	1996
John D. Stewart, II, M.D.	1997
W. Lisle Dalton, M.D.	1998
J. Michael Moore, M.D.	1999

Index of Names

A

Abernethy, John (1764-1831) 139
Allen, John R. (1837-1877) 125, 136
Auenbrugger, Leopold (1722-1809) 137

B

Bache, Franklin (1792-1864) 80
Barkley, A. H. (1872-1937) 266, 286, 300
Barrow, David (1858-1932) 241, 294, 308
Barrow, Woolfolk (1883-1923) 294
Bell, John (1796-1872) 80
Bichat, Marie-Francois (1771-1802) 137, 255
Black, Joseph (1728-1799) 30
Boerhaave, Hermann (1668-1738) 176
Bond, Thomas (1712-1784) 132
Boone, Daniel (1734-1820) 168
Bowditch, Henry Pickering (1840-1911) 178
Bradford, John (1749-1830) 25-26, 41, 106, 108
Bradley, Ernest B. (1877-1946) 291, 294
Brashear, Walter (1776-1860) 33, 83, 91, 172
Breckinridge, General John C. (1821-1875) 230-232
Britton, Mary E. (1857-1925) 246
Broussais, Joseph Victor (1772-1838) 255
Brown, James (1766-1836) 31
Brown, John (1757-1837) 30
Brown, John (Scotland) (1735-1788) 97
Brown, Orlando (1801-1867) 116
Brown, Samuel (1769-1830) 28, 30-32, 34, 37-38, 40-44, 48, 65-66, 68, 70-73, 76-80, 82, 94-95, 98, 100,105-107,109-112,143,169, 181-182, 188-189, 198, 203, 208, 210, 264
Buchanan, Joseph (1785-1829) 91
Bullock, Waller (1875-1953) 43, 253, 274-275, 294, 300
Bush, James Miller (1808-1875) 118, 227-228

C

Caldwell, Charles (1772-1853) 38, 44, 53-54, 65, 98, 186, 193, 198, 203, 205, 208-212
Chambers, John S. (1889-1971) 122, 290
Chapman, Nathaniel (1778-1853) 203
Chipley, W. S. (1810-1880) 134, 150, 152
Clay, Henry (1777-1852) 33, 108, 136, 203, 206, 208, 285-286, 305
Clay, Thomas Wythe (1802-1869) 136
Cooke, John Esten (1783-1853) 98-99, 208, 212
Cooper, Sir Astley (1768-1841) 130
Cromwell, Elizabeth (Circa 1860's) 242
Cullen, William (1710-1790) 97

D

Davidge, John B. (1768-1829) 30
Davis, Nathan Smith (1817-1904) 71, 77, 80, 167, 179, 247, 314
Delafield, Edward 76, 79-80
Desha, John (1804-1878) 231, 233, 235
Drake, Daniel (1785-1852) 48, 51, 53, 82, 98, 145, 150, 169-170, 172-174, 179, 183, 185, 187-198, 205, 208, 210, 264, 287
Dudley, Benjamin (1785-1870) 33, 43, 48-49, 53, 65, 98, 118, 137, 139, 141-147, 172, 182-183, 185, 187-198, 207, 210, 212, 221, 228, 264
Dudley, Ethelbert L. (1818-1862) 142, 228-230
Duke, Basil (1766-1828) 91, 95, 110

E

Earle, Benjamin Prince (1846-1918) 233-234
Eliot, Charles (1834-1926) 179
Estill, Julian (1877-1952) 271, 291

F

Filson, John (1753-Circa 1788) 168
Fishback, James (1776-1845) 42, 44, 91, 112, 139, 181-182
Flexner, Abraham (1866-1959) 175
Flexner, James Thomas (1908-) 64
Fracastoro, Girolamo (1484-1553) 145

G

Goforth William (1766-1817) 38, 169-170
Gross, Samuel David (1805-1884) 80, 203, 221, 232, 247, 250, 287

H

Halsted, William Stewart (1852-1922) 272
Hays, Isaac (1796-1872) 71-72, 80
Hippocrates (460-377 B.C.) 127
Hodge, Hugh (1796-1873) 80
Holley, Horace (1781-1827) 198, 206, 210

Holloway, Thomas C. (1873-1925) 269, 279, 292-293
Holmes, Oliver W. (1809-1894) 256
Hosack, David (1769-1835) 28, 30, 40, 105, 112
Humphreys, Alexander (Circa 1751-Circa 1798) 28
Hunt, Josephine (1878-1962) 247
Hunter, Bush (1894-1983) 250, 304
Hunter, John E. (Kentucky) (1863-1956) 248, 250, 279

J

Jackson, Samuel (1787-1872) 80
Jefferson, Thomas (1743-1826) 32, 40, 83, 105, 203-204
Jenner, Edward (1749-1823) 100, 110-111

K

Knight, Jonathan (1789-1864) 80
Koch, Robert (1843-1910) 132

L

Laennec, Rene T. H. (1781-1826) 137
Larrey, Dominique Jean (1766-1842) 139
Leake, Chauncey (1896-1978) 65-66, 70-71, 77
Lister, Joseph (1827-1912) 133, 256, 264
Long, Crawford W. (1815-1878) 132, 256
Louis, Pierre (1787-1872) 256

M

Mather, Cotton (1662-1728) 91
McClellan, George (1796-1847) 73
McClure, William B. (1858-1947) 241, 266, 268, 285
McCormack, Joseph (1847-1922) 292
McCreery, Charles (1785-1826) 83
McCullough, John Lawson (Circa 1793-1825) 183, 192
McDowell, Ephraim (1771-1830) 83, 221, 285-286
McVey, Frank (1869-1953) 290
Meigs, Charles (1792-1869) 80
Michaux, F. A. (1770-1855) 105, 109
Miller, Henry (1800-1874) 46, 48, 50, 80, 235
Mondeville, Henri de (1260-1320) 145
Monro, Alexander "Secunders" (1733-1817) 30
Morgagni, Giovanni Battista (1682-1771) 136
Morgan, John (1735-1789) 93, 176-178, 226
Morton, William (1819-1868) 27, 49, 108, 132
Mott, Valentine (1785-1865) 74, 143

N

Nightingale, Florence (1820-1910) 132, 250, 252

O

Osler, Sir William (1849-1919) 198
Overton, James (1785-1865) 182-183, 185, 187, 189-191

P

Pancoast, Joseph (1805-1882) 80
Paré, Ambrose (1510-1590) 144
Parrish, Joseph (1779-1840) 80
Pasteur, Louis (1822-1895) 132, 256
Percival, Thomas (1740-1894) 32, 66, 71-72, 78
Peter, Francis Dallam (1843-1864) 226, 228-229
Peter, Robert (1805-1894) 31, 187, 226, 230
Physick, Philip Syng (1768-1837) 143
Pinel, Philippe (1755-1826) 133, 255
Poteau, Claude (1725-1775) 145
Pryor, J. W. (1856-1956) 237-239, 241-242, 283-285, 288-289

R

Rafinesque, Constantine (1784-1840) 198
Rhorer, Melvin (n a) 294
Richardson, William Hall (1785-1844) 49, 65, 98, 182-183, 185, 187-192, 196, 198, 207
Ridgely, Frederick (1756-1824) 28, 31-33, 38, 40, 42, 44, 95, 106-107, 139, 172, 181-182
Roche, René de la (1769-1830) 66, 73, 78-80
Roentgen, William (1845-1922) 256, 264
Rogers, Coleman (1781-1855) 43, 48, 189-191
Roosevelt, Theodore (1858-1919) 278
Rush, Benjamin (1745-1813) 28, 32, 38, 97-98, 105, 166, 203

S

Schleiden, Matthias Jacob
(1804-1881) 137
Schwann, Theodore (1810-1882) 137
Scott, John (1875-1966) 274, 279,
282, 304, 306
Semmelweiss, Ignaz Philip
(1818-1865) 256
Shippen, William (1736-1808) 96
Short, Charles Wilkins (1794-1863) 116, 121,
189, 208, 212
Sigerist, Henry Ernest (1891-1957) 175
Simpson, James Young (1811-1875) 235
Solomon, William "King"
(1775-1854) 119, 121
Sprague, George (1863-1942) 266, 274,
279, 290-294
Stevens, Alexander H. (1789-1869) 76, 80
Stillé, Alfred (1813-1900) 243-244
Stucky, Joseph A. (1857-1931) 271, 282,
286, 290, 292-293
Sutton, William L. (1797-1862) 221, 262
Sydenham, Thomas (1624-1689) 127

T

Todd, Levi (1755-1807) 94

V

Van Meter, Benjamin Franklin
(1873-1934) 266, 270-
271, 279, 294
Virchow, Rudolph (1821-1902) 137, 255
von Bergmann, Ernst (1836-1907) 256

W

Warfield, Walter (Circa 1760-1826) 181
Washburn, Julia (1861-1949) 246
Waterhouse, Benjamin (1754-1846) 105, 110,
112
Wilkinson, James (1757-1825) 91, 95
Wood, George Bacon (1797-1879) 80

Y

Yandell, David W. (1826-1898) 198, 245
Yandell, Lunsford P. (1805-1878) 53, 98,
114, 128, 130-131, 208, 212
Young, F. O. (1850-1931) 292-294

Index of Subjects

A

African-American Physicians 246-250, 304
AMA 76-83, 247, 296, 298
  Code of Ethics 32, 66, 71-72, 77-78, 80
  Delegates (1846-47) 71, 79-80
  First President 203
  Founding 77, 179
  National Convention (1846-47) 71, 76-80, 167
  Preamble 79
American Philosophical Society 32
Antisepsis 132-133, 144-145, 252, 256, 264
Appendicitis Mortality 300
Apprenticeship 37-38, 48-49, 96, 168-175, 178, 204-205
Athens of the West 22, 113, 122, 222

B

Baltimore 72-73, 263
Banqueted (1891) 239-242
Bloodletting 97-98
Bloody Flux (see Dysentery)

C

Calomel 96, 98-99, 115, 118, 128-131, 148-149, 234
Cardinal Hill Hospital 305
Carnegie Report 179
Cars 276, 278, 280-281
Cholera 98, 113-127, 210, 264
  Epidemic (1833) 113-123
  Epidemic (1849) 123-127
  Firing of Cannon 125-126
  Frankfort Commonwealth 116
  Niles Weekly Register 117-118
  Orphan Asylum 122-123
  Solomon, William "King" 119-121
  Victims 113-114
  Victims
   (Physicians and medical students)
   126-127
Cincinnati 23, 82, 113
  Ft. Washington 105
  Population 23, 209
Civil War 54, 222-223, 231-232
  Diary 226-228
Coca-Cola 290
Criminal Abortion 291-294

D

Depression, The Great 301
Disease Specificity 137
Dysentery 126-131, 210

E

Eastern State Hospital (see Lunatic Asylum)
Edinburgh University Medical School 30, 42, 48, 93, 97, 177
Education
    Pioneer Lexington 167-168
    Pre-Civil War 175-179, 210-212

F

Fayette County Medical Society 24, 233, 242,266, 274
    Lost "minutes" 284-285
    Minutes (Good of the Order-1907)
    264-271
    Why Belong? 314
Federal Subsidies to Medicine 301-302
Fevers 148, 150, 210
Flexner Report 272
Flu Epidemic of 1918-19 282-284
    Quarantine 283

H

Halsted Revolution 272

J

Jefferson Medical College 64, 73
Julius Marks Sanatorium 304-305

K

Kappa Lambda Society of Hippocrates 64-83
    Antimasonic Movement 74-75
    Code of Medical Ethics 32, 66, 71-72, 76
    Conspiracy 74
    Constitution 1821 69
    Demise of Kappa Lambda 72-77
    Founding 42, 66, 82
    Secrecy 72, 74-76
    Spurious Link to the Lexington Medical Society
    68
Kentucke Gazette 25-26
Kentucke Society for Useful Knowledge
    24-27
Kentucky Gazette 43

L

Breckinridge (General John C.), Last Illness
    230-233
Late Eighteenth-and Early Nineteenth-Century Medicine
    90-91

Lexington
    City Hospital and the Work House
        112, 131-132
    Dying Century 263-264
    National Medical Meeting 282
    Population 23, 95, 135, 209, 239, 288
Lexington and Fayette County Medical Society
        235, 242
    First Woman Officer 247
Lexington and Ohio Railroad 209
Lexington Clinic 294-295, 298-299
Lexington College of Physicians and Surgeons
        53-54
Lexington Medical Society 42-54, 65, 68, 70, 82
    Debates 53
    Ends 23, 51, 53, 208-210
    Founding 22, 27-28, 41-43, 50, 82, 180
    Members 37, 42, 44, 181
    Preamble 1821 37
    Student and Physician Officers 46, 48-49, 82
Licensing 37, 39, 66, 70, 73
Lithotomy 141, 146-147
Louisville 112
    Population 23, 209
Lunatic Asylum
    Eastern State Hospital 124, 133-136, 283
    Williamsburg, VA 134

M

Medical College in Lexington 287-290
Medical Practice in the 1860s 233-235
Medical Schools
    First American 176-178
    Founding 176-177
Medical Societies in America 27, 40
Medical Societies, Post-Civil War 235-237
Medical Theorists 97-99
MEDICUS 70, 74

N

National Medical Insurance 278
New York City 71, 73-77, 263
New York City Medical and Physical Journal
        74
Niles Weekly Register 116-117
North American Medical and Surgical Journal
        74, 78, 82
Nursing and Hospitals 250-255
    Good Samaritan 252-254, 283
    St. Joseph 252-253

P

Paris, France 90
Philadelphia 32, 46, 64-66, 73-74, 76, 90, 93, 263

Philadelphia Medical College 38, 206
Physicians
 Early Lexington 91, 95-96
 First American 91
 Irregular 72, 96
 Regular 96, 146
Preceptor 37-38, 40, 48, 169, 172-175, 178-179, 181, 204, 207
Prevailing Diseases 147-151, 282
Progressive Party 278
Pryor's (Dr.) Reminiscences 237-239, 283-285

Q

Quacks 39, 41, 96, 210

R

Respect 41, 255, 317

S

San Francisco Earthquake 274
Scientific Societies 24
Shriners Hospital 305
Smallpox 99-113
 Act Regulating Inoculation of Smallpox (Kentucky) 101-103
 Cowpox "Thread" 105, 109-110
 Inoculation and Vaccination 42, 100, 105
 Inoculation in Lexington 100, 104
 Jenner 100, 105
 Newspaper Reports of the "Pox" 104-108
 Quarantine 99
 The Pox Returns (1849) 112-113
Spanish-American War 308
Specialization 256, 295-298
Statuary Hall Tribute to Drs. McDowell and Drake 285-286
Steamboat 115, 209
Study Abroad 175-176
Surgery 136-147
 Cleanliness 144-146

T

Telephone 237, 276, 278-280, 297-298
Transylvania University 28, 65, 264
 Bond with Lexington 186
 Closure of Medical Department 222
 Demise of Medical School 208-210, 212, 221-222
 Dudley's (Ethelbert) Valedictory Address 142
 Enrollment and Graduation 206
 First Medical School Graduate 192
 Founding of Medical Department 22, 27-28, 33, 42, 82, 181-182

Grave Robbers 207-208
Loss of Faculty Members to Louisville 23, 212
Medical Department 31, 33, 113, 180-182
Medical Faculty Duels 187-198
Medical Library 205-206, 210
New President and Medical Faculty 198-204
Reorganization of the Transylvania Medical School 182-184
School of Medicine 23, 37
The Medical Hall 223
The Transylvania Journal of Medicine and the Associate Sciences 151-152
Transylvania Medical Journal 229
Tribute to Members of the Transylvania Faculty by Students 183-186
Tuberculosis 150, 282, 290-291, 304-305

U

University of Kentucky 24, 283, 287-289
University of Kentucky Medical School 42
Early Attempt 288
Founded 290

V

Veterans Medical Center 306
Vital Statistics of Lexington and Kentucky 151-152

W

Women Admitted into Medical Societies 246
Women in Medicine 242-246
Women Physicians in Lexington 246-247
Women's Auxiliary 302
World War I 278, 308-309
World War II 290, 295, 308, 310-311